DEVELOPMENTAL ASSESSMENT CLINIC

Comprehensive Management of
Cerebral Palsy

Comprehensive Management of Cerebral Palsy

Edited by
George H. Thompson, M.D.

Assistant Professor of
Orthopaedic Surgery and Pediatrics
Case Western Reserve University
Cleveland, Ohio

Isadore Leslie Rubin, M.B.B.Ch.,B.Sc.

Instructor in Pediatrics
Harvard University
Children's Hospital Medical Center
Boston, Massachusetts

Robert M. Bilenker, M.D.

Assistant Professor of Pediatrics
Case Western Reserve University
Cleveland, Ohio

Grune & Stratton
A Subsidiary of Harcourt Brace Jovanovich, Publishers
New York   London
Paris   San Diego   San Francisco   São Paulo
Sydney   Tokyo   Toronto

Library of Congress Cataloging in Publication Data
Main entry under title:

Comprehensive management of cerebral palsy.

　　Includes bibliographies and index.
　　1. Cerebral palsy.　2. Cerebral palsied children—
Rehabilitation.　I. Thompson, George H. (George Harman),
1944–　　.　II. Rubin, Isadore Leslie.　III. Bilenker,
Robert M.
RJ496.C4C56　1982　　　616.8'36　　　82-15827
ISBN 0-8089-1504-5

Grune & Stratton, Inc.
111 Fifth Avenue
New York, New York 10003

Distributed in the United Kingdom by
Academic Press Inc. (London) Ltd.
24/28 Oval Road, London NW 1

Library of Congress Catalog Number 82-15827
International Standard Book Number 0-8089-1504-5
Printed in the United States of America

*This book is dedicated to all children:
may they always be provided with the
best possible attention for the attainment of
physical, emotional, and social well-being.*

Contents

Part V   **Social, Educational, and**
              Maturational Considerations

Acknowledgment

We would like to express our sincere gratitude and thanks to Ann Daniels, Cynthia Bates and her secretarial staff at the D.E.C. at Wrentham State School, Wrentham, Massachusetts, and most importantly Deborah Such at Cleveland Metropolitan General Hospital for typing and retyping the manuscript.

We would also like to offer our sincere gratitude and thanks to our wives and children who patiently tolerated our prolonged spells of absence in the preparation of this book.

Preface

For many years the care for children with cerebral palsy has been fragmented. Nearly all the components necessary for the evaluation and management were available, but communication between each discipline was limited in most cases. Over the last decade there has been an evolution toward improved coordination of services for these children and their families. This process has resulted in the concept of the "interdisciplinary" approach and has culminated in this book.

The chapters in this text represent contributions from several major centers and reflect approaches to the clinical entity of cerebral palsy that are somewhat individualized. Each center has its own unique personality, and the focus and functions of one may be quite different from the other. Nonetheless what is offered is the opportunity to sample various aspects involved in the understanding of cerebral palsy and in the practical aspects of long-term management as well as prevention.

In the spirit of the appreciation of the multiple and complex needs of the child with a life-long disability, this book was designed to fill in the missing pieces of the puzzle for each discipline. By so doing it is hoped that the child and family will benefit from the awareness of as many facets as possible so as to ensure optimal physical, emotional, and social development.

We are deeply indebted to all our colleagues and teachers whose names could fill this book, but in the final analysis we are most grateful to our patients, the children, their parents, brothers and sisters, grandparents, and friends, because they made us look, listen, and apply our knowledge to what they were saying and asking.

Contributors

Norberto Alvarez, M.D.
Director, Seizure Control
and Neurology Program
Wrentham State School
Wrentham, Massachusetts
Assistant in Neurology
Children's Hospital Medical Center
Instructor in Neurology
Harvard Medical School
Boston, Massachusetts

Estelle M. Argie, M.Ed.
Child Life Specialist
Cleveland Metropolitan General Hospital
Cleveland, Ohio

Betty Q. Banker, M.D.
Professor of Pathology
Case Western Reserve University
Director, Division of Neuropathology
Cleveland Metropolitan General Hospital
Cleveland, Ohio

Robert M. Bilenker, M.D.
Assistant Professor of Pediatrics
Case Western Reserve University
Director, Comprehensive Care Program
Cleveland Metropolitan General Hospital
Cleveland, Ohio

Naomi Breslau, Ph.D.
Associate Professor of
Epidemiology and Community Health
Assistant Professor of
Pediatrics in Sociology
Case Western Reserve University
Cleveland, Ohio

Arnold J. Capute, M.D.
Associate Professor of Pediatrics
Johns Hopkins University
Deputy Medical Director
John F. Kennedy Institute
Baltimore, Maryland

Mary Cassidy-Conway, M.S., R.P.T.
Physical Therapy Department
Children's Hospital Medical Center
Boston, Massachusetts

Allen C. Crocker, M.D.
Associate Professor in Pediatrics
Harvard Medical School
Director, Developmental Evaluation Clinic
Children's Hospital Medical Center
Boston, Massachusetts

Leroy J. Dierker, M.D.
Assistant Professor
Department of Obstetrics and Gynecology
Case Western Reserve University
Cleveland Metropolitan General Hospital
Cleveland, Ohio

James C. Drennan, M.D.
Director, Orthopaedic Surgery
Newington Children's Hospital
Newington, Connecticut

Robert M. Eiben, M.D.
Professor of Pediatrics
Associate Professor of Neurology
Case Western Reserve University
Assistant Director
Department of Pediatrics
Cleveland Metropolitan General Hospital
Cleveland, Ohio

James R. Gage, M.D.
Director of Research
Newington Children's Hospital
Newington, Connecticut

Nancy L. Golden, M.D.
Assistant Professor of Pediatrics
Case Western Reserve University
Cleveland, Ohio

Jocelyn Bruce–Gregorios, M.D.
Fellow in Neuropathology
Cleveland Clinic Foundation
Cleveland, Ohio

Roger H. Hertz, M.D.
Associate Professor
Case Western Reserve University
Director, Antenatal Drug Unit
Cleveland Metropolitan General Hospital
Cleveland, Ohio

Irwin B. Jacobs, M.D.
Assistant Professor of
Pediatrics and Neurology
Case Western Reserve University
Cleveland, Ohio

William E. Kiernan, Ph.D.
Clinical Associate
Boston University
Instructor
Assumption College
Director of Rehabilitation
Developmental Evaluation Clinic
Children's Hospital Medical Center
Boston, Massachusetts

William C. Kim, M.D.
Fellow in Pediatric Orthopaedic Surgery
Case Western Reserve University
Cleveland, Ohio

Mary C. Lawlor, Ed. M., O.T.R.
Director of Occupational Therapy
University of Massachusetts Medical Center
Worcester, Massachusetts

E. Byron Marsolais, M.D., Ph.D.
Assistant Professor of Orthopaedic Surgery
Case Western Reserve University
Cleveland, Ohio

Pamella McMillan, M.A.
Clinical Instructor
Case Western Reserve University
Senior Audiologist
Cleveland Metropolitan General Hospital
Cleveland, Ohio

John T. Makley, M.D.
Associate Professor of Orthopaedics
Case Western Reserve University
Cleveland, Ohio

Paul R. Mitchell, M.D.
Assistant Clinical Professor of
Ophthalmology
University of Connecticut Medical School
Farmington, Connecticut
Pediatric Ophthalmologist
Newington Children's Hospital
Newington, Connecticut

Priscilla R. Morrison
Adult with Cerebral Palsy
Boston, Massachusetts

Hugo W. Moser, M.D.
Professor of Neurology and Pediatrics
Johns Hopkins University
Director
John F. Kennedy Institute
Baltimore, Maryland

Clyde L. Nash, M.D.
Associate Professor of Orthopaedic Surgery
Director, University Youth Spine Center
Case Western Reserve University
Cleveland, Ohio

Nancy Neuer, A.C.S.W.
Social Worker
Comprehensive Care Program
Cleveland Metropolitan General Hospital
Cleveland, Ohio

Stephanie Neuman, Ph.D.
Assistant Professor in Pediatrics
Case Western Reserve University
Cleveland, Ohio

Carolyn Oppenheimer, M.A.
Sex Educator and
Family Planning Coordinator
Comprehensive Care Program
Cleveland Metropolitan General Hospital
Cleveland, Ohio

Frederick B. Palmer, M.D.
Assistant Professor of Pediatrics
The Johns Hopkins University
    School of Medicine
Developmental Pediatrician
John F. Kennedy Institute
Baltimore, Maryland

Harold Rekate, M.D.
Assistant Professor of Neurosurgery
Assistant Clinical Professor of Pediatrics
Case Western Reserve University
Cleveland, Ohio

Ronald R. Riso, Ph.D.
Neurophysiologist
Rehabilitation Engineering Center
Departments of Orthopaedics and
    Biomedical Engineering
Case Western Reserve University
Cleveland, Ohio

Isadore Leslie Rubin, M.B.B.Ch., B.Sc.
Instructor in Pediatrics
Harvard Medical School
Pediatrician
Developmental Evaluation Clinic
Children's Hospital Medical Center
Boston, Massachusetts

Irwin A. Schafer, M.D.
Professor of Pediatrics
Case Western Reserve University
Director, Medical Genetics
Cleveland Metropolitan General Hospital
Cleveland, Ohio

John W. Shaffer, M.D.
Assistant Professor of Orthopaedic Surgery
Case Western Reserve University
Cleveland, Ohio

Bruce K. Shapiro, M.D.
Assistant Professor of Pediatrics
Johns Hopkins University
Developmental Pediatrician
John F. Kennedy Institute
Baltimore, Maryland

Bernard H. Shulman, J.D., D.Ed.
Superintendent of Livingston Schools
Livingston, New Jersey

Gerald A. Strom, A.C.S.W.
Social Work Supervisor
Comprehensive Care Program
Cleveland Metropolitan General Hospital
Cleveland, Ohio

George H. Thompson, M.D.
Assistant Professor of
Orthopaedic Surgery and Pediatrics
Case Western Reserve University
Chief, Pediatric Orthopaedic Surgery Service
Cleveland Metropolitan General Hospital
Cleveland, Ohio

Renee C. Wachtel, M.D.
Assistant Professor of Pediatrics
Johns Hopkins University
Developmental Pediatrician
John F. Kennedy Institute
Baltimore, Maryland

Janet Yost, M.A.
Speech Pathologist
Comprehensive Care Program
Cleveland Metropolitan General Hospital
Cleveland, Ohio

Jean M. Zadig, Ph.D.
Director, Special Education
Developmental Evaluation Clinic
Children's Hospital Medical Center
Boston, Massachusetts

Richard M. Zawacki, M.S., R.P.T.
Director, Physical Therapy Services
Wrentham State School
Wrentham, Massachusetts

Anita Zielinski, O.T.R.
Clinical Supervisor
Department of Occupational Therapy
Children's Hospital Medical Center
Wrentham State School
Wrentham, Massachusetts

Comprehensive Management of
Cerebral Palsy

PART I

Coordination of Comprehensive Care

Robert M. Bilenker

1

Coordination of Services

The availability of services for the developmentally disabled has increased greatly over the past 20 yr. In most disciplines, evaluation and therapeutic services have been provided to handicapped children and their families. Training programs in diverse disciplines have been established. These activities exist to enable developmentally disabled persons to achieve maximum potential, yet some children remain unidentified and unserved. Many others' problems have been identified, but they remain underserved by one or more disciplines. Coordination of care is a method to secure those services most appropriate for a given child. This chapter describes coordinated care and discusses the adaptational strategies of patients and families. Finally, coordination of care by parent and worker skills to improve adaptation will be explained.

A useful definition of coordinated care has been provided by Wallace:

> By coordinated care we mean that the various health services which are described for individual children and their families are integrated into a single system, which provides these services either in one geographic location, or in a chain of services so structured that easy referral of patients and interchange of information will be carried out. Not all services need to be provided in one location, but services of specialists or supporting programs must be easily available to children who need them.[12]

Health services includes the social, psychological, hearing, speech, vocational, and other community services required throughout a person's life. There is a difference between *coordinated care,* which has just been defined, and the *coordination of care.* The latter term implies that a particular person is involved in procuring services for a developmentally disabled

person. A coordinator might be a physician, nurse, or social worker who coordinates efforts among disciplines, involved agencies, and the individual or family. Within a particular interdisciplinary program or service network the discipline of the coordinator might change based on the child's age, developmental status, and nature of the problem and family needs. Other terms have been suggested for the concept of coordinated care. One such term is *direction service,* which Brewer and Kakalik have argued should not be affiliated with existing service providers.[2] Zeller has suggested that such services be based within the school setting.[13] The legal rationale for such a location would be derived from Public Law 94-142 and Section 504 of The Rehabilitation Act of 1973. At present, in many areas of the country, there are more coordinators than there are coordinated services.

ROLE OF THE COORDINATOR

Studies such as that by Kanthor and associates seek to determine areas of responsibility in the provision of health care to multiply handicapped children.[6] The results of their interviews with families of 44 children with spina bifida enrolled in the Birth Defects Clinic at the University of Rochester indicated large gaps in the provision of certain services to these families. One area was *advice,* such as information on special schooling, the child's adjustment to the handicap, discipline, and behavior. In addition, families did not feel that *future planning,* such as information on school and vocational activities, marriage, and sexual functioning, had been ad-

3

equately provided. A rough measure of "comprehensiveness" was scored for each child, and the lack of such comprehensiveness for the vast majority of children was demonstrated. The authors concluded that someone must be designated to provide effective care for children with complex chronic disabilities, whether that person is the primary physician, the specialty clinic, or a coordinating pediatrician in the community.

Many skills are required of the designated professional. A thorough understanding of the disability, the patient, and the family is mandatory. Effective communication skills are needed to explain and interpret. Thorough knowledge of both available and unavailable community resources is needed. The physician who becomes involved has to stay involved on a continuous basis whenever possible.

The physician's availability to provide continuity of care appears to correlate strongly with consumer satisfaction. Breslau and Mortimer have recently examined the effect of physician continuity on satisfaction with speciality care for disabled children.[1] They performed multiple regression analyses in which source of care, continuity of care, waiting time, and patient and family characteristics were used as predictors of satisfaction. Continuity of care accounted for a large part of the observed association.

ADAPTATIONAL STRATEGIES

The effective coordinator determines needed services and helps the family gain access to them. The information derived from each service is interpreted by the individual provider. The coordinator helps the patient and family to integrate new information on a continuing basis. To perform this task well, the coordinator must know that family's adaptational process. Family members may be at different stages in their adaptation to the disability; moreover, intellectual and emotional adaptation occur at different rates. Each family member is conditioned by earlier life experiences. Individual coping styles evident during earlier times may again be employed.[8] Lipowski describes the coping process very well:

Physical illness or disability can be conceived of as a form of psychological stress involving threat of suffering and losses. But it is just as cogent to view them as giving rise to a set of adaptational tasks, challenges and goals to be mastered or attained, where success may result in psychological growth. Illness has one crucial characteristic; the primary source of psychological stress lies within and not outside the person's body boundaries. Thus, it both imposes tasks to be dealt with and impairs in some degree the subjects capacity to meet life's demands and follow his goals.[7]

The coordinator's role can differ based on the type of health care delivery system used. An integrated system at a single site allows for informal interaction between disciplines. When only a few disciplines are represented in one location, however, the need for prompt oral and written communication is even greater. The coordinator must know the basic language of each discipline. Helping the family articulate important questions prepares them for visits with other providers. Even then, the patient may not fully understand information received. At times the family and the consultant may perceive the same interaction quite differently. The coordinator can quickly see the disparity and act to narrow the difference. This activity often requires a great deal of energy from the family, coordinator, and consultant. The thorough integration of new information may require a great deal of time.

COMPREHENSIVE CARE

Thus far, this chapter has dealt with those health services provided to evaluate and treat the developmentally disabled child or adolescent. The care has been focused on the disability itself and the family's adaptation. Well child services and health care for siblings provide additional opportunities to address the disability. Wallace's definition of comprehensive care continues to be of value:

Comprehensive care requires the integration of preventive, curative and rehabilitative services and includes care of both acute and chronic illness. Such preventive services as immunizations anticipatory guidance and accident prevention must be provided for along with case finding and the treatment of minor/major illnesses and social problems.[12]

The addition of primary care services provides added challenge and opportunity for coordinated care. These services are frequently unavailable within the specialty setting itself. Primary care most often remains with the referring physician, whether located in the hospital or community. This is often as it should be. A trust relationship with that provider has been established over time. Siblings often receive care from the same provider. Again, the role of coordinator as communicator is emphasized. The ways in which the

Table 1-1
Coordination of Care Sequence

With assistance of case manager, family is able to schedule, cancel, and reschedule planned appointments for multiple services

Family is able to schedule, cancel, and reschedule planned multiple service appointments independently

Family in collaboration with case manager will gather and review information from multiple service providers and will begin appointment diary

Family will record in diary anecdotes of child's responses to interventions

Family understands medical, psychosocial history, and current plans and goals to meet child's needs

Family understands content of planned service visits and records impressions and recommendations in diary

Family reviews medical, social, educational, and rehabilitational records in collaboration with case manager and maintains current collection of records independently

Quarterly collaboration and review by parents and case manager to coordinate multiple service plans and goals

Family conveys information and coordinates goal setting among multiple service providers and integrates new information independently

---

disabled child resembles other children frequently must be emphasized. Well child care provides a setting that allows the physician to work with the family under relatively nonstressful conditions.

A child's cognitive, physical, and psychosocial development evolves over a long period. Specific phases of development and identity tasks must be mastered to enable future development. Parents generally foster normal patterns of development as the child progresses toward independence. The presence of a developmental disability interferes with this normal process. Lack of self-esteem and social opportunities has been shown to impede emotional growth in adolescents with physical handicaps.[5,10]

PARENT AND WORKER COORDINATION SKILLS

The person who has adapted well to a disability does not allow that disability to become the focus of all activity.[4,9,11] The disability continues to affect the patient's development, but a balance can be sought. The coordinator can help the family and patient to develop their own coordination skills, thus adding to their sense of mastery, even if all fears and anxieties are not allayed. An open relationship with providers is begun and encouraged. Understandably, not all patients or families are capable of functioning in this capacity. Developing levels of coordination skills within the family can make coordination of care a treatment modality. An example of such a coordination of care scale is shown in Table 1-1.[3]

Coordination of care is integral to providing good care. The more the patient and family understand and participate in the process, the greater the chance for successful adaptation.

The objective of those who work with the disabled is to help them live as normally as possible with their disabilities. This may require work with children, adolescents, adults, family members, and significant others. In the future, advances in maternal–fetal medicine may limit or eliminate disabilities now faced daily. The following chapters present current concepts in assessment and management of cerebral palsy and developmental disabilities. The scope of the field is wide. The success of the effort depends on the cooperation and understanding of all involved.

REFERENCES

1. Breslau N, Mortimer EA: Seeing the same doctor: Determinants of satisfaction with specialty care for disabled children. Med Care 19:741, 1981
2. Brewer G, Kakalik J: Handicapped Children: Strategies for Improving Services. New York, McGraw-Hill, 1979
3. Croucher DA, Hull P, Neuman S, et al: Unpublished data, 1981
4. Drotar D, Baskiewicz A, Irvin N, et al: The adaptation of parents to the birth of an infant with a congenital malformation: A hypothetical model. Pediatrics 56:710, 1975

5. Hayden PW, Davenport SCH, Campbell MM: Adolescents with myelodysplasia: Impact of physical disability on emotional maturation. Pediatrics 64:53, 1979

6. Kanthor H, Pless B, Satterwhite B, et al: Areas of responsibility with health care of multiply handicapped children. Pediatrics 54:779, 1974

7. Lipowski ZJ: Physical illness, the individual and the coping process. Psychiat Med 1:91, 1970

8. Mattson A: Long-term physical illness in childhood: A challenge to psychosocial adaptation. Pediatrics 50:801, 1972

9. Miller L: Toward a greater understanding of the parents of the mentally retarded child. J Pediatr 73:699, 1968

10. Richardson SA: People with cerebral palsy talk for themselves. Dev Med Child Neurol 14:524, 1972

11. Tew BJ, Payne H, Laurence KM: Must a family with a handicapped child be a handicapped family? Dev Med Child Neurol (suppl 32) 16:95, 1974

12. Wallace HM, Dooley SW, Thiele SL, et al: Comprehensive health care of children. Am J Public Health 58:1839, 1968

13. Zeller RW: Direction service: Collaboration one care at a time, in Elder JO, Magrab PR (eds): Coordinating Services to Handicapped Children. Baltimore, Brookes, 1980

Leslie Rubin

2
The Role of the Pediatrician

It was William John Little who first described the clinical entity of what has become known as cerebral palsy. Little had learned to perform the procedure of Achilles tenotomy after it was successfully performed on him.[9] Since that time the management of cerebral palsy has been primarily the domain of orthopaedic surgeons, later to be supplemented by physical and occupational therapists, while neurologists wrestled with pathophysiologic mechanisms. The role that the pediatrician played has traditionally been in the provision of primary care. This is not to underestimate the valuable contributions made in the prevention of cerebral palsy by improved obstetric management, neonatal care, and health and safety measures during infancy and childhood.[10] The decline in infant mortality is a tribute to these preventive measures (Figure 2-1).[5,25]

The major thrust toward comprehensive management of the child with cerebral palsy came about with the growth of the sciences relating to child development. Awareness of neurologic maturation and the development of motor, cognitive, and social skills gave rise to the concept that each child should be encouraged to achieve full developmental potential.

The custodial institutional model of the management of children with severe cerebral palsy and related developmental disabilities has given way to a more enlightened and positive approach. The revised World Health Organization (WHO) definition of health as being not only freedom from disease but promotion of physical, emotional, and social well-being implies the multifaceted nature of health and well-being. One need only to examine the contents of this book, be involved in a cerebral palsy clinic, or closely follow an involved child to realize the multiplicity of problems that occur as well as the number of medical and allied specialities involved in managing these problems. Orthopaedic surgeons, neurologists, ophthalmologists, and neurosurgeons may all be involved with a child at a particular point, as may social workers, physical therapists, speech pathologists, psychologists, and educators.

What, then, is the pediatrician's role in the management of children with cerebral palsy and related developmental disabilities? The provision of basic primary health care should be seen as an immutable priority. This role and service is pervasive across a wide spectrum of disabilities and for all ages. For the most part, the primary health problems encountered do not differ greatly from similar clinical problems in the general population; however, some challenges may arise in special clinical problems that occur with increased frequency (Table 2-1) or as complicating factors of one or more associated disabilities (Table 2-2) and their treatment.[20,21] Other aspects of the pediatrician's role should then be appropriately addressed depending on the patient's age, family and social situation, clinical setting, and availability of services.

An attempt is made in this book to include as many aspects as possible within the scope of clinical involvement and to present the contents with a developmental theme in order to indicate the changing involvement with age from birth through childhood, adolescence, and adulthood and thus to complete the cycle (Figure 2-2).

7

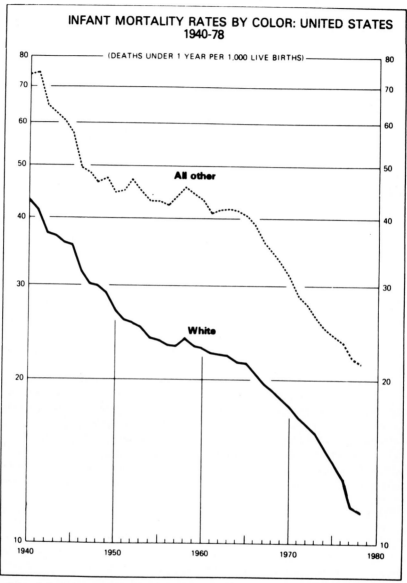

Figure 2-1. Infant mortality in the United States, 1940 - 1978. Data from the National Center for Health Statistics. (Reprinted with permission from Wegman ME: The decline in infant mortality in the United States. Pediatrics 66:823-833, 1980.)

PREVENTION

The area of prevention has been the greatest in terms of pediatric contributions to health care.[10] As the medical profession becomes more and more involved in sociocultural and politicoeconomic issues in relation to health care, so must awareness of pre-

ventive measures become a pervasive part of medical practice.[16]

Pregnancy and Birth Control

The pregnant woman's need for good obstetric care is actually intermediate in the prevention of ce-

Table 2-1

Distribution of Primary Care Visits (%)

Problem	Study Group	General Population
General medical examination	16	5
Skin infections	15	—*
Traumatic injuries	12	3
Earache and infection	9	6
Seizure disorder	8	—
Sore throat and cold	5	10
Allergic skin reactions	5	3
Behavior problems	2	—

Reprinted with permission from Schor EE, Smalky KA, Neff JM: Primary care for previously institutionalized mentally retarded children. Pediatrics 67:536, 1981.

*<1 percent or no comparable data available.

rebral palsy and other congenital and developmental abnormalities. The high rate of adolescent pregnancies and their association with increased risk of disabled children speaks to the need for early education on sexuality and birth control. In addition, the advantages of "intensive care" for this group of young mothers demonstrates an improved outcome for their infants.[17] The responsibility for education or "anticipatory guidance" not only for parents but also for the growing child falls into the hands of the pediatrician in day-to-day practice.[3] The problems are obviously interwoven with many other sociocultural and environmental factors, but patient education should be attempted as part of clinic contact.

Genetics

It should also be the pediatrician's responsibility to be aware of genetic and other factors that are potentially harmful to the developing fetus.[8,19] Here patient education and antenatal and neonatal screening for potentially preventable or treatable conditions are shared with the obstetrician.[14,15]

Low Birth Weight Infants

Awareness of the perinatal and neonatal factors, particularly as they affect the high-risk low birth weight infant, form, after all, the rationale for the establishment and maintenance of neonatal intensive care units (ICUs). The focus is not solely the management of infants with respiratory distress and metabolic disturbances, but how these conditions may cause brain damage and what can be done to prevent it.

IDENTIFICATION OF DISABILITY

Prenatal and neonatal screening procedures will obviously help to identify a number of potentially disabling conditions and thus help to prevent them or minimize their effects. Nothing, however, can substitute for a thorough physical examination for signs of possible congenital anomalies, neurologic problems, or other disturbing neurobehavioral signs.[2,18]

It may not be realistic to expect all pediatricians to be skilled in neonatal screening or the screening for the follow-up study of high-risk infants, but careful attention should be given to the developmental

Table 2-2

Prevalence of Selected Chronic Problems of Children (%)

Problem	Study Group (N = 48)	State Institution (N = 308)	General Population
Behavior disturbances	56	17	17
Allergic diathesis	56	NA	15–20
Convulsive disorder	31	21	0.34
Oculomotor abnormality	25	10	6.7
Acne	21	NA	1.7
Hearing loss	19	3	4–5
Cerebral palsy	12	34	0.13
Obesity	10	NA	2–15

Reprinted with permission from Schor EE, Smalky KA, Neff, JM: Primary care for previously institutionalized mentally retarded children. Pediatrics 67:536, 1981

SEQUENTIAL PROGRAM NEEDS OF AN INDIVIDUAL WITH
MENTAL RETARDATION AND OTHER DEVELOPMENTAL DISABILITIES

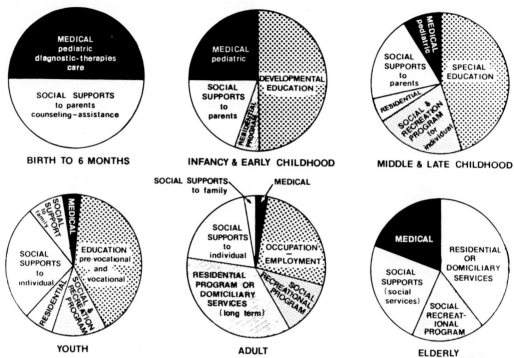

Figure 2-2. Pattern of changing needs with age for an individual with retardation and/or developmental disabilities. Developed by M. Cullinane and presented by A. C. Crocker at "Training in Developmental Pediatrics," a transdisciplinary national symposium. Gloucester, Massachusetts, 1978.

progress of all infants and children.[1] Screening guides are readily available, but most important of all may be careful attention to parental concerns, particularly if the parents are comparing the achievements of their child with another, be it a sibling or a comparable-age child.[6] An awareness of the problems relating to development, as well as their various modes of management, will help to identify children with developmental disabilities, particularly those who are more severely affected.

The importance of early detection cannot be overemphasized. With recognition, appropriate early intervention can be addressed, and parents can be counseled on their child's disability and so help the child to attain maximum potential.[22]

Within the school-age group, children will most likely be identified because of lack of academic progress. The pediatrician should be aware of these prob-

lems, since they occur in a larger number of children than do the more severe disabilities.[13]

DETERMINATION OF ETIOLOGY

One of the most frequent questions a parent asks is "Why? What causes this to happen? Was it something I did or did not do or something someone else did?" The legal implications, particularly in the United States, will not be addressed in this book, since the physician's role in any clinical setting is understood to be in the patient's best interests.

Etiologic considerations are vital, not only for the consideration of parental concerns, but also, realistically, in terms of the natural history of the particular disability, the issues of management, prevention of a similar problem in future pregnancies, and, of course, genetic counseling where appropriate. These etiologic considerations can be divided into three broad categories: prenatal, perinatal, and postnatal.

Prenatal. Prenatal etiologies usually reflect chromosomal abnormalities, genetically determined disorders, and the group of nonchromosomal "syndromes" that are spontaneous or caused by environmental factors such as infectious disease, medication, and alcohol.[8,11,19]

Perinatal. Perinatal etiologies reflect injuries sustained by the fetus immediately before delivery, during the birth process, and in the immediate neonatal period.

Postnatal. Postnatal factors are represented by illnesses, injuries, toxins, and psychosocial environment and their effects on the developing central nervous system (CNS).

Accurate and detailed history of pregnancy, birth, and development, examination with references to genetics, atlases of syndromes, and laboratory examination is the general approach to determination of etiology. Even in situations where etiologic diagnoses are vigorously pursued, however, there remains a group in whom a firm etiologic diagnosis cannot be established. This number tends to diminish slowly as advances in knowledge become applied to the delineation of congenital syndromes and the identification of biochemical and chromosomal abnormalities and other antenatal factors.

Although an etiologic diagnosis may not be made at first clinic contact, later identification may be facilitated as clinical progress is observed or as newer diagnostic techniques become available. By the same token, diagnoses may also be revised. One should therefore always bear in mind the need to pursue, confirm, or reconsider etiologic diagnoses.

CLINICAL ASSESSMENT

The clinical assessment, which includes a detailed neurologic examination, is directed toward (1) determining the nature of the lesion by appropriate diagnostic tests or procedure such as computed tomography (CT) scans of the brain, chromosome analysis, or metabolic evaluations and (2) determining the extent to which the pathologic condition affects physical, emotional, and social function.

It is frequently helpful for the pediatrician to consider and use the evaluative services provided by the various disciplines as special investigations that help delineate and quantify vital clinical information, e.g., referral to a psychologist to determine the level of cognitive function, to a physical therapist for gross motor function, to an occupational therapist for fine motor function, to an orthopaedist for overall musculoskeletal assessment, to an ophthalmologist for visual and occular function, and to a speech pathologist for receptive and expressive communication skills.

As with other clinical investigations, the pediatrician must be familiar with at least the principles of the investigation and, more important, with the interpretation of the results as they relate to a particular patient. As to developmental evaluation, instruments may not be precise, and their value depends to a far greater extent on the skills and experience of the person who performs the test. A pediatrician should therefore become familiar with available services.

The patient's and family's emotional and social status should be assessed, since the diagnosis and its life-long consequences must be presented and interpreted to the family. Here, social service and psychologic or psychiatric assessments will help to provide the the family with necessary support.

What has been outlined above constitutes the interdisciplinary evaluation process. This process can occur at many different levels and in many different ways. The major determinants relate to clinical setting, team composition, and the professional relationships between team members. The sum of the various evaluations comprises the clinical assessment, which is then synthesized into a unifying diagnosis and long-term goal-oriented plan of management.

THERAPY AND FOLLOW-UP EVALUATIONS

The results of the clinical assessment will determine the plan for therapy. Orthopaedic, ophthalmologic, and neurosurgical consultations will be considered where appropriate, as will specific therapeutic interventions from physical and occupational therapists, speech pathologists and audiologists, and other pediatric health care providers.

Regular follow-up care is essential in the management of developmental disabilities such as cerebral palsy to determine progress, effects of therapy, complications, or the appearance of new problems. Team evaluation with input from all members is very important if complications are to be minimized and maximum physical, emotional, and social development obtained. These evaluation or reevaluation processes should occur after a defined period to determine more objectively the nature of progress. The time interval will vary according to the clinical picture, the degree of severity, the presence or absence of progress, or the appearance of complications.

MANAGEMENT OF ASSOCIATED PROBLEMS

The child with cerebral palsy is a child with multiple handicaps and special needs. Some of these needs, which are discussed in detail in this book, include the need for orthopaedic surgery, seizure management, and management of visual disorders and behavior problems—all of which require identification and management or appropriate referral. Here, the pediatrician's role is that of a coordinator assuming a long-term relationship with the child and family.

MANAGEMENT OF INTERCURRENT PROBLEMS

The diagnosis and management of intercurrent illnesses can be complicated by underlying physical problems as well as by medications, such as anticonvulsants or psychotropic agents. Specific problems that occur in the general population may be more difficult to manage because of underlying physical and emotional disabilities including dental problems, constipation, sleep disorders, or behavior problems. Trauma is another problem that can occur with increased frequency. Because of problems with balance, movement disorders, and seizures, these children are likely to fall and sustain contusions, lacerations, and fractures. Some fractures may even occur with overzealous physical therapy by an inexperienced person in a child with severe spasticity. The issue of child abuse should also be borne in mind, since there is evidence that it occurs with increased frequency in children with developmental disabilities.[7,23] Available statistics on primary health and intercurrent problems usually relate to groups of retarded children in residential setting but can serve as

a guide to the kinds of problems one is likely to encounter.[20,21]

Developmental issues are frequently raised by parents with anxious expectancy. Basic motor functions such as sitting and walking will be delayed, but the more significant issues such as eating of solid foods, problems of poor or excessive weight gain, and toilet training—all the questions generally asked of pediatricians—will be asked regarding this group of children. They will naturally be more difficult to answer, and they will be based on the child's developmental status and degree of disability.

MANAGEMENT OF PARENTAL CONCERNS

Parents' emotional reactions vary with many factors, including age, family structure and stability, socioeconomic status, cultural background, and presence of support systems. It is very difficult to predict accurately how any one family will react, but basically, because of an increased investment in the child, the parents will have greater needs. These needs may appear in more frequent calls to the pediatrician, exaggerated concern over minor problems, or more time required to talk in the physician's office. The spectrum of family pathologic states is great in the general population, and it may be greater in this potentially stressful situation. Marital disharmony, divorce, depression, neglect, and even child abuse are very important clinical entities to bear in mind.[7,23] It may well be the pediatrician who will have the opportunity to identify a pathologic family situation and, by early recognition and referral, prevent potentially serious consequences.

SIBLINGS

Pediatricians usually have the opportunity of managing siblings of developmentally disabled children in a routine health care situation. These siblings too may experience the emotional stress that parents feel.[4] As a result of parental overinvolvement in the affected child, other children may feel or actually be neglected. Children may also feel some measure of guilt and responsibility for their affected sibling's condition. As a result of these and other social issues, siblings may have emotional, behavioral, or psychosomatic problems. They may also manifest a surprising interest in etiologic factors, and their own interpretation may be more frightening to them than the reality. Concern may also arise in older siblings approaching childbearing age about the genetics of the disability.

GENETIC COUNSELING

Although cerebral palsy per se is not a genetically determined disorder, many other causes of developmental disabilities may be. Families do tend to be concerned about recurrence. Where a diagnosis can be made, referral to a geneticist may help as well—if not to establish a diagnosis, then perhaps to reassure the family.[26]

PEDIATRIC INVOLVEMENT AT DIFFERENT AGES AND STAGES

The pediatrician's role in management follows growth and development. At each stage the involvement is different and changes quite rapidly. albeit at times imperceptibly.

Perinatal Period

Pediatricians are often involved while the mother is still pregnant. This may be because of previous involvement with siblings or because parents are anxious to have someone identified ahead of time to care for their as yet unborn infant. In addition, and more significantly, particularly with newer techniques in antenatal care and prenatal diagnosis, pediatricians may be involved because of anticipated problems with the birth. The management of high-risk infants requiring resuscitation and intensive care can be very demanding. Parental concerns, anxieties, and reactions to this situation also require careful consideration.[12] The importance of clinical responsibility toward parents at this stage can not be overemphasized, since it represents the beginning of a long-term relationship, not only between parents and infant, but also between family and professionals. Difficult questions, such as prognosis for life or prognosis for normal development, may or may not be expressed by the parents but must be addressed. Improved perinatal and neonatal care has resulted in the reduction of the incidence of cerebral palsy, even for low birth weight premature infants. It is this latter group that has come to represent the highest risk for the development of cerebral palsy in developed countries.[5]

Infancy

Routine health care issues and special problems should include special attention to neuromotor development. Other routine issues such as feeding, sleeping, intercurrent illnesses, immunizations, and so on should be dealt with appropriately. One must remember, however, that parents' usual anxieties may be accentuated, and they may require more time for discussion.

Preschool and School-age Child

When issues of socialization and assimilation into peer groups arise, the needs of the child and family change, and the pediatrician's role naturally changes as well. Visits may become less frequent, but the relationship that has been established will greatly facilitate the management of the child and family during these years. The pediatrician's role as leader in team assessment and long-term management becomes more important during this time, since there is increased use and participation of the various specialists involved in patient care.

Questions about surgery, hospitalization, seizures, physical handicaps, intellectual disability, and all other associated problems must be evaluated, since they now begin to relate to the school setting. They should be evaluated not only with respect to physical problems but also to problems of learning, across a spectrum from mild disabilities to more significant intellectual impairment as well as to hearing, behavior, and socialization.

Built into this clinical relationship is always the anticipation of the future. For parents it is often related to independence, vocation, and potential for family life. For the clinician, it should relate to the imminent problems attendant with puberty and adolescence.

The Adolescent and Young Adult

Within the sphere of the clinical diagnosis of cerebral palsy there exists a spectrum of differences in severity as well as in the nature of problems. Generalizations may help to establish a conceptual framework from which to operate, but the individual must always be appreciated for his or her own personality, both in strengths and in weaknesses. Nowhere is this issue more sensitive than in adolescence.

Emotional Problems

Adolescents' acute self-awareness tends to be exaggerated in the presence of recognizable differences. The adolescent with cerebral palsy therefore requires a great amount of support and encouragement to develop self-esteem. Psychologists, psychiatrists, social workers, or counselors can help them realize this.

Behavioral Problems

Behavioral problems may arise as a result of the emotional disturbances associated with adolescence or may be aggravated in the person with an underlying behavior disorder. Again, consultation with psychiatrists or psychologists may be required to help deal with these problems.

Emerging Sexuality

Careful monitoring of puberty is important, and appropriate issues relating to sexuality, including birth control, should be discussed.

Physical Growth

For the individual with a mild disability, physical growth will present no real problem, since it is merely an aspect of growing to adulthood. There are, however, two situations in which it may present a problem. The first situation concerns patients with the more severe physical disabilities. The functioning of an individual who is physically dependent on crutches or wheelchairs or on a caregiver for am-

bulation or transport may be compromised by an increase in size and weight. Weight control is important but, all too often, difficult. The pediatrician's knowledge of nutrition, exercise, dieting, and other weight control measures, even those involving behavior management, are important for early identification and prevention, which may greatly facilitate later management.

The second situation concerns patients with the more difficult behavior problems. Whereas the younger and smaller child can be more readily controlled by a larger and stronger adult, the adolescent has now grown and, coupled with the aggravation of behavior problems that can occur during adolescence, may be very difficult to manage. This particularly applies to parents who may not be as young, strong, or tolerant as they were when the child was younger. It is at this point, with the more severely affected individuals, that parents often begin to look at residential placement. Consultation with a psychiatrist with a view toward behavior management with or without psychotropic medication may be necessary.[24] Awareness of community residential programs is also important.

Independence

The goal, as stated at the beginning of this chapter, is to encourage each child to attain his or her maximum functioning potential to gain as independent a living and working situation as possible. For most children, this will be attainable. The achievement for each individual will depend on self-potential, on professional help and preparation, and on the security and support of family and society.

REFERENCES

1. Amiel-Tison C: A method of neurological examination within the first year of life. Curr Probl Pediatr 2:, 1976.
2. Brazelton TB: Neonatal behavioral assessment scale. Clin Dev Med 50:, 1973.
3. Brazelton TB: Anticipatory guidance. Pediatr Clin North Am 22:533, 1975.
4. Crocker AC:, in Milunsky A (ed): Involvement of Siblings of Children with Handicaps. Coping with Crisis and Handicap. New York, Plenum, 1981, pp 219–223.
5. Dale A, Stanley FJ: An epidemiological study of cerebral palsy in western Australia. Dev Med Child Neurol 22:12, 1975.
6. Frankenberg WK, Goldstein AD, Camp BW: The revised Denver developmental screening test: Its accuracy as a screening instrument. J Pediatr 79:988, 1971
7. Frodi AM: Contribution of infant characteristics to child abuse. Am J Ment Defic 85:341, 1981
8. Grossman III JH: Perinatal viral infections. Clin Perinatol 7:257, 1980
9. Green WT: Historical notes—the past generation in orthopedic aspects of cerebral palsy, in Samilson RL: Clinics in Developmental Medicine, no. 52/53. London, William Heineman, 1975
10. Henderson DA: Expanding horizons on a diminishing planet. Pediatrics 67:771, 1981

11. Iosub S, Fuchs M, Bingol N, et al: Fetal Alcohol Syndrome Revisited. Pediatrics 68:475, 1981
12. Klaus MH, Kennell JH: Maternal–Infant Bonding. St. Louis, Mosby, 1976
13. Levine MD, Brooks R, Shonkoff JP: A Pediatric Approach to Learning Disorders. New York, Wiley, 1980
14. Mamunes P: Neonatal screening tests. Pediatr Clin North Am 27:733, 1980
15. Miles JH, Kaback MM: Prenatal diagnosis of hereditary disorders. Pediatr Clin North Am 25:593, 1978
16. Nader PR, Ray L, Brink SG: The new morbidity: Use of school and community health care resources for behavioral, educational, and social family problems. Pediatrics 67:53, 1981
17. Perkins RP, Nakashima II, Mullin, M et al: Intensive care in adolescent pregnancy. Obstet Gynecol 52:179, 1978
18. Prechtl HFE: The neurological examination of the full-term newborn infant, in Samilson RL: Clinics in Developmental Medicine, no. 63. London, William Heineman, 1977
19. Redmond GP: Effects of drugs on intrauterine growth. Clin Perinatol 6:5, 1979
20. Schor EE, Smalky KA, Neff JM: Primary care for previously institutionalized mentally retarded children. Pediatrics 67:536, 1981
21. Smith DC, Decker HA, Herberg EN, et al: Medical needs of children in institutions for the mentally retarded. Am J Public Health 59:1376, 1969
22. Soboloff HR: Early intervention—fact or fiction. Dev Med Child Neurol 23:261, 1981
23. Solomons G: Child abuse and developmental disabilities. Dev Med Child Neurol 21:101, 1979
24. Szymanski LS, Tanguay PE: Emotional Disorders of Mentally Retarded Persons. Baltimore, University Park Press, 1980
25. Wegman ME: Annual summary of vital statistics—1979: With some 1930 comparisons. Pediatrics 66:823, 1980
26. Wood JW: The pediatrician as genetic counsellor. Pediatr Clin North Am 21:401, 1974

PART II

Etiology and Prevention

Robert M. Eiben
Allen C. Crocker

3

Cerebral Palsy Within the Spectrum of Developmental Disabilities

Conceptualization of the comprehensive aspects of cerebral palsy requires an understanding of its current definition, classification, etiologic factors, and integration and relationship within the spectrum of other developmental disabilities.

GENERAL ORIENTATION

Cerebral palsy is a term applied to a number of disabilities resulting from developmental or perinatal injury to the central nervous system (CNS) (Table 3-1). No single definition of cerebral palsy will satisfy all interested in the clinical management of handicapping disorders. Generally, major congenital malformations of the nervous system that are clinically recognizable would not be included. Most, however, would apply the term to individuals whose nervous system dysfunction resulted from prenatal and perinatal events. The term implies a nonprogressive disturbance of nervous system function characterized by an abnormality of motor function and posture or an aberrant movement disorder.

The classification of the disorders included is made on the basis of the distribution and character of motor dysfunction or movement disorder; unfortunately, the etiologic basis of the disability is not considered. In addition, the problem of mental subnormality and seizures, which represent other manifestations of CNS dysfunction, although related etiologically to the motor disability, are often dealt with quite separately from the motor problem. It must be emphasized that the diagnosis of cerebral palsy implies a nonprogressive disorder; in general, the cerebral palsies are not considered among the heredofamilial diseases. There are, however, developmental disorders associated with spastic states that have proven familial occurrence.[9]

As is true with most handicapping conditions, the management of these patients is best accomplished through a multidisciplinary approach. As a result of a lack of consistency in the criteria for diagnosis, the estimated frequency of occurrence of cerebral palsy in the general population is difficult to ascertain. Fairly reasonable estimates suggest an incidence of approximately 7:1000 live births and a prevalence of nearly 500 cases:100,000 population.

The results of a prospective study of 54,000 pregnant women conducted between 1959 and 1966 in the National Institutes of Health Collaborative Perinatal Project (NCPP), has provided the most recent and possibly the most accurate prevalence figures of the occurrence of cerebral palsy in a defined population for the United States (Table 3-2).[10]

Remarkable advances in the clinical management of low birth weight and sick neonates have been achieved, and there has been concern that the infant graduates of neonatal intensive care units (ICUs), many having experienced major stress, would significantly increase the prevalence of cerebral palsy. The results of the NCPP study do not indicate that this is the case. Our experience in postmortem examination of infants dying in the neonatal ICU has not shown the lesions of brain that are felt to char-

19

Table 3-1

Etiologic Classification of Cerebral Palsy

Developmental anomalies[9,13]
  Disorders of neuronal migration (polymicrogyria)
    Spastic Diplegia
  Schizencephalies (double symmetric porencephalies)
    Double or bilateral hemiplegia
Perinatal trauma[6]
  Intracerebral hemorrhage, cerebral infarction, or both
    Spastic states
Metabolic disorders in perinatal period[2,3]
  Hypoxia
    Premature infant
      Spastic diplegia
    Full-term infant
      Spastic states
      Choreoathetosis
      Ataxia
  Hypoglycemia
    Spastic states
  Hyperbilirubinemia
    Choreoathetosis

Table 3-3

Clinical Presentation of Cerebral Palsy

Symptom	Percentage
Hemiplegia	25–40
Spastic diplegia	10–33
Spastic quadriplegia	9–43
Extrapyramidal (including athetoid, ataxic, and dystonic forms)	9–22
Mixed	9–22

acterize asphyxia in the same frequency that had been observed before the rapid advances in neonatology occurred.

Because of the multiple etiologies of these conditions, predisposing factors vary. Maternal infection appears etiologically connected to a number of developmental abnormalities considered among these disorders. High birth weight predisposes to trauma and intracerebral bleeding and clearly accounts for a number of patients with spastic states.[6] The metabolic disturbances encountered in the perinatal period probably account for the greatest number of patients with "cerebral palsy," and particularly vulnerable is the low-birth-weight child. The metabolic conditions of anoxia, hypoglycemia, and hyperbilirubinemia can

be shown to be associated with rather stereotyped pathologic states and clinical manifestations.[3–5] The classification and distribution of the varied clinical presentation of cerebral palsy is shown in Table 3-3.[10]

Anoxic encephalopathy warrants a particular emphasis in view of the apparent differences seen in full-term newborns as compared to those prematurely born. The writings of Little in 1843 emphasized the relationship of low birth weight and poor socioeconomic circumstances to the type of cerebral palsy often identified with his name.[8] Little's disease is now described as the spastic diplegic form of cerebral palsy.

It would be highly desirable to recognize cerebral palsy at an early age. Physicians are certainly in a position to identify the individual at risk, but in the NCPP project none of the 60 prenatal factors distinguished the type of cerebral palsy in the study group from control participants. Neonatal characteristics identified only severely handicapped persons with intracranial hemorrhage and neonatal seizures, the major discriminators between severely handicapped and control children.[11] The estimated average life span of an individual with cerebral palsy is 30 yr; a disproportionate number of the severely handicapped die by 5 yr, and most of the severely handicapped die by 15 yr.

Table 3-2

Prevalence of Cerebral Palsy at 7 Yr of Age (in 1000 Children)

Diagnosis	No.	Low Estimate*	High Estimate†
Definite	202	4.0	5.2
Congenital	178	3.5	4.6
Moderate and severe congenital	101	2.0	2.6

*Based on 50,805 live births.
†Based on 38,533 live births with known 7-yr outcome.

It has long been recognized that the newborn exhibits primarily instinctive and reflex behaviors and that many infants appear to grow into their disability, an observation that obscures the origin of the developmental problem and raises the question of progressive disease in what is in fact a static disorder.

LOCATION IN A SPECTRUM OF DEVELOPMENTAL DISABILITIES

Quest for Causation

In addressing the situation of a child with a handicap, early attention inevitably rests on the issue of causation. The drive in this regard has many motivations, including the need to be able to provide (1) parental counseling, (2) guidance on prognosis, (3) office or clinic statistics as these relate to agency function, (4) a base for public health concerns in prevention, and (5) the simple intellectual satisfaction of understanding what has apparently happened clinically. As any worker who has spent time coding the records of developmentally disabled children can vouch, however, establishment of the presumed base for the cortical (or other) handicap is a tenuous operation. Classification on symptomatic (qualitative) or functional (quantitative) grounds is relatively satisfactory, although it must be admitted that the medical, federal, and even international systems in this regard have often been confounding. When it comes to affirmations of causation, however, one enters an area of fractious judgment, arbitrary conviction, potential vested interest, data gaps, and tests of fairness. It could be claimed that when etiologic discussion involves the role of a single gene or a single virus, the road is smooth, but even here are issues of variable expression and effect. It becomes more complicated with seemingly discrete events, e.g., a chromosomal aberration or a cranial trauma, where universality of outcome cannot be assumed. When one gets beyond these relatively deterministic circumstances, the inductive process becomes notably more confused.

One of the obvious deterrents to proceeding with classification schemes for the origin of handicaps is the implication that there is "a" cause for the problem. This downgrades the reality of multifactorial sources working in combination and especially of the role of altered vulnerability in an organism. The American Association on Mental Deficiency's 1982 *Manual on Terminology and Classification* will incorporate a tier system for causational language, which will assist in this regard.

Organizational Approach to Developmental Disabilities

The experience of the Developmental Evaluation Clinic at the Children's Hospital Medical Center in Boston, a study unit for children with multiple handicaps mental retardation, or both, has led to the adoption of a modified chart of "etiology."[7,14] In this plan one prepares a basic inventory of developmental hazards, organized in chronologic sequence, and uses the best judgment available to weight the circumstantial evidence surrounding each child's presentation. In this fashion it is usually possible to declare an ascendant mechanism for the exceptionality. If a determination cannot be made or competitive multiple issues exist, the "unknown" category is used. This schema is illustrated in Table 3-4. It is apparent that this classification is only partially one of "causation," since the true etiology remains obscure for chromosomal changes, the vast majority of prenatal influence syndromes, most fetal malnutrition, the variable impact of hypoxia, and the route for childhood psychosis and autism. It is justified, however, to declare the child with sporadic occurrence of multiple congenital anomalies to have incurred a first-trimester stress and the child who is small for dates and accompanied by placental infarcts to have had late-pregnancy deprivation. In this sense, one is identifying a mechanism if not an etiology.

A few additional comments are appropriate regarding the inevitable "unknown" category. The Developmental Evaluation Clinic findings portray three groups of children with mental retardation, each probably heterogeneous. In one, there were indeed abnormal events of interest, but generally of low degree and in tandem with other circumstances that also could have had effect; no single mechanism could be defended. Another group had interesting neurologic abnormalities, often mild, but did not have other signs or a history of prenatal or perinatal difficulties. Yet others had no clues or accompanying pathologic states (beyond mental retardation) and represented a group of real "unknown unknowns." The distribution of degree of intellectual handicap among the unknown-mechanism children was similar to that in the more familiar categories. As knowledge grows about markers and other discriptive elements in "new" syndromes, it is reasonable to assume that some children with previously obscure presentations will be taken

Table 3-4
Mechanisms of Developmental Disabilities*

Disorder	Total Mentally Retarded Group (%)
Hereditary disorders: preconceptual origin, variable expression, multiple somatic effects, frequently a progressive course	4
Inborn errors of metabolism, e.g., Tay-Sachs disease, Hurler's disease, phenylketonuria	
Other single gene abnormalities, e.g., muscular dystrophy, neurofibromatosis, tuberous sclerosis	
Chromosomal aberrations, including translocation	
Polygenic familial syndromes	
Early alterations of embryonic development: sporadic events affecting embryogenesis, phenotypic changes, usually a stable developmental handicap	32
Chromosomal changes, including trisomy, e.g., Down's syndrome	
Prenatal influence syndromes, e.g., intrauterine infectins, drugs, unknown forces	
Other pregnancy problems and perinatal morbidity: impingement on progress of fetus during last two trimesters or on newborn, neurologic abnormalities frequent, handicap stable or occasionally worsening	12
Fetal malnutrition and placental insufficiency	
Perinatal difficulties, e.g., prematurity, hypoxia, trauma	
Acquired childhood diseases: acute modification of developmental status, variable potential for functional recovery	4
Infection, e.g., encephalitis, meningitis	
Cranial trauma	
Other, e.g., cardiac arrest, intoxications	
Environmental and social problems: dynamic influences, operational throughout development, commonly combined with other handicaps	17
Deprivation	
Parental neurosis, psychosis	
Childhood neurosis	
Childhood psychosis	
Unknown causes: no definite hereditary, gestational, perinatal, acquired, or environmental issues or else multiple elements present	31

*Mental retardation, cerebral palsy, seizure disorders, and sensory handicaps.
†Hospital referral experience.

out of the unknown category. Recent examples include those with fetal alcohol effects and with the fragile-X-chromosome syndrome, although phenotypic clues in those instances could sometimes have suggested first-trimester or constitutional mechanisms.

Changing Concepts

A decade ago, formulation was made of a more general "developmental disabilities" concept, first speaking to the common service needs across the varied types of expression of early cortical handicap.

It is certainly clear that symptomatic and functional overlapping is conspicuous in children who have cerebral palsy, mental retardation, epilepsy, and other chronic neurologic disorders.[1] Common neurogenic pathways may underly these disabilities. In hospital-based cerebral palsy clinics about half to two thirds of the children will also have significant mental retardation, and similar figures are found in hospital seizure clinics. In the Developmental Evaluation Clinic the population selected primarily for presumed mental retardation had other widespread problems, e.g., motor function difficulties, seizures, and language and sensory handicaps. The motor function problems, present in well over half the children, commonly involve abnormalities in tone, strength, balance, coordination, motor planning, and visual motor perception.

The conventional definition of cerebral palsy (nonprogressive abnormality of motor function and posture, or aberrant movement disorder) is selected to give special concern to the effects of prenatal or perinatal events. This obviously focuses on the prenatal influence syndromes, fetal malnutrition and placental insufficiency, and perinatal difficulties noted in Table 3-4. Gross malformations of the CNS, also an element of the prenatal influence syndromes, are viewed as a separate issue. It must be admitted, however, that compelling phenocopies of cerebral palsy can be produced in some of the hereditary syndromes and early acquired disorders.

Identification of an etiology for the handicap of cerebral palsy is as complex as is that exercise for mental retardation. That a reliance on traditional views is not satisfactory is well shown in the recent report by Nelson and Ellenberg on the large prospective experience of the NCPP study.[12] They have analyzed childhood outcomes as coordinated with the parameter of Apgar scoring, which can be used as one index of perinatal difficulties (either from obstetric complications or special vulnerability). In their findings, 73 percent of the children who subsequently developed cerebral palsy had Apgar scores of 7 to 10 at 5 min, and of the surviving infants who had had late low (0 to 3) scores, only 12 percent went on to develop cerebral palsy. It must be assumed that the majority of the children in their project who developed cerebral palsy had relatively inconspicuous CNS malformations with adequate status in the immediate birth period.

The right-hand column of Table 3-4 presents incidence data for apparent mechanisms of mental retardation in a hospital referral population, the Developmental Evaluation Clinic.[14] It is suggested that this scheme of settings, arranged in a developmental sequence, can also serve as a guide for consideration for all handicapped children when one is pursuing the quest for causation. The quantitative assignments for the various categories will obviously differ based on the nature of the clinical and demographic sample and the codifier's judgmental criteria. In the final analysis, children with cerebral palsy, or those eligible for the services of a cerebral palsy clinic, could derive the origin of their multifaceted exceptionality from any of the mechanisms of developmental compromise.

REFERENCES

1. Accardo PJ, Capute AJ: Epidemiology, in Acardo PJ, Capute AJ (eds): The Pediatrician and the Developmentally Delayed Child. Baltimore, University Park Press, 1979, pp 13–19
2. Banker B, Larroche J: Periventricular leukomalacia of infancy. Arch Neurol 7:386, 1962
3. Banker B: The neuropathological effects of anoxia and hypoglycemia in the newborn. Dev Med Child Neurol 9:544, 1967
4. Byers RK, Paine RS, Crothers B: Extrapyramidal cerebral palsy with hearing loss following erythroblasts. Pediatrics 15:248, 1955
5. Churchill JA, Colfert RH: Etiologic factors in athetoid cerebral palsy. Arch Neurol 9:400, 1963
6. Craig W: Intracranial hemorrhage in the newborn. A study of diagnosis and differential diagnosis based upon pathological and clinical findings in 126 cases. Arch Dis Child 13:89, 1938
7. Crocker AC: The biologic components of mental retardation, In Szymanski LS, Tanguay PE (eds): Emotional Disorders of Mentally Retarded Persons; Assessment, Treatment, and Consultation. Baltimore, University Park Press, 1980, pp 51–59
8. Little WJ: Course of lectures on the deformities of the human frame: Lecture VIII. Lancet 1:318, 1843
9. Miller JQ: Lissencephaly in 2 siblings. Neurology 13:841, 1963
10. Nelson KB, Ellenberg JH: Epidemiology of cerebral palsy. Adv Neurol 19:421, 1978
11. Nelson KB, Ellenberg JH: Neonatal signs as predictors of cerebral palsy. Pediatrics 64:225, 1979
12. Nelson KB, Ellenberg JH: Apgar scores as predictors of chronic neurologic disability. Pediatrics 68:36, 1981
13. Yakovlev PI, Wadsworth RC: Double symmetrical porencephalies (Schizencephalies). Presented at the 67th annual meeting of the Trans American Neurological Society, 1941
14. Zadig JM, Crocker AC: A center for study of the young child with developmental delay, In Friedlander BZ, Sterritt GM, Kirk GE (eds): Exceptional Infant, vol. 3. New York, Brunner/Mazel, 1975, pp 5–39

Betty Q. Banker
Jocelyn Bruce-Gregorios

4

Neuropathology

DEFINITION AND BACKGROUND

More than 100 yr ago, Little linked abnormal parturition, difficult labor, premature birth, and asphyxia neonatorum with a spastic rigidity of the limbs.[10–12] Since then, numerous clinical and pathologic studies have confirmed this concept, yet many factors concerning the pathogeneses of these conditions are poorly understood.[1,4,17–20] In the last 15 yr, studies of monkey fetuses that were subjected to episodes of asphyxia by mechanisms simulating those in humans and then resuscitated have contributed to an understanding of the pathologic bases of so-called cerebral palsy.[14] Studies with modern techniques such as computerized axial tomography (CAT) scans and ultrasound studies of the brain have enabled the clinician to visualize the topography, extent, and nature of the destructive processes in many infants.[13,21] These techniques have provided a window into the brain and have resulted in an understanding of many diseases before a postmortem examination. Still other contributions may lead to an understanding of the pathogenesis of some of these entities.

NEUROPATHOLOGIC LESIONS

Experimental

Recently, animal models of neonatal intraventricular hemorrhage have been produced.[5,16] In the 24- to 72-hr-old beagle, intraventricular hemorrhage has been induced by a hypercapric insult coupled with elevated systemic arterial blood pressure, after moderate phenylephrine-induced hypertension, and after volume expansion following hemorrhagic hypotension. Goddard et al. have suggested that the increased cerebral blood flow in all regions in response to phenylephrine-induced hypertension and the increased cerebral blood flow in the subcortical region and brain stem in response to hypotension followed by a rapid volume expansion appear to contribute to subependymal and intraventricular hemorrhages in the neonatal beagle.[5] In the subependymal hemorrhage of the premature rabbit, the vessels of the germinal matrix either do not possess a basal lamina or, if they do, it is ill defined and appears to be discontinuous; in comparison, the cortical vessels were well enclosed by a basal lamina.[16] These authors suggested that such incomplete formation of basement membrane could make the germinal matrix more vulnerable to hemorrhage in this very young age group. Grunnet has compared the capillaries of the germinal matrix in premature rats and humans with the vessels of adjacent structures.[7] In each case the capillaries in the germinal plate had thicker and less regular endothelium, more endothelial microvilli, and a less dense basement membrane than vessels of similar size in the adjacent structures. On the basis of these studies, Grunnet has stressed the importance of immaturity of vessel structure in the pathogenesis of subependymal hemorrhage in the very young infant.

Many studies are thus contributing to an understanding of the clinical, pathologic, and radiologic features of the multiplicity of conditions that hide under the umbrella of cerebral palsy. More recently, experimental studies have been directed toward an understanding of the pathogenesis of individual conditions.

Table 4-1
Estimated Gestational Age at Birth (914 Infants)

Gestation (wk)	No. of Infants	Percentage
<24	105	12.0
24–28	252	28.9
28–30	104	11.9
30–32	89	10.2
32–34	62	7.1
34–36	70	8.0
36–38	76	8.7
38–40	81	9.3
40–42	18	2.0
>42	15	1.7
Subtotal	872	
Unspecified	42	
Total	914	

Table 4-3
Birth Weight

Weight (g)	No. of Infants	Incidence (%)
1000	314	35.6
1000–2000	297	33.7
2000–2500	109	12.4
2500–3000	66	7.5
3000–3500	53	6.0
3500–4000	28	3.2
4000	14	1.6
Subtotal	881	
Unspecified	33	
Total	914	

Infant

This chapter focuses on the neuropathologic incidence of various conditions in the first year of life. An understanding of the topography and frequency of the changes in the nervous system and the complications that may follow the insult will undoubtedly aid in more accurate diagnosis as well as in the appreciation of the structural defects in children who have had a major nonprogressive disturbance of motor function since birth. Such an understanding can only result in better patient care.

The material presented here is based on the study of the central nervous system (CNS) of 914 infants (506 male and 408 female) under the age of one year, obtained from consecutive autopsies at the Cleveland Metropolitan General Hospital. All tissues were examined at autopsy over a period of nine and one half years. The estimated gestational age at birth, the mode of delivery, and the infants' birth weight are listed in Tables 4-1 to 4-3. The vast majority of neuro-

pathologic changes in these autopsied infants could be divided into three distinct groups: subependymal hemorrhage, anoxic encephalopathy, and developmental anomalies (Table 4-4).

Subependymal Hemorrhage

Subependymal hemorrhage was the most common neuropathologic change encountered in our autopsy material (see Table 4-4). This abnormality was found in 43.6 percent of all infants who were autopsied in the first week of life. In 75.3 percent of the subependymal hemorrhages the blood had ruptured into the lateral ventricle. Almost all these infants were of low birth weight, the vast majority being under 28 wk of gestational age.

Pulmonary hemorrhages of varying sizes were found in 39.3 percent of infants with subependymal hemorrhage and in 36.1 percent of infants without subependymal hemorrhage. Hyaline membrane disease of the lung was present in 54 percent of infants with subependymal hemorrhage but in only 32.1 percent of infants without subependymal bleeding. Periventricular leukomalacia was present in 10.7 percent of infants with subependymal hemorrhage and in 9.3 percent of infants without such hemorrhages.

The characteristic change in the brain consists of a small lake of blood in the subependymal germinal matrix near the caudate nucleus at the level of the mammillary bodies (Fig. 4-1). The bleeding is frequently bilateral. In 24.7 percent of infants the blood remains loculated (Fig. 4-2), while in others it ruptures through the adjacent ependyma, resulting in an intraventricular hemorrhage (Fig. 4-3). It is not unusual to find a cast of blood distending the entire ventricular system. In those infants who survive the bleeding, there is proliferation of connective tissue

Table 4-2
Mode of Delivery

Mode	No. of Infants	Percentage
Spontaneous	583	73.8
Cesarian section	153	19.4
Forceps	54	6.8
Subtotal	790	
Unspecified	124	
Total	914	

Table 4-4

Incidence of Neuropathologic Changes in Relation to Age of Infant

Age at death (days)	Stillborn	1–7	8–28	29–84	85–180	181–365	Total number of infants
Number of infants	263	514	77	38	10	12	914
Neuropathologic change*							
Anoxic encephalopathy							
Cortical and subcortical changes	43	148	28	18	8	5	250
Subependymal gliosis	55	123	16	14	2	1	211
Periventricular leukomalacia	0	51	14	8	1	0	74
Subependymal hemorrhage	27	224	27	6	0	0	284
Developmental anomalies	24	54	6	7	0	2	93
Other intracranial hemorrhages	11	28	8	2	0	0	49
Kernicterus	1	18	0	0	0	0	19
Meningitis	1	18	15	8	0	3	45
Encephalitis	2	6	6	6	0	0	20
Infarction	1	10	7	1	0	0	19
Tentorial tears	2	11	0	0	0	0	13
Contusions, lacerations, or both	0	4	0	0	0	0	4
No abnormalities	122	73	6	0	1	2	204

*More than one neuropathologic change could be present in a single infant.

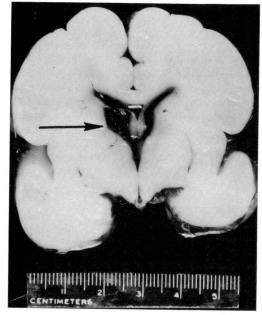

Figure 4-1. A subependymal hemorrhage *(arrow)* has ruptured into the lateral ventricle and filled and distended the lateral and third ventricles with blood. The brain is from an infant born after 22 wk of gestation.

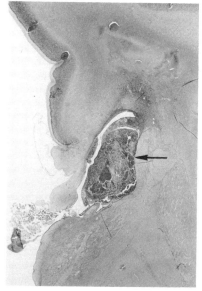

Figure 4-2. This subependymal hemorrhage *(arrow)* is well loculated within the germinal matrix of the lateral ventricle.

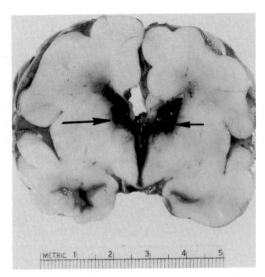

Figure 4-3. Bilateral subependymal hemorrhages *(arrows)* have ruptured into the lateral ventricles.

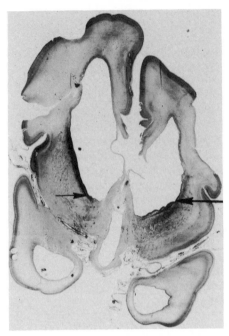

Figure 4-4. This infant died at two months of age. Old blood and gliosis obstructed the foramina of Luschka, resulting in the hydrocephalus. The scars of the previous bilateral subependymal hemorrhages *(arrows)* are located in the characteristic zone.

in the subarachnoid space as well as glia traversing and obstructing the foramina of Luschka. This obstruction to the flow of cerebrospinal fluid (CSF) results in the development of hydrocephalus (Fig. 4-4).

Subependymal hemorrhage results in the death of many of the afflicted infants and in spasticity and hydrocephalus in those who survive. These disastrous effects are the result of the rupture of blood into the ventricle; the source of the hemorrhage is represented by only a small scar, consisting of pigment-laden macrophages and surrounded by a glial wall adjacent to the lateral ventricle. The tracts in the corona radiata may degenerate as a result of the sudden distension of the ventricle by blood. The point to be stressed is that a small bleed close to the ventricle in a small infant will penetrate into the ventricle, distend the ventricular system, and be handled very poorly by the immature nervous system; yet, very little of the nervous tissue lies in the path of the bleeding, and it is damaged only as a result of the casting within the ventricles and the obstruction to the iters.

In correlating the clinical signs with the pathologic changes, it is obvious that the decrease in hematocrit reflects the severity of the bleeding. The disturbances of consciousness ranging from lethargy to coma and the hyporeflexia, flaccidity, incomplete Moro's reflex, and signs of increased intracranial pressure also reflect the severity of the hemorrhage. The sudden worsening of the clinical state presum-

ably corresponds to the penetration of the subependymal blood into the ventricle.

The pathogenesis of the subependymal hemorrhage is not understood. Any theory of pathogenesis must take into consideration the infant's immaturity and the stereotyped topography of the hemorrhage. The selective vulnerability of the immature vessels (Fig. 4-5) in the germinal matrix in the designated zone has been suggested for many years to represent a key factor.[2] It has been postulated that the lack of adequate supporting fibers in the subependymal matrix facilitates venous rupture when stasis occurs. The zone of periventricular matrix persists until 34 wk of gestation and usually has disappeared by 40 wk.[7] Furthermore, the dense collection of immature cells provides a poor supporting stroma.[7] This factor plus the presence of immature veins in the subependymal zone would logically explain the consistent localization of the lesion and its high incidence in the immature infant. An all-embracing theory of the pathogenesis of subependymal hemorrhage would also have to consider the distribution and regulation of cerebral blood flow in the premature infant, the el-

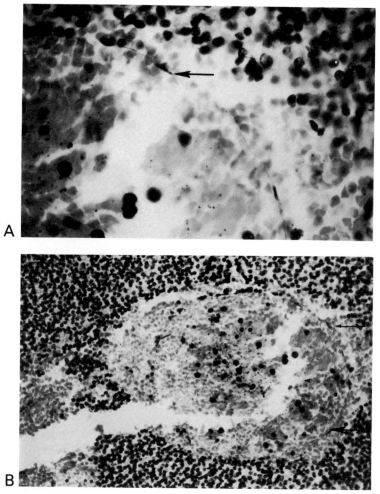

Figure 4-5 (A and B).   The wall of this vein is unusually thin *(arrows)*, and blood has escaped into the germinal matrix. Hematoxylin and eosin (H and E) stain.

evation of venous pressure, the lack of integrity of the immature blood vessels in the germinal matrix, and the extravascular supporting structures. Recent studies in both animals and humans support this concept.[5,7,16] More definitive studies are necessary, however, and an understanding of the precipitating factors is essential before one can prevent this very common disease entity.

Anoxic Encephalopathy

Of the many conditions affecting the neonate, anoxia is of prime importance because of its frequency and its potential for severe disruption of the CNS. The very common neuropathologic abnormal-

ity in the newborn is anoxic encephalopathy. In the encephalopathy that results, the gray matter may be severely and diffusely damaged or the white matter may be selectively affected in one of three characteristic patterns.[1,2] Each of these lesions possesses a number of unique features. The topography and the histologic characteristics of the alterations in this age group differ from those in the more mature brain.

Gray matter lesions.   In the newborn infant, the changes in the gray matter are diffusely present throughout cortex, basal ganglia and thalamus, brain stem, and spinal cord. Involvement of the subcortical white matter (Fig. 4-6) and lower layers of cortex is

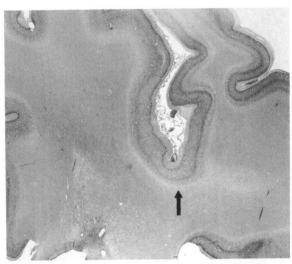

Figure 4-6.   A zone of pallor *(arrow)* outlines the area of subcortical necrosis.
H and E stain.

prominent, while in the more mature patient a pseu-
dolaminar necrosis of cortex is the more characteristic
change. Another feature detected only in the neonate
is the karyorrhexis of neurons. This degeneration of
neurons is characterized by eosinophilia and swelling
of the cytoplasm and fragmentation of the nucleus.
A paucity of tissue reaction accompanies this degeneration. It is the tissue reaction that guides one in the
appreciation of cell loss.

As a result, neuronal loss cannot be assessed
with any degree of certainty after the acute stage of
the insult. This lack of reaction presents a major
problem for the pathologist who examines the CNS
of a child who has been mentally retarded and spastic
since birth. When studying the microscopic sections
of the CNS, one has the impression that there are too
few neurons and that the alignment of neurons in
columns and layers is defective, yet a glial proliferation in these zones is absent. The counting of
neurons to substantiate a change is too laborious and
time consuming. Grossly, the brain is usually small,
the ventricles symmetrically enlarged, and the white
matter decreased.

White matter lesions.   Lesions in the white matter
are often observed in the periventricular zone as small
areas of coagulation necrosis (periventricular leukomalacia) or as ischemic changes in the subcortical
white matter. Grossly, these latter changes appear as
dark linear bands that outline and accentuate the deep
layers of the cerebral cortex (see Fig. 4-6). The microscopic appearance varies in accordance with the

duration of the lesion. The mildest and most frequent
change detected in the neonate's white matter is periventricular gliosis. This increase in astrocytes is frequently accompanied by a pallor of tissue and a deposition of small calcific material in perivascular
distribution. This form of gliosis is often a subtle
change and rarely interrupts the architecture of the
white matter. It is a very nonspecific change and may
exist alone or in association with other manifestations
of anoxic encephalopathy.

Any or all of the changes in the gray or white
matter may follow an anoxic insult to the neonate.
In infants who survive for any length of time, the
result is similar: the brain is small, and there is frequently a reduction in the white matter and an en-
largement of the ventricular system. This is the pathologic change that characterizes so many of the children
who are mentally retarded and have a spastic gait. It
appears that anoxic encephalopathy is the basis of the
alterations in the brain in the majority of the children
who are classified as having cerebral palsy. Myers
has subjected monkey fetuses at term to total or to
partial asphyxia followed by resuscitative measures.[14]
After total asphyxia and the monkey's extended survival, the major pathologic changes have been localized to the brain stem. After partial asphyxia, the
major alterations are in the cerebral hemispheres. The
changes are characterized by cortical necrosis that,
in the monkeys that have survived for some time, is
manifested as areas of cerebral cortical atrophy, white
matter sclerosis, and status marmoratus of basal ganglia. It is of interest that the changes following both

complete and partial asphyxia resemble closely some forms of anoxic encephalopathy in the human fetus.

Developmental Anomalies

The previous groups of alterations represent destructive changes to the developed CNS tissue. The developmental abnormalities, on the other hand, represent alterations in which the program of development has been curtailed at one or more of the three basic stages of CNS development. These three periods are marked by (1) the fusion of the lips of the neural plate into the neural tube, (2) the cleavage and evagination of the prosencephalon into the paired optic vesicles, olfactory buds, and cerebral hemispheres, and (3) the migration of neuroblasts from the neuromedullary zone to their permanent residence.

The most common developmental defect in this study is the arrest in migration of neuroblasts. Such collections of cells are termed *heterotopias* or *ectopic neurons*. When the migratory pattern is not complete, the cortex is depleted of nerve cells and the architecture of those remaining is frequently defective.

Multiple factors may cause developmental defects. Drugs ingested by the pregnant woman, e.g., alcohol, diphenylhydantoin (Dilantin), and thalidomide, and irradiation have arrested CNS development.[6,8,15] The type of defect is governed by the stage of CNS development when the exposure occurs. A virus that infects the CNS early in its development can also arrest the developmental pattern as well as destroy tissue.[3,9] Such examples include infections by cytomegalic, rubella, and herpes simplex viruses.[3,9] Polymicrogyria, heterotopias, and microcephaly have been described in these infants.

REFERENCES

1. Banker BQ, Larroche J-C: Periventricular leukomalacia of infancy. A form of neonatal anoxic encephalopathy. Arch Neurol 7:386, 1962
2. Banker BQ: The neuropathological effects of anoxia and hypoglycemia in the newborn. Dev Med Child Neurol 9:544, 1967
3. Bray P: Personal communication
4. Fujimura M, Salisbury DM, Robinson RO, et al: Clinical events relating to intraventricular haemorrhage in the newborn. Arch Dis Child 54:409, 1979
5. Goddard J, Armstrong DL, Michael LH: Regional cerebral blood flow (RCBF) in an experimental model of intraventricular hemorrhage. J Neuropathol Exp Neurol 40:344, 1981
6. Golbus MS: Teratology for the obstetrician: Current status. Obstet Gynecol 55:269, 1980
7. Grunnet ML: Relative immaturity of germinal plate blood vessels: An ultrastructural study. J Neuropathol Exp Neurol 40:345, 1981
8. Hanson JW, Smith DW: The fetal hydantoin syndrome. J Pediatr 87:285, 1975
9. Larroche J-C: Developmental Pathology of the Neonate. Amsterdam, Excerpta Medica, 1977
10. Little WJ: Course of lectures on the deformities of the human frame: Lecture VIII. Lancet 1:318, 1843
11. Little WJ: Lectures on the nature and treatment of the deformities of the human frame. Longmans, Green and Co., London, 1853, pp 1–402
12. Little WJ: The influence of abnormal parturition, difficult labours, premature birth, and asphyxia neonatorum on the mental and physical condition of the child, especially in relation to deformities. Trans Obstet Soc London 3:293, 1861
13. Krishnamoorthy KS, Fernandez RA, Momose KJ, et al: Evaluation of neonatal intracranial hemorrhage by computerized tomography. Pediatrics 59:165, 1977
14. Myers RE: Two patterns of perinatal brain damage and their conditions of occurrence. Am J Obstet Gynecol 112:246, 1972
15. Smithells RW: Environmental teratogens of man. Br Med Bull 32:27, 1976
16. Sotrel A, Lorenzo AV, Welch K: Ultrastructure of germinal matrix vessels in preterm rabbits with spontaneous IVH. J Neuropathol Exp Neurol 40:344, 1981
17. Terplan KL: Histopathologic brain changes in 1152 cases of the perinatal and early infancy period. Biol Neonate 11:348, 1967
18. Towbin A: Mental retardation due to germinal matrix infarction. Science 164:156, 1969
19. Towbin A: Central nervous system damage in the human fetus and newborn infant. Am J Dis Child 119:529, 1970
20. Towbin A: Organic causes of minimal brain dysfunction. Perinatal origin of minimal cerebral lesions. JAMA 217:1207, 1971
21. Volpe JJ: Current concepts in neonatal medicine. N Engl J Med 304:886, 1981.

Nancy L. Golden
Leslie Rubin

5

Intrauterine Factors and the Risk for the Development of Cerebral Palsy

Crothers and Paine make the following opening statement about the etiology of cerebral palsy: "Ever since Little published his classic paper in 1861 concerning the connection between abnormal birth histories and cerebral palsies, debate has continued as to whether such factors are of major causative importance or whether the majority of cases may be due to antenatal influences or other unrecognised factors."[1] The list of factors in their series includes illness in the first three months of pregnancy, toxemia, minor illnesses, abdominal surgery, other trauma, and bleeding and threatened miscarriage.

A decade later, after the thalidamide experience led to experiments in teratology and the rubella epidemic created awareness of the harmful effects of viral infections on the developing fetus, Aladjim tried to express the relationship between fetomaternal exchange and fetal outcome.[2] The 1970s saw a greater appreciation of the vulnerability of the fetus, not only to the hazards of the perinatal period, but also to environmental agents operating in utero, e.g., chemicals, pharmaceuticals, roentgenograms, infectious agents, and maternal pathophysiology.[3] Yet although the last 20 yr have resulted, to some extent, in the resolution of the dilemma presented by Crothers and Paine, a significant number of children remain with cerebral palsy or mental retardation in whom an etiologic factor cannot be established. O'Reilly and Walentynowicz could not establish an etiologic diagnosis in 27 percent of the children with cerebral palsy in their clinic between 1940–1949.[4] Between 1970–1979 the figure was 16 percent. The decrease in proportion may represent an improvement in ability to make diagnoses based on increased knowledge and

information, or it may represent a relative increase in proportion of other etiologic factors, e.g., prematurity (see Chap. 7). Crocker failed to establish a firm etiologial diagnosis in 30 percent of children with mental retardation (see Chap. 3).

Holm goes a step further and includes the 28 percent of children in whom there was a negative birth and postnatal history with the 25 percent in whom a prenatal cause could be established and classified them all as prenatal.[5] If this group with unknown etiologies for their disability can, justifiably, be assumed to be prenatal in origin, then there is all the more reason to examine potential intrauterine insults.

In order to do so, one must appreciate that the embryo and fetus are undergoing rapid changes and that the effect of any insult will depend to some extent, on the developmental stage during which the insult occurs.

CENTRAL NERVOUS SYSTEM DEVELOPMENT

Major events in the development of the central nervous system (CNS) can be divided into six stages[6] (Figures 5-1–5-5).

Dorsal Induction

Dorsal induction begins at about the third week of gestation with the development of the neural plate and ends at about the fourth week with the formation of the neural tube. Defects that can occur during this phase result in problems of neural tube closure. The

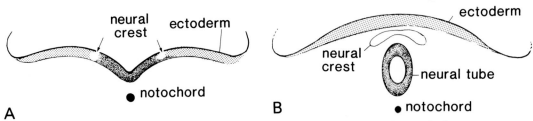

Figure 5-1 (A and B). Dorsal induction and the formation of the neural tube

more severe malformations will result in spontaneous abortion, accounting for about 1–3 percent of all aborted fetuses.[7] Most of the fetuses that go to term will be found to have some form of myelodysplasia.

Ventral Induction

Ventral induction takes place between the fifth and sixth weeks of gestation and involves the formation of the face and brain. Neural crest cells play a major role during this phase, and studies suggest that defects in crest cell migration may be responsible for the spectrum of mid-face and holoprosencephalic malformations.[8]

Neural Proliferation

Neural proliferation occurs maximally between the second and fourth months and takes place in the periventricular or periluminal zones. This phase is

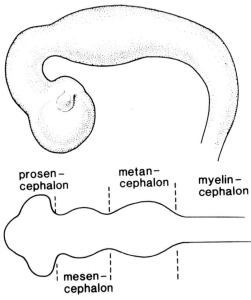

Figure 5-2. Ventral induction

critical for the determination of eventual cell number. A number of drugs and environmental agents are known to interfere with this proliferative activity, e.g., roentgenograms, viral infections, zinc deficiency, excess vitamin A, and prenatal and postnatal malnutrition in the mammalian embryo.[9]

Decreases in absolute cell number can result in microcephaly; however, it is likely that, because different parts of the brain proliferate at different rates and at different times, the timing of the insult will determine which area is affected. The resulting defects will therefore reflect dysfunction of the affected area.[9]

Neuronal Migration

Neuronal migration, wherein cells, having proliferated in the periventricular zones, now migrate to their definitive anatomic positions in the cortex or in the bodies of specific nuclei, takes place maximally between the third and sixth months of gestation. As Rakic notes: "It is generally recognised that neuronal migration in the brain serves the special purpose of allowing synaptic junctions to develop between specific cell classes, which are the structural basis for the function of the mature brain. It is in this sense that neuronal migration in the developing brain is to be considered as a 'biological necessity.' "[10]

Several abnormalities can occur during this phase.

Complete Failure of Migration

In complete failure of migration the cells remain close to their site of origin; they then degenerate, possibly as a result of the absence of proper synaptic input. The final outcome will be a decrease in cell number, which will be indistinguishable from the result of a failure of proliferation.

Curtailment of Migration

Curtailment of migration is seen when neurons become arrested in their migratory pathway. It probably occurs between the 10th and 16th weeks of fetal life. It has been demonstrated in the heterogeneous

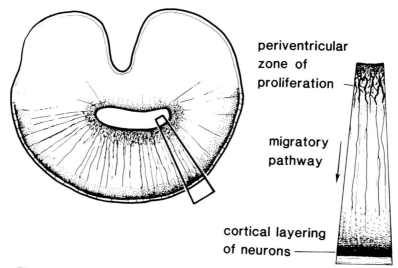

periventricular
zone of
proliferation

migratory
pathway

cortical layering
of neurons

Figure 5-3. Neuronal proliferation and migration from the periventricular zone to the cortical area.

group of disorders such as lissencephaly and pachygyria as well as in the cerebrohepatorenal syndrome of Zellweger and in trisomy 18.

Aberrant Neurons in Target Structures

Aberrant neurons in target structures represent a later developmental phenomenon. The cells have left their site of origin and have undergone the migratory process but do not quite reach their predetermined destination. Some factor operating at this point prevents the final migratory phase, and the neurons are found in a truly ectopic position.

The roles of viruses, irradiation, and various drugs in the pathogenesis of this abnormality have been established in experimental animals.[10] This pathology has also been demonstrated in the fetal alcohol syndrome.[11]

Rakic points out that the above-mentioned factors can interfere either with the production of neurons or with their migration and stresses that the determining factor of which abnormality occurs is critically dependent on the developmental stage at which the agent exerts its biological effect.[10]

Disorders of cell migration were the most common developmental abnormality reported by Banker and Bruce–Gregorios in their neuropathologic survey (see Chapter 4).

Organization

Organization occurs from six months of gestation to birth and continues for some time postnatally. It involves the orientation of neurons, the elaboration

of dendritic processes (with arborization and the formation of dendritic spines), and the establishment of synaptic contacts. Differentiation and proliferation of glia also occur at this stage. Pathologic findings referrable to this stage are associated with a variety of etiologic factors, e.g., chromosome abnormalities, metabolic disturbances, intrauterine asphyxia, and other perinatal insults.[12]

Myelination

Myelination occurs from birth and continues through adult life. Although the major disturbances are related to inborn errors of metabolism, some effects have been suggested to occur in congenital rubella and have been reported in the Rubinstein–Taybi syndrome.[6]

FETOPLACENTOMATERNAL UNIT

In considering intrauterine factors that result in cerebral palsy, it is not sufficient to view the fetus in isolation and the insult as a discreet causative agent. As Crocker suggests in Chapter 3, the reality is probably "of multifactorial sources, working in combination, and especially of the role of the altered vulnerability of the organism." (Figure 5-5) The disciples of Little, who held that cerebral palsy was the direct result of birth injury, were countered by others like Freud, who postulated "the existance of some underlying intrinsic abnormality of maternal reproduc-

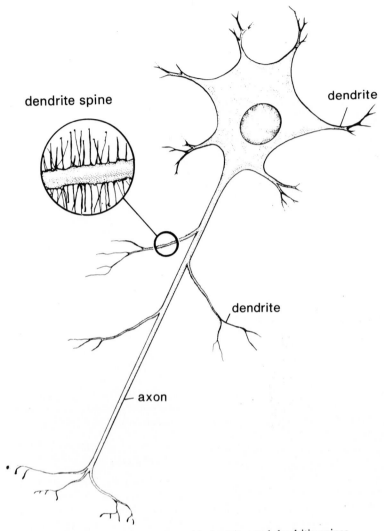

Figure 5-4. Mature neuron with dendrites and dendritic spines

tive capacity causing both disorders of parturition and abnormalities of the fetus."[13,14] Ingram and Russell in Scotland examined the reproductive histories of 278 mothers of diplegic patients and found that they were older, had more problems with fertility, and had more problems with other pregnancies than the general population.[15] This led them to postulate that these infants were more vulnerable and would be predisposed to suffer from the adverse effects of even minor degrees of hypoxia during the perinatal period.

Intrauterine Growth Retardation

Hagberg et al. examined the prenatal and perinatal factors in a series of 560 children with cerebral palsy born in Sweden between 1954–1970 and compared these to the general population. They found a highly significant correlation with maternal toxemia, antepartum bleeding, and multiple births in those children who developed cerebral palsy. In addition, in analyzing the trend of causative factors in cerebral palsy over that 16-yr period, they found that (1) the incidence of asphyxia–cerebral hemorrhage alone (i.e., without any adverse maternal factors) decreased significantly, (2) the incidence of infants who had been exposed to adverse maternal factors (fetal deprivation of supply [FDS]) (Table 5-1) with or without asphyxia–cerebral hemorrhage remained unchanged, and (3) the association between FDS and asphyxia–cerebral hemorrhage was highly significant, suggesting the additive effect of perinatal insults on prenatal stress. Pathologic correlates of intrauterine

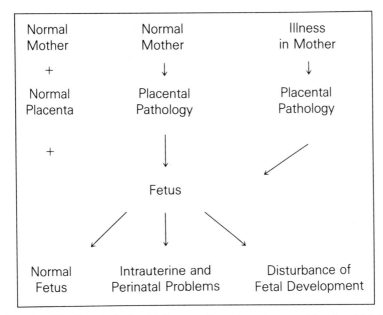

Figure 5-5.   Simplification of relationship between feto–placento–maternal unit and fetal outcome

growth retardation (IUGR) help illustrate this vulnerability (Table 5-2). Some of the clinical features described in both the above-mentioned studies can be appreciated with an understanding of placental pathophysiology. Placental pathology has been well correlated with fetal outcome, but further investigation is required to determine directly the relationship with developmental outcome.[17] Nevertheless, there is indirect evidence; e.g., the placentas of toxemic mothers show a much greater frequency of infarcts, and the presence of maternal toxemia is associated with the increased risk of the child developing cerebral palsy.[16,17] This is also true with multiple births and antepartum hemorrhage.

The Premature Infant who is also Small-for-Gestational Age

The situation of prematurity is of interest when considering the group of infants who are of low birthweight, which includes those who are appropriate-for-gestational age (AGA) and small-for-gestational age (SGA). The increased risk for the development of cerebral palsy in low birthweight infants is well recognized (see Chapter 7). In a report on children with cerebral palsy from the National Collaborative Perinatal Project, however, Ellenberg and Nelson found that there was a significantly increased risk for those infants who were of low birthweight even for their gestational age.[18]

Bennett et al. examined the perinatal factors in

preterm infants and compared those infants who went on to develop cerebral palsy with those who did not.[19] They found a significant difference (even for small numbers) in birthweight, head circumference, and low one-minute Apgar scores. (Birthweight and head circumference did not necessarily fall in the SGA range but clustered around the 20th and 10th percentiles, respectively.) They felt that their findings represented the adverse effects of intrauterine influences on growth as well as on the ability of the infant to adapt to the extrauterine environment (as is reflected in the low one-minute Apgar scores). Fitzhardinge and Pape had a larger number of infants in a similar study, but they matched their preterm SGA infants with AGA infants by weight and by neonatal problems.[20] At 18 mo the SGA infants (by implication,

Table 5-1
Clinical Evidence for Fetal Deprivation of Supply

Bleeding during pregnancy

Infarction of the placenta

Toxemia

Small for dates

Diabetes in the mother

Adapted from Hagberg G, Hagberg B, Olow I: The changing panorama of cerebral palsey in Sweden: 1954–1970. III. The importance of foetal deprivation of supply. Acta Paediatr Scand 65:403, 1976. With permission.

Table 5-2

A Comparison of the Brains of AGA and SGA Infants*

	Cerebral Weight (g)	Cerebral Cellularity (%)	Cerebellar Weight (g)	Cerebellar Cellularity (%)
AGA*	430	100	27.6	100
SGA**	333	81	17.5	65

*AGA: Appropriate for gestational age
**SGA: Small for gestational age

those who had IUGR) were significantly smaller had significantly more neurologic problems and had lower Bayley mental scores, suggesting that the "complication of IUGR significantly increases the risk of serious sequelae in the tiny premature infant."[20]

Risk Factors in Pregnancy

In a follow-up study of preterm SGA infants, Commey and Fitzhardinge found an extremely high incidence of severe handicap (49 percent), but more interesting was the presence of high-risk factors in 75 of the 103 pregnancies (Table 5-3).[21]

The likely conclusion is that there are factors operating during pregnancy that may not be readily recognized as such but that nonetheless have a significant role to play in the long-term outcome of all infants. This also has an important implication in terms of prevention, as was shown by Perkins et al., who studied the pregnancies in adolescent mothers.[22] The outcome of the pregnancies was no different from

Table 5-3

The Frequency of the Major High-Risk Categories in the 103 Pregnancies

Category	Percentage
Multiple pregnancy	25
Toxemia	16
Chronic maternal disease	16
Poor obstetric history	13
Young mothers (18 yr)	11
Older mothers (35 yr) or elderly primigravida (30 yr)	9
Excessive smoking	2

Reprinted with permission from Commey JOO, Fitzhardinge PM: Handicap in the preterm small-for-gestational age infant. Pediatr 94:781, 1979.

that of the general population when the principles of "intensive care" were applied to the antenatal management.

SPECIFIC ETIOLOGIC AGENTS

Although specific etiologic agents are well recognized as resulting in severe and sometimes devastating consequences, they occur in a relatively small percentage of children with cerebral palsy and other developmental disabilities. Nonetheless, the importance of the awareness of these agents and how they affect the outcome must be appreciated for at least three reasons:

1. As discreet causative factors, they provide a model for the understanding of how prenatal influences exert their effects.
2. By the awareness of this mechanism, the agents can be identified, and thus, where possible, consequences can be prevented.
3. Although they may be relatively few, their effects are often severe, and multiple handicaps are frequent.

Congenital Infections

Congenital infections are often referred to as TORCH infections (Table 5-4). Although each of these infectious agents has specific characteristics and

Table 5-4

Intrauterine (TORCH) Infections

Infections		Etiologic Agent
To	Toxoplasmosis	One-celled animal
R	Rubella	Virus
C	CMV	Virus
H	Herpes simplex	Virus
S	Syphilis	Spirochete

results in specific clinical syndromes, there is some overlap, particularly in the manifestation of rubella, CMV, and toxoplasomosis (Figure 5-6). These agents cause a relatively mild infection in the pregnant mother yet have severe effects upon the fetus. In addition, the timing of the infection is important in terms of outcome.[23] An infection very early in pregnancy can result in abortion; during embryogenesis, congenital malformations may result, particularly cardiac and CNS. Cataracts, chrorioretinitis, and deafness may result, with later infections. Perinatal infections can result in hepatitis, thrombocytopenia, and meningoencephalitis. Latent manifestations include diabetes, thyroid disease, and even degenerative CNS disease.[24]

Rubella

In a follow-up study on the course and early sequelae of congenital rubella encephalitis, Desmond et al. reported that as many as 80 percent of patients had neurologic manifestations and 50 percent were diagnosed as having cerebral palsy.[25] The clinical symptoms included hypotonia, hypertonia, movement disorders, and varying disability from monoparesis to quadriparesis. Pathologic changes at autopsy revealed leptomeningitis, vasculitis, multifocal parenchymal necrosis, perivascular calcification, and delayed myelinization.

In a further follow-up study of 29 nonretarded children with congenital rubella, Desmond et al. found that 70 percent had neurologic abnormalities during infancy that persisted as poor balance and muscle weakness.[26] Three children (10 percent) were diagnosed as having cerebral palsy.

CMV

Berenberg and Nankervis reported that 6 of their 12 patients with congenital CMV infections developed cerebral palsy.[27] Hanshaw et al. reported school failure, mental retardation, microcephaly, hearing loss, and chorioretinitis in a significant number of infants in whom CMV was detected at birth.[28] They also found that CMV was the most common congenital infection in the United States. Viruria was found in approximately 1 percent of all infants routinely tested, thus placing it in an important role in the etiology of CNS impairment.

Toxoplasmosis

Desmonts and Couvreur found that of 64 infants with congenital toxoplasmosis, 72 percent were asymptomatic, 17 percent had mild disease, and 11

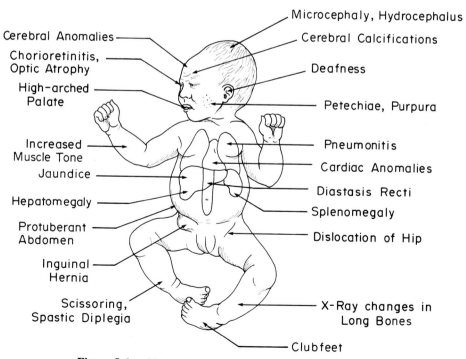

Figure 5-6. Clinical features common to intrauterine infections

percent were severely disabled.[29] Those more se-verely disabled tended to have been infected earlier in pregnancy.

Alford et al. found abnormalities in cerebrospinal fluid (CSF) even in the infants who were asymptomatic.[30] In those who were symptomatic, 69 percent had predominantly neurologic features, and these features tended to manifest themselves later than in those infants with systemic disease.

Herpes

Herpes simplex virus infections have a devastating effect on the CNS whether aquired prenatally or perinatally. Prevention is obviously important, and adenine arabinoside may be used to treat infants who are infected or where the risk of infection is high.[31]

Syphilis

Although the incidence of congenital syphilis has decreased with screening tests on pregnant women and with the use of penicillin, it is still a significant problem and should be considered in the neonatal period where clinical features are suggestive. Taber and Huber suggest that infants should be followed, since treatment may not prevent long-term sequelae.[32]

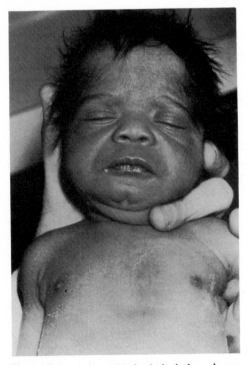

Figure 5-7. Infant with fetal alcohol syndrome

Maternal Hyperthermia

Although many other infections in the first trimester have been implicated in causing fetopathy, the common denominator in some may well be that of maternal hyperthermia. Pleet et al. have implicated maternal hyperthermia occurring between 4–14 wk of gestation as a causative agent in some children with dysmorphic features and neurologic sequelae.[33]

Chemical Toxins

Chemical toxins to which pregnant women are exposed constitute another risk category for the development of cerebral palsy. Many of these substances cross the placental barrier unchanged, are present in the fetus in high concentrations, and can injure the developing brain. Alcohol, phencyclidine (angel dust), and methyl mercury are examples of agents that have been implicated in causing damage to the fetal brain and resulting in cerebral palsy.

Fetal Alcohol Syndrome

In 1975, Jones and Smith described several infants of alcoholic mothers, who were small at birth and had dysmorphic features.[34] These infants went on to have developmental delays (Figure 5-7). The fetal alcohol syndrome has come to represent a significant preventable cause of developmental pathology.

The characteristics include midface hypoplasia, short palpebral fissures, absence of the "cupids bow" of the upper lip, and cardiac anomalies. Neurologic features in the neonatal period include hypotonia, jitteriness, and seizures, which may represent withdrawal symptoms.[35] Persistent neurologic findings of spasticity, gross motor delay, poor fine motor coordination, hyperactivity, and mental retardation are also seen. These findings are secondary to the abnormalities of brain development. Autopsy studies confirm the low brain weight consistent with microcephaly due either to decreased cell production or to loss of neurons (see above). Other findings include a spectrum of abnormalities from ancephaly, meningomyelocele, and absent corpus callosum to abnormalities of neuronal migration.

Phencyclidine

Phencyclidine (angel dust) has also been implicated as a possible cause of cerebral palsy. Originally developed as an anesthetic agent similar to ketamine, it is now licensed for use only in animals. It remains one of a widely used street drug, especially among adolescents. Phencylidine causes drowsiness, altered perception, and hallucinations, which make it desirable as a drug of abuse. Recently we reported the case of a male infant with abnormal neurobehavioral features, an unusual physical appearance, and spastic quadriplegia.[36] His mother had used large amounts of phencyclidine throughout her pregnancy. The child had a triangular shaped face with pointed chin and narrow mandibular angle (Figure 5-8). His eyes had an antimongoloid slant. There was a widened anterior fontanelle and patent metopic suture. Soon after birth his behavior was noted to be abnormal. He was hypertonic, jittery, and tremulous with stimulation but hypotonic and lethargic at rest. He had poor head control and nystagmus, did not track visually, and fed poorly. He was diagnosed as having spastic quadriparesis at two months and continues to have developmental delay.

The possibility that maternal phencyclidine use was responsible for the infant's problems was not suspected until a week after his birth, so placental transfer of phencyclidine was not confirmed. The lesson to be learned from this is that a detailed drug history should be obtained from all mothers when an infant is found to have dysmorphic features or abnormal neurologic signs.

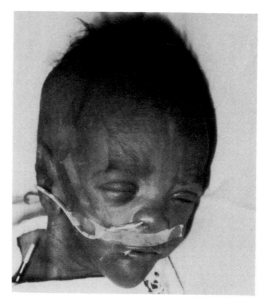

Figure 5-8. Male infant whose mother had taken phencyclidine throughout gestation.

Methyl Mercury

Methyl mercury, a fungicide, has been found to cause cerebral palsy in infants exposed in utero. In the early 1970s, widespread methyl mercury poisoning occurred in rural Iraq.[37] Wheat treated with methyl mercury was made into bread, and 32 women were poisoned shortly before or during pregnancy. Their symptoms and those of their children varied directly with the amount of methyl mercury to which they were exposed (as measured by longitudinal analysis of hair samples). Fourteen of these infants were symptomatic at birth, and 10 of them were diagnosed as having cerebral palsy. Six infants were blind, two had poor vision, and five were microcephalic and retarded.

Pharmacologic Agents

Ever since the establishment of the relationship between thalidomide and birth defects, there has been a growing awareness of the medications that can cause birth defects and CNS malformations when ingested during pregnancy. The best known of these include aminopterin, warfarin, trimethadione, and diphenylhydantoin.[38] Many other agents have been shown to cause embryopathies and fetopathies in experimental animals.[39]

PREVENTION

Although the identification of prenatal factors in the etiology of cerebral palsy and related developmental disabilities has improved, there still remains a significant percentage of infants and children in whom no etiological factor can be established. As yet the evidence points to undiscovered intrauterine events. It is only through constant scrutiny, vigilance, and careful analysis that these factors can be discovered and can lead to preventive measures. At present, we do have knowledge of specific agents, e.g., rubella, which specific public health measures have been able to overcome. We are also aware of specific adverse chemical and physical agents, e.g., X-rays and alcohol, which can be prevented, and we are also aware of the general health needs of the pregnant mother, which should be carefully monitored with as much "intensive care" as is given to their infants after birth.

REFERENCES

1. Crothers B, Paine RS: The Natural History of Cerebral Palsy. Cambridge, Harvard University Press, 1959
2. Aladjam S: The Early placenta, in Fraser FC, McKusick VA (eds): Structure and Function in Congenital Malformations. Amsterdam, Exerpta Medica, 1970, pp 117–146

3. Melnick M: Current concepts in the etiology of central nervous system malformations, in Myrianthopoulos NC, Bergsma D (eds): Recent Advances in the Developmental Biology of Central Nervous System Malformations. New York, The National Foundation of the March of Dimes, 1979, pp 19–41

4. O'Reilly DE, Walentynowicz JE: Etiological factors in cerebral palsy: An historical review. Dev Med Child Neurol 23:633, 1981

5. Holm VA: The etiology of cerebral palsy in the seventies. Dev Med Child Neurol 21:117, 1979

6. Volpe JJ: Normal and abnormal human brain development. Clin Perinatol 4:3, 1977

7. Myrianthopoloulos NC: Our load of central nervous system malformations, in Myrianthopoulos NC, Bergsma D (eds): Recent Advances in the Developmental Biology of Central Nervous System Malformations. New York, The National Foundation of the March of Dimes, 1979, pp 1–18

8. Johnston MC: The neural crest in abnormalities of face and brain, in Bergsma D (ed): Morphogenesis and Malformation of the Face and Brain. New York, The National Foundation of the March of Dimes, 1975

9. Langman J, Rodier P, Webster W: Interference with proliferative activity in the CNS and its relation to facial abnormalities, in Bergsma D (ed): Morphogenesis and Malformation of the Face and Brain. New York, The National Foundation of the March of Dimes, 1975

10. Rakic P: Cell migration and neuronal ectopias in the brain, in Bergsma D (ed): Morphogenesis and Malformation of the Face and Brain. New York, The National Foundation of the March of Dimes, 1975

11. Jones KL: Aberrant neuronal migration in the fetal alcohol syndrome, in Bergsma D (ed): Morphogenesis and Malformation in the Face and Brain. New York, The National Foundation of the March of Dimes, 1975

12. Purpura DP: Developmental pathology of cortical neurons in immature human brain, in Gluck L (ed): Intrauterine Asphyxia and the Developing Fetal Brain. Chicago, Year Book Medical Publishers, 1977

13. Little WJ: On the influence of abnormal parturition, difficult labours, premature birth, asphyxia neonatorum on the mental and physical condition of the child, especially in relation to deformities. Trans Obstet Soc Lond 3:293, 1862

14. Freud S: Infantile cerebral palsies (trans Russin LA). Coral Gables, University of Miami Press, 1897

15. Ingram TTS, Russell EM: The reproductive histories of mothers of patients suffering from congenital diplegia. Arch Dis Child 36:34, 1961

16. Hagberg G, Hagberg B, Olow I: The changing panorama of cerebral palsy in Sweden: 1954–1970. Acta Paediatr Scand 65:403, 1976

17. Benirschke K, Gille J: Placental pathology and asphyxia, in Gluck L (ed): Intrauterine Asphyxia and the Developing Fetal Brain. Chicago, Year Book Medical Publishers, 1977

18. Ellenberg JH, Nelson KB: Birthweight and gestational age in children with cerebral palsy or seizure disorders. Am J Dis Child 133:1044, 1979

19. Bennett FC, Chandler LS, Robinson NM, et al: Spastic diplegia in premature infants. Am J Dis Child 135:732, 1981

20. Fitzhardinge PM, Pape KE: Intrauterine growth retardation (IUGR): An added risk to the preterm infant. Pediatr Res 11:562, 1979

21. Commey JOO, Fitzhardinge PM: Handicap in the preterm small-for-gestational age infant. J Pediatr 94:799, 1979

22. Perkins RP, Nakashima II, Mullin J, et al: Intensive care in adolescent pregnancy. Obstet Gynecol 52:179, 1978

23. Dudgeon JA: Congenital rubella in the United Kingdom of Great Britain. Prog Clin Biol Res 3:23, 1975

24. Cooper LZ: Congenital rubella in the United States. Prog Clin Biol Res 3:1, 1975

25. Desmond MM, Wilson GS, Melnick JL, et al: Congenital rubella encephalitis: Course and early sequelae. J Pediatr 71:311, 1967

26. Desmond MM, Fisher ES, Vordeman AL, et al: The longitudinal course of congenital rubella encephalitis in non-retarded children. J Pediatr 93:584, 1978

27. Berenberg W, Nankervis G: Long term follow up of cytomegalic inclusion disease of infancy. Pediatrics 46:403, 1970

28. Hanshaw JB, Sheiner AP, Moxley AW, et al: CNS sequelae of congenital cytomegalovirus infection. Prog Clin Biol Res 3:47, 1975

29. Desmonts G, Couvreur J: Toxoplasmosis: Epidemiologic and serologic aspects of perinatal infection. Prog Clin Biol Res 3:115, 1975

30. Alford CA, Stagno S, Reynolds DW: Toxoplasmosis: Silent congenital infection. Prog Clin Biol Res 3:133, 1975

31. Committee on Fetus and Newborn and Committee on Infectious Diseases: Perinatal herpes simplex infections. Pediatrics 66:147, 1980

32. Taber LH, Huber TW: Congenital syphilis. Prog Clin Biol Res 3:183, 1975

33. Pleet H, Graham JM, Smith DW: Central nervous system and facial defects associated with maternal hyperthermia at 4–14 weeks of gestation. Pediatrics 67:785, 1981

34. Clarren SK, Smith DW: The fetal alcohol syndrome. N Engl J Med 298:1063, 1978

35. Golden NL, Sokol R, Rubin IL: Angel dust: Possible effects on the fetus. Pediatrics 65:18, 1980

36. Amin–Zaki L, Majeed MA, Elhas–Sani SB, et al: Prenatal methyl mercury poisoning. Am J Dis Child 133:172, 1979

37. Smith DW: Recognizable Patterns in Human Malformation. (ed 2). Philadelphia, Saunders, 1976, pp 340–347

38. Tuchman–Duplessis H: Drug Effects on the Fetus. Sydney, Adis Press, 1975

Leroy J. Dierker
Roger H. Hertz

6

Intrapartum Prevention of Brain Damage

The obstetrician's role is unique in at least two respects. First, the obstetrician is charged with the responsibility for delivering optimal medical care to two distinct yet intimately interrelated patients—the mother and the fetus. Second, one of these patients, the fetus, is physically isolated within the confines of the mother's uterus, limiting the physician's ability to evaluate its clinical growth and health. In no other area of medicine are clinicians required to diagnose and treat a patient who can neither communicate nor be directly seen or examined and still be expected to deliver a healthy patient with full intellectual and physical potential for 70+ productive years. Although this chapter aims to review current methods used to minimize the risk of cerebral injury, it must be remembered that much of the recognized cerebral dysfunction occurs either before labor or in the neonatal period. The day of delivery is probably the single most important day of fetal life, but it is certainly not the only hazardous period.

In treating their two patients, obstetricians must frequently make clinical decisions that are in the best interests of one patient while potentially compromising the interests (health) of the other. For example, optimal care of a pregnant woman with toxemia (severe preeclampsia or eclampsia) may require delivery of a very premature infant in the absence of any sign of fetal distress. Such a delicate decision is made in the mother's best interests in order to prevent or treat a potential maternal life-threatening complication in the knowledge that premature delivery subjects the infant to a different, although equally significant, potential set of risks. In another example, when the fetal

membranes rupture well before the fetus is mature, the mother's health may be jeopardized if the pregnancy is allowed to continue.

FACTORS ASSOCIATED WITH FETAL BRAIN DAMAGE

Congenital Malformations

The obstetrician's ability to diagnose and prevent fetal brain damage remains extraordinarily limited. Except in fetuses with major structural congenital malformations involving the central nervous system (CNS) (such as anencephaly, hydrocephaly, mental retardation as a consequence of specific inherited [genetic] metabolic diseases [e.g., Tay-Sachs], or chromosomal abnormalities such as Down's syndrome [Trisomy 21]) that are diagnosable by amniotic fluid analysis early in pregnancy or by ultrasound, obstetricians are still searching for means of diagnosing brain damage antenatally. The diagnosis of the limited groups of diseases mentioned above is done in partnership with geneticists, biochemists, and sonographers. Today, as the technology for improved diagnostic techniques is being developed, the obstetrician's concern is to diagnose and develop effective therapeutic interventions for conditions associated with premature delivery, fetal distress in utero, asphyxia neonatorum, and mechanical birth trauma, conditions that are all associated with an increased incidence of cerebral palsy and mental retardation.

43

Prematurity

Premature birth is, by itself, a major etiologic factor in the development of brain dysfunction. In addition, it is a major contributing factor when associated with metabolic or physical fetal insults that are also etiologic factors in brain damage and mental retardation. In recent years much research has been directed toward developing effective therapeutic methods of inhibiting labor, thereby preventing premature delivery. These efforts have met with significant success, and during 1980 the Food and Drug Administration (FDA) approved the use of ritodrine hydrochloride (a beta-sympathomimetic drug) for the pharmacologic inhibition of premature labor. The effect of pharmacologic inhibition of labor on brain damage and mental retardation will be a major area of academic interest during the coming decade.

Clinical methods of antepartum fetal evaluation include auscultation of fetal heart rate, analysis of the mother's perception of fetal activity, and measurement of fetal growth by recording serial growth of the uterus. Although these techniques provide valuable data, they are of limited value in predicting either fetal outcome or brain damage. Modern techniques of fetal evaluation include sonographic measurement of fetal physical growth as well as assessments of fetal cardiac activity patterns that have largely evolved from continuous electron fetal monitoring during labor. Accurate knowledge of gestational age is of great importance in the management of a number of obstetric complications involving the premature fetus.

Abnormal Physiologic Labor

The association of prematurity and abnormal physiologic labor with neonatal outcome has resulted in several major changes over the past 10–15 yr in the way labor is managed and delivery is accomplished. The goal of preventing birth trauma and, in particular, brain injury, and the association of abnormalities in the normal physiologic process of labor with poor neonatal outcome, have led clinicians to describe and document the normal course of labor, normal heart rate patterns, normal biochemical status of mother and fetus, and the pitfalls associated with "difficult" (forceps and breech) deliveries.

The strong association between prolonged labor and increased perinatal morbidity and mortality is now well recognized. The definition of *prolonged labor* was not universally accepted until Friedman described the normal progress of labor in terms of the time course of cervical dilatation and descent of the presenting part through the maternal pelvis in both nulliparous and multiparous patients.[4] In describing norms for labor progress, he also defined abnormal labor progress in simple mathematic terms and clearly demonstrated that it was associated with an increased perinatal morbidity and mortality based on intelligent quotient (IQ) scores and poor performance on developmental tests.

Using a simple technique for graphing labor progress, Friedman was able to identify mothers at risk for delivering infants who would subsequently develop neurologic abnormalities, presumably secondary to their labor experience.[4] Today, "Friedman curves" are widely used for early identification and treatment of abnormal labor progress in order to minimize risk of birth injury and brain damage and to alert physicians to potential mechanical problems associated with certain types of labor abnormalities so that they can undertake appropriate therapeutic interventions.

FETAL MONITORING

In order for the fetal metabolic condition to remain stable, nutrient blood flow in both maternal and fetal compartments must remain sufficient to meet normal fetal requirements. Major physiologic alterations take place during labor in both the mother and fetus. Before the onset of labor, the relatively stable steady-state flow dynamics in the "relaxed" antepartum uterus are modified by increasing uterine tone, periodic interruption of placental blood flow by uterine contractions, and a shortening of contraction-free intervals, during which time metabolic recovery can take place. When these acute intrapartum events are imposed on a chronically stressed fetus, e.g., a fetus suffering from intrauterine growth retardation, there is a high risk for physiologic decompensation with significant morbidity or even mortality.

The increasing awareness that intrapartum events are related to perinatal outcome and Benson's demonstration that intermittent auscultation of the fetal heart rate (FHR) during labor did not significantly improve neonatal outcome led Hon and others to develop a technology for continuous electronic monitoring of the uterine pressure (the physiologic stress) and the FHR.[2,5] Hon and Mendez-Bauer et al. defined the classification system for describing normal and abnormal FHR baseline and periodic changes in the FHR pattern, which can be used to discriminate between fetuses at low risk and those at high risk for fetal distress and asphyxia neonatorum.[5,7] Their original contributions form the basis of the classification system in clinical use today.

Intrauterine Pressure

Intrauterine pressure is recorded by indirect (external monitoring) or direct (internal monitoring) techniques. External monitoring involves placing a strain–gauge (tocodynamometer) on the maternal abdomen over the uterus. Internal pressure monitoring is accomplished by passing a fluid-filled catheter through the cervix into the amniotic cavity. Although external monitoring provides poorer quality information and records only relative changes in uterine pressure, it carries no risk. Internal monitoring provides reliable, actual intrauterine pressure data but requires rupture of the fetal membranes. Internal monitoring may carry a small risk of maternal infection from the catheter and fetal scalp injury or infection from the electrocardiographic (ECG) electrode. Internal techniques also require the use of high-level medical personnel. When fetal monitoring is indicated, the type of monitoring technique used will depend on the status of membranes, the stage of labor, the specific information required, and the relative risks and benefits of monitoring in each individual circumstance.

Heart Rate

During labor, the FHR is usually detected using one of three techniques: (1) an external Doppler ultrasound transducer placed on the maternal abdomen and directed at the fetal heart, (2) a directly acquired fetal ECG obtained from an electrode attached to the fetal presenting part, or (3) an indirect fetal ECG obtained from the mother's abdominal wall, which requires equipment capable of sophisticated signal processing.

Evaluation

The baseline FHR is defined as the mean heart rate between uterine contractions. The normal baseline FHR falls between 120 and 160 beats/min (bpm). A baseline FHR greater than 160 bpm for over 10 min is called fetal tachycardia and is considered abnormal. A baseline FHR under 120 bpm is called fetal bradycardia and is also considered abnormal. Sustained fetal tachycardia or bradycardia requires close observation and a search for a potentially adverse etiology. In addition to the absolute value of the FHR, short- and long-term beat-to-beat FHR variability as well as periodic FHR changes provide useful information on fetal condition. FHR variability refers to changes in heart rate both on a beat-to-beat basis (short term) and over longer periods, generally over one minute (long term). Short-term FHR variability appears to be controlled by the parasympathetic nervous system and may be diminished in response to drugs (e.g., atropine) or increased in association with such fetal activity as breathing movements.[11] Long-term variability appears to represent input from both the sympathetic and the parasympathetic nervous systems. Long-term fluctuations usually occur with a frequency of 3–6 cycles/min (cpm) with an amplitude of 6–10 bpm.

Periodic FHR changes (accelerations or decelerations) refer to changes in the baseline FHR associated with uterine contractions. Some of the periodic changes are reflex in origin, while others are associated with hypoxia, acidosis, or both.

Normal short- and long-term variability are associated with normal acid–base status at birth. Loss of variability, on the other hand, may be associated with fetal acidosis but may also be seen in association with various medications (e.g., meperidine, diazepam, methyldopa). Cyclic loss of variability for short periods in association with decreased fetal movements is frequently noted and may be related to periods of fetal sleep.[12]

FHR decelerations are of greatest concern because of a greater association with fetal distress. There are three basic FHR deceleration patterns based on Hon's original work; they are characterized by the relationship of the onset of the deceleration with the onset of the uterine contraction.

Early Decelerations

Early decelerations (Fig. 6-1) begin at or near the onset of the associated uterine contraction, are symmetric (usually mirroring the contraction), and recover to baseline by the end of the uterine contraction. The nadir usually coincides with the peak of the contraction. The early deceleration pattern has been ascribed to fetal head compression and is mediated by a vagal reflex, since it can be abolished with atropine or vagal nerve transection. This deceleration pattern is not associated with cardiorespiratory depression (asphyxia) at birth.

Late Decelerations

Late decelerations (see Fig. 6-1) begin well after the onset of the contraction (often after the peak of the contraction), appear uniform, and are often proportional to the strength and duration of the contrac-

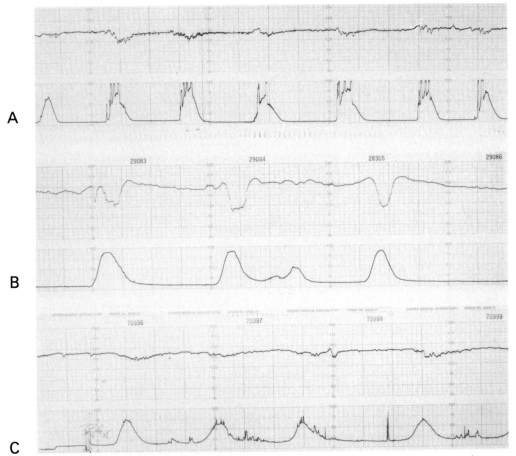

Figure 6-1.   Three FHR and intrauterine pressure tracings. The upper portion of each panel displays the FHR; the lower portion displays the intrauterine pressure. (A): Early decelerations characterized by recurrent FHR decelerations, which begin early in relation to the uterine contraction and recover to baseline by the end of the contraction. (B): Variable FHR decelerations of variable shape and occurring at various times with respect to the uterine contraction. (C): Late FHR decelerations that begin after the peak of the uterine contraction and do not recover to the previous baseline rate until the contraction has been completed.

tion. Late decelerations reach their nadir well after the peak of the contraction and usually do not return to baseline until the contraction is over. This type of pattern is sometimes associated with slow return to the baseline FHR. Among other etiologies, late decelerations may be due to CNS depression or a direct hypoxic effect on the fetal myocardium.[6] Myers and associates have demonstrated FHR decelerations associated with a paO$_2$ of less than 15 mm Hg in experimental animal models.[8]

The late deceleration is the most worrisome type of periodic FHR deceleration, particularly when associated with decreased FHR variability, baseline fetal bradycardia, or both. Hypoxia severe enough to

cause FHR decelerations may lead to profound fetal acidosis as a result of anaerobic glycolysis. Late repetitive decelerations, even when quite mild, should be evaluated by fetal microblood sampling (described below) if they cannot be abolished by changing maternal position (e.g., alleviate supine hypotension), administering oxygen, or discontinuing oxytocin infusion, modifications that are designed to maximize oxygenated flow to the fetus.

Variable Decelerations

Variable decelerations (see Fig. 6-1) are, as their name implies, variable in onset with respect to the uterine contraction, have a variable shape, and are frequently preceded or followed by an FHR acceleration. The variable deceleration is classically ascribed to umbilical cord compression, is mediated by the vagal nerve, and may be modified or abolished by the administration of atropine. Variable decelerations, when severe (under 60 bpm) or prolonged (30 sec), may be associated with the development of fetal acidosis. They require further evaluation (e.g., microblood analysis), particularly when associated with the loss of FHR variability.

Accelerations

FHR accelerations associated with uterine contractions are felt by some to represent an early sign of fetal distress. It is thought that the FHR acceleration may represent the fetus's attempt to increase cardiac output. Extrinsic pressure on the umbilical cord may result in partial compression of the relatively thin-walled umbilical vein, resulting in a decreased return of oxygenated fetal blood from the placenta to the fetus. This venous occlusion may be followed by sympathetic stimulation of the fetal heart, clinically evident as an acceleration associated with the contraction. In such circumstances, the FHR returns to baseline shortly after the compression is relieved. These accelerations may sometimes be differentiated from accelerations occurring in association with fetal movements; the latter are usually short and are related specifically to fetal movement rather than to uterine contractions. Short FHR accelerations associated with fetal movement (rather than contraction) are felt to be a reliable sign of fetal well-being and do not represent fetal distress.

FHR monitoring should be considered a screening technique for detecting fetal distress. When the FHR pattern is normal, i.e., there is a normal baseline FHR with normal variability and no periodic FHR decelerations, neonatal condition at birth (based on Apgar scores) is almost uniformly good. This association is not nearly as reliable, however, in the event of abnormalities in the baseline FHR, FHR variability, or appearance of periodic FHR changes. Even in cases where there are ominous-appearing late decelerations, the association with fetal acidosis, neonatal depression, or both only approaches 50 percent. The association between FHR deceleration and fetal status is even less impressive for variable decelerations and the generally benign early deceleration pattern. Accurate assessment of those fetuses who are not tolerating labor well and who require active intervention can best be accomplished with fetal biochemical (microblood) evaluation where the association exceeds 80 percent.

pH Assessment

The normal fetal pH is lower than that of the mother (7.34 versus 7.44), a finding largely due to the fetal–maternal differences in the partial pressure of carbon dioxide in the blood. The placenta is relatively impermeable to the bicarbonate ion, which crosses the placenta very slowly. Under conditions of relative fetal hypoxemia, fetal energy production is derived from anaerobic glycolysis. Anaerobic metabolism is associated with the accumulation of lactic acid and the development of a metabolic acidosis.

Saling's original description for obtaining fetal microblood samples during labor is still used in an essentially unchanged form.[9] Fetal microblood samples can be obtained only after rupture of the membranes. Samples are obtained transvaginally and transcervically from the presenting fetal part, which is usually the scalp. Using a clinical endoscope, a small area of presenting part is isolated, cleaned, and carefully incised under aseptic conditions. A fetal blood sample is collected in heparinized capillary tubes, which are promptly sealed (to prevent diffusion of blood gases) and analyzed as quickly as possible.

The correlation of fetal capillary blood with Apgar scores at birth is better than any other method available today but is still not perfect. Beard et al. have shown that up to 10 percent of infants with a capillary blood pH below 7.10 will be clinically normal at birth.[1] This 10 percent false-positive rate can be reduced by obtaining a simultaneous maternal "free-flowing" antecubital vein pH value rather than an intrinsic fetal metabolic acidosis. When normal maternal "free-flowing" venous pH has been documented (7.34–7.45), a fetal capillary pH of 7.25 is considered normal. A fetal capillary pH of 7.25–7.20 is defined as preacidosis, and a fetal pH under 7.20 is considered acidotic. The lower the pH in the acidotic range, the higher the incidence of neonatal depression.

Indications for fetal microblood analysis include FHR patterns that are of concern, particularly when accompanied by meconium-stained amniotic fluid. These FHR patterns include persistent loss of FHR variability, recurrent decelerations (regardless of degree), and recurrent, severe, variable decelerations. Once undertaken, biochemical monitoring is a primary monitoring method that will determine the ongoing management of labor.

Despite the sensitivity and specificity of fetal microblood sampling techniques in predicting true fetal distress and neonatal depression, fetal microblood analysis is not widely used, possibly because a physician must collect the sample and because relatively sophisticated technical assistance is needed to analyze the specimen. In order to provide the highest level of fetal care, however, this modality of fetal monitoring should be available, especially for fetuses at risk for birth asphyxia and its long-term complications, including brain damage.

DELIVERY

Midforceps Delivery

Taylor, Friedman, and others have demonstrated that midforceps delivery is associated with increased perinatal morbidity and mortality when compared to either low forceps or spontaneous vaginal delivery.[4,10] The frequency with which midforceps deliveries are performed in teaching institutions has dramatically decreased over the past 10 yr in an attempt to minimize traumatic birth and neonatal depression, which may be associated with later evidence of brain damage. This trend is in part related to the increasing safety of cesarean birth for both mother and fetus. The current trend is to use oxytocin to allow vaginal delivery from a lower pelvic station or, failing that, to deliver by cesarean section rather than risk a difficult midforceps delivery. This change in management is not specifically directed toward those infants who would otherwise be injured but to a much larger group at increased risk for birth trauma.

Breech Presentation

The management of breech presentation is another aspect of perinatal care that has recently undergone major changes because of the desire to reduce the occurrence of traumatic and hypoxic brain damage. Before 1970 the vast majority of breech presentations were delivered vaginally. During the past decade, the incidence of cesarean birth for breech presentation has risen dramatically; it now approaches 100 percent in some institutions. Physicians thought that excessive perinatal mortality and morbidity were related to the mode of delivery and could be precluded by cesarean section in breech presentations. Clinicians' rationale for the marked increase in the cesarean birth rate was that studies of deliveries with breech presentations seemed to show both uncorrected and corrected perinatal mortality and morbidity statistics that were higher in breech presentations delivered

vaginally but that approached the statistics of vertex presentations delivered vaginally when cesarean section was used. Those data are difficult to interpret accurately, however, since they were derived from retrospective studies with major design problems. Most important among those design problems were the nonrandom indications for the choice of cesarean versus vaginal birth. Other reasons for difficulty based on data interpretation arise from the fact that breech presentation is more commonly associated with congenital malformation, intrauterine growth retardation, multiple pregnancy, uterine anomalies, and, especially, prematurity, a condition that itself has a strong correlation with morbidity, mortality, and brain damage.

Neonatal morbidity and mortality with breech presentations relate to traumatic birth injuries due to fetal size, maternal pelvic capacity, entrapment of the fetal head, and the increased incidence of umbilical cord prolapse, factors that are significantly affected by the type of breech presentation (e.g., footling versus frank breech). Prolapse of the umbilical cord may be responsible for hypoxic and traumatic damage to the fetal CNS. Attempts to minimize hypoxic insult to the fetal brain may result in limb, skull, or spinal injury. Cruikshank and Pitkin reviewed existing retrospective studies and concluded that there was no scientific foundation for the concept that cesarean birth was the optimal route of delivery with breech presentation.[3] The subject was subsequently retrospectively reviewed by a number of authors, and data from these reviews, as well as the New York City data presented in the draft report of the Task Force on Cesarean Childbirth, supported the thesis that there is no proof that prophylactic cesarean birth in *all* premature breech presentations results in significantly better outcome for the fetus.[13] Cesarean childbirth certainly does *not* improve outcome for the mother and indeed may result in major morbidity or mortality.

The literature is quite clear in documenting that cesarean birth is advantageous for footling (single or double) and incomplete breech presentations, however. Furthermore, cesarean section is clearly beneficial in breech presentation for large (over 4000 g) and small (under 1000–1500 g) fetuses, for those presenting with a hyperextended head, or when the maternal pelvis is small, even when the fetus is of normal size. Clearly, the risk of poor neonatal outcome is greatest in those patients who have combinations of factors such as prematurity, breech presentation, and abnormal FHR patterns.

REFERENCES

1. Beard RW, Morris ED, Clayton SG: pH of foetal capillary blood as an indicator of the condition of the foetus. J Obstet Gnyecol Br Commonwealth 74:812, 1967

2. Benson RC, Shubek R, Deutschberger WW, et al: Fetal heart rate as a predicator of fetal distress. Obstet Gynecol 32:259, 1968

3. Cruikshank DP, Pitkin RM: Delivery of the premature breech. Obstet Gynecol 50:367, 1977

4. Friedman EA: Labor: Clinical Evaluation and Management. New York, Appleton-Century-Crofts, 1978

5. Hon EH: Detection of fetal distress, in Wood C (ed): Fifth World Congress of Gynecology and Obstetrics. London, Butterworths, 1967

6. James LS, Morishima HD, Daniel SS, et al: Mechanisms of late deceleration of the fetal heart rate. Am J Obstet Gynecol 113:578, 1972

7. Mendez-Bauer C, Arnt IC, Gulin L, et al: Relationship between blood pH and heart rate in the human fetus during labor. Am J Obstet Gynecol 97:530, 1967

8. Myers RE, Mueller-Heubach E, Adamsons K: Predictability of the state of fetal oxygenation from a quantitative analysis of the components of late deceleration. Am J Obstet Gynecol 115:1083, 1973

9. Saling E: A new method for examination of the child during labor: Introduction, technique and principles. Arch Gynaekol 197:108, 1962

10. Taylor ES: Can midforceps operations be eliminated? Obstet Gynecol 2:203, 1953

11. Timor-Tritsch IE, Zador I, Hertz RH, et al: Human fetal respiratory arrhythmia. Am J Obstet Gynecol 127:622, 1977

12. Timor-Tritsch IE, Dierker LJ, Hertz RH, et al: Studies of antepartum behavioral state in the human fetus at term. Am J Obstet Gynecol 132:524, 1978

13. Draft Report of the Task Force on Cesarean Childbirth: Presented at the Consensus Development Conference on Cesarean Childbirth, National Institutes of Health, Bethesda, September 1980

Leslie Rubin

7

Perinatal Factors

More than 100 yr ago, Little identified that adverse perinatal factors were causally related to the physical disabilities he was seeing in his professional practice as an orthopaedic surgeon.[1] In a recent review of neuropediatric handicaps, Hagberg et al. reported that 45–65 percent of children with cerebral palsy had etiologic factors referrable to the perinatal period.[2] For those with mild mental retardation, the figure was 10–15 percent, and for those with severe mental retardation, it was 10–17 percent.*

PERINATAL MORTALITY

As a result of advances in the management of pregnancy and labor and in neonatal intensive care practices, there has been a dramatic decline in perinatal mortality. Statistics from the United States show the mortality to have decreased from 1930, when the figure was 21.1:1000 to 12.8:1000 in 1970 and 6.2:1000 in 1980.[3,4] Similar trends have been reported from many parts of the United States as well as from other countries.[5–8]

PREVALENCE OF CEREBRAL PALSY

It is of interest to compare the prevalence of cerebral palsy with the decline in neonatal and perinatal mortality (see Table 7-1). Hagberg in Sweden and Stanley in western Australia both examined the

*None of the statistics included congenital anomalies. The first percentage figure is for birth to 7 days of age; the second, for 28 wk of gestation to 4 wk of age.

period from the 1950s to the 1970s.[7,8] The relationship between perinatal mortality and the prevalence of cerebral palsy is, however, not a simple one. Whereas Hagberg demonstrated a steady decline from the early 1950s to the mid-1960s and stabilization with a slight increase in the 1970s, Stanley's data initially showed a rise with peaks in the 1960s before falling in the early 1970s but then rising again in the mid 1970s (see Figure 7-1). This pattern of inconsistency is found to be greater when results from other centers are examined as well.[9] There is no doubt that neonatal intensive care practices have played a major role in the outcome for survival and handicap, and may well explain the discrepancies in relationship between mortality and morbidity.

INFLUENCE OF BIRTHWEIGHT

The greatest impact on the reduction in neonatal mortality has come from the increased survival of low birthweight infants (less than 2500 g) and very low birthweight infants (less than 1500 g). Philip et al. combined data from several centers in England and North America and showed that for infants of 1000–1500 g, mortality improved from 44 percent in the 1960s to 18 percent in the 1970s; for those 500–1000 g, mortality decreased from 91 to 58 percent.[11]

Lee et al. compared birthweight-specific neonatal mortality at the Bronx Municipal Hospital Center, New York, between 1966–1973 and 1974–1977 and found a statistically significant improvement in survival for those infants of 1501–2000 g.[12] They also demonstrated that the low birthweight rate significantly affected statistics of neonatal mortality. This in part explains the variations in reports from different

Table 7-1
The Rates of Perinatal Mortality, Infant Mortality, Stillbirths, and Cerebral Palsy in Sweden, 1951–1975

Category	1951–1955	1956–1960	1961–1965	1966–1970	1971–1975
Perinatal mortality (stillbirths and deaths within 7 days): 1000 births	30.1	26.7	22.2	17.7	13.8
Infant mortality (death within 1 yr): 100 live births	19.3	16.9	14.8	12.3	10.0
Stillbirths (deaths before and during delivery): 1000 births	17.7	15.1	11.5	8.9	6.9
Cerebral palsy: 1000 live births	2.3	1.9	1.8	1.4	1.5

Reprinted with permission from Hagberg B: Epidemiological and preventive aspects of cerebral palsey and severe mental retardation in Sweden. Eur J Pediatr 130:71, 1979.

centers and different countries: those centers with higher LBW rates will tend to have higher mortality.

Although the rate of birth of infants weighing less than 2500 g is only about 7–10 percent of total live births, the mortality of these infants accounts for almost 90 percent of neonatal deaths. By the same token, this group is more likely to develop cerebral palsy and other handicapping conditions.

Britton et al. examined the outcome of infants less than 801 g born in 1974–1977.[13] There were no survivors below 500 g. From 500–700 g the survival rate was 17 percent, and all the survivors had residual handicaps. Between 700–749 g the survival rate was 24 percent, and between 750–800 g it was 41 percent. The incidence of handicap in these 2 groups was 39 percent. As birthweight increases, mortality and risks of handicap thus decrease.

There are numerous reports on the changing incidence of handicaps in low birthweight survivors[14–16] (Fig. 7-2). All reflect an improvement in outcome,

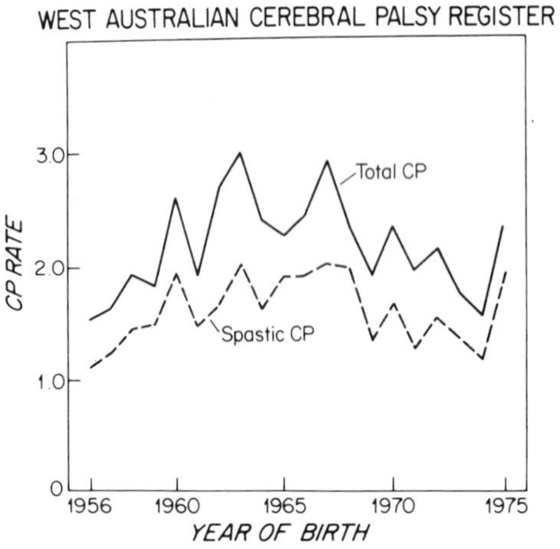

WEST AUSTRALIAN CEREBRAL PALSY REGISTER

Figure 7-1. Prevalence of cerebral palsy per 1,000 live births in western Australia. As a period of time elapses from birth to the diagnosis of cerebral palsy, the data obtained tends to reflect perinatal statistics and practices that have changed and do not necessarily have relevance in terms of current perinatal statistics and practices. This condition is not an uncommon problem in trying to evaluate outcome data of innovations in perinatal care. It is nevertheless extremely useful in trying to determine how changing patterns of perinatal care tend to affect the prevalence of handicap and how these patterns might be improved. (Data obtained by personal communication from Dr. Fiona J. Stanley.)

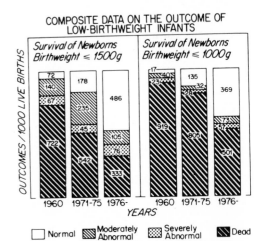

Figure 7-2. Composite data on the outcome on low-birthweight infants. (From Budetti P, Barrand N, McManus P, et al: The costs and effectiveness of neonatal intensive care. Washington, D.C., Office of Technology Assessment, U.S. Government Printing Office, P. 38, 1981).

but the results vary. The variations are a result of many factors, e.g., characteristics of the study population, the type of assessment performed, and the rigor with which criteria are applied. Important variables that have been identified include whether the infant was born in a tertiary perinatal center or required transportation and the importance of the relationship between birthweight and gestational age.[5,11,14,16] Synthesis of the results of numerous studies of "high-risk" survivors shows a median rate of cerebral palsy at 7 percent and of mental retardation at 15 percent.[5]

There is no question that this group of infants contributes to a significant proportion of children with cerebral palsy, and there are suggestions that the relative representation is increasing. O'Reilly and Walentynowicz examined the etiologic factors of cerebral palsy in their clinic.[17] They found an increased proportion of children who had been premature: from 12 percent before the 1940s, with a steady increase to 29 percent in the 1970s. There was a corresponding decrease in factors that were more likely to involve larger infants; e.g., dystocia decreased from 14.6–4.4 percent.

Dale and Stanley examined the incidence of spastic cerebral palsy between 1968–1970 and 1971–1975 and found a statistically significant reduction for birthweights greater than 2500 g.[18] There was no reduction for birthweights less than 2500 g between these 2 periods.

The pattern that seems to emerge is as follows:

1. There is a decrease in the incidence of cerebral palsy for infants born at term with birthweights greater than 2500 g.
2. There is an increased survival rate for infants with birthweights less than 2500 g as well as for those less than 1500 g.
3. The risk for the development of cerebral palsy in the low birthweight and very low birthweight infants is relatively high.

Kiely et al. commented that "no consideration of the net effect of newborn intensive care on handicaps can ignore this important demographic shift."

PATHOLOGY

In 1862, Little said that "pathology has gradually taught [us about] diseases incidental to the act of birth."[1] This provides a framework for an understanding of the perinatal factors involved in the pathogenesis of cerebral palsy.

The neuropathologic survey of 914 infants by Banker and Bruce–Gregorios offers the opportunity to examine these factors (see Chap. 4). The largest group in their study was represented by lesions of anoxic encephalopathy (535); subependymal hemorrhages were the most common discreet lesion (284). These lesions and the spectrum of other pathologic entities in their series is representative, in nature and proportion, of the clinical syndromes that are associated with central nervous system (CNS) insults in the neonatal period and the permanent damage that results in the clinical picture of cerebral palsy.

The clinical diagnosis of these conditions in the perinatal period has been facilitated with the use of electroencephalograms (EEGs), computed tomography (CT) scans, and ultrasound techniques (see Chap. 11). In addition, studies from animal models have greatly contributed to understanding the pathogenetic mechanisms.[19,20]

It is important to bear in mind that more than one neuropathologic lesion can be present in the same infant. This is particularly relevant in the situation of multiple hemorrhages and in the finding of minor periventricular lesions.

PERINATAL INSULTS

Hypoxic–Ischemic Encephalopathy

Hypoxic–ischemic encephalopathy is the most common insult, accounting for more than 50 percent of all findings at autopsy. More than half, however, were represented by the lesions of periventricular leukomalacia and gliosis; these lesions are relatively nonspecific and may be present with other manifestations of anoxic encephalopathy (see Chap. 4).

The question that may be asked is, What factors determine whether an infant will develop the minor periventricular lesions or the more extensive lesions of grey matter necrosis? It appears that this is not merely a question of degree. The experimental work of Myers on animals has furnished a possible explanation.[19,20] The presence of glucose during the period of oxygen deprivation is highly correlated with the development of cerebral edema. In the absence of oxygen, glucose is metabolized into lactic acid. The lactic acid is toxic to the neurons and causes tissue damage. In this context, the issue of degree is important. The duration of hypoxia, the amount of glucose available, and the consequent concentration of lactic acid are the determining factors in this model.

Experimental studies show that accumulations of lactate in brain tissue in excess of 25 μmol/g lead to changes in membrane physiologic properties, breakdown of blood–brain barrier (BBB), shifts of fluid into the intracellular compartment (leading to tissue edema), and widespread destruction of brain tissue.[20] This may well explain the clinical finding that full-term infants tend to have a more dramatic immediate and long-term outcome directly attributable to the consequences of hypoxia. Full-term infants are more likely to have adequate blood glucose levels and glycogen stores. Preterm and small-for-gestational age (SGA) infants, on the other hand, do not have adequate glycogen stores and are, in fact, more likely to suffer from hypoglycemia and therefore, are less likely to develop generalized tissue necrosis and cerebral edema. Consequently, they tend to have local tissue necrosis directly related to hypoxia and ischemia. The lesions of periventricular leukomalacia and gliosis being more common in the low birthweight infant.

The clinical syndromes of the child with cerebral palsy can be viewed in this light. The larger infant with the more generalized and destructive process will develop the quadriplegic syndrome with significant intellectual impairment, while the smaller infant with periventricular lesions will tend to develop the diplegic syndrome.[23] Davies and Tizard demonstrated the latter clinical relationship in their analysis of Little's original paper.[1,22]

Clinical Correlates

Neonatal hypoxic–ischemic injuries are due to intrauterine or intrapartum asphyxia in 90 percent of cases and when present clinically at birth, reflect significant CNS insult.[23] The newborn infant with low Apgar scores requires immediate attention and resuscitation. Once this has taken place, it is the neurologic picture in this critical period that will determine whether there are ongoing problems in the CNS. The evolution of the clinical picture through the stages of initial shock, irritability, lethargy, seizures, and coma have been well described by Volpe, who stresses that observation of the infant in the early hours after asphyxia is crucial for optimal management.[23] Dubowitz and Dubowitz have devised a system for the comprehensive neurologic evaluation of term and preterm infants that promises to be a valuable guide for immediate as well as long-term assessment.[24]

Quality of Survival

Determination of the Apgar score as an index of cardiorespiratory and CNS well-being is generally accepted. It is extremely valuable for the immediate assessment and management of the newborn, but there are some questions on its long-term prognostic value. Nelson and Ellenberg reviewed Apgar scores as predictors of neurologic impairment in the National Collaborative Perinatal Project.[25] The mortality of infants with low scores (0–3) was high, particularly if the scores remained low. For low-birthweight infants the mortality was 48.2 percent, with Apgar scores of 0–3 at 1 min and 95.7 percent if the score remained low at 20 min. For full-term infants, the corresponding mortality was 5.6 percent and 59 percent, respectively. When they examined long-term outcome, however, they found that only 27 percent of infants with Apgar scores of less than 7 at 5 min had cerebral palsy. The remaining 73 percent were free of handicap. A poor prognosis could be predicted for those term infants who developed seizures between 4–24 hr after birth and had low Apgar scores at 10 and 20 min.

The importance of the clinical course after asphyxia cannot be overemphasized for its importance for immediate management as well as for predicting long-term outcome. Minkowski et al. analyzed the outcome of birth asphyxia by clinical course:[26]

1. Those infants who recover within the first week are unlikely to have abnormal sequelae.
2. Of those who persist with symptoms after the first week, 20–30 percent are likely to have a serious outcome.
3. Of those who persist with neurologic abnormalities and uncontrollable seizures, 70 percent will have subsequent handicap.

Intraventricular Hemorrhage

In the pathologic situation, "almost all infants with these hemorrhages are of low birthweight, the vast majority being under 28 weeks gestation" (see Chap. 4). Before the advent of CT scans, intraventricular hemorrhage (IVH) was thought to be uniformly fatal in premature infants. The clinical course was almost always identified by a sudden deterioration, with a drop in blood pressure and hematocrit, and the ominous bulging fontanelle. Attempts at resuscitation often failed, and the diagnosis was confirmed at autopsy. A gloomy outlook was predicted for those infants who survived.

The ability to diagnose IVH clinically has been greatly enhanced with the use of CT scans and ultrasound. New perceptions in the care of low birthweight infants have been appreciated, especially in IVH:

- IVH has been found to be more common than previously thought. Papile et al. found IVH in 20 of 46 infants less than 1500 g who were subjected to routine CT scan.[28]
- IVH is not necessarily fatal. In Papile's series, the mortality was 55 percent. (This was, however, greater than the 23 percent for control infants without IVH.)
- Not all infants with IVH were symptomatic. The presence of IVH was confirmed in those who demonstrated the classic clinical picture, and these tended to be the larger bleeds. The asymptomatic lesions tended to be smaller or to develop more slowly.
- The association of IVH with the development of hydrocephalus was confirmed. It was also found that ventricular dilatation occurred well before the increase in head size became clinically evident.[29]

In an attempt to describe the natural history, Papile et al. devised a grading system:[28]

Hemorrhages without dilatation of the ventricles
    Grade 1: localized to the subependymal area (SEH) or germinal matrix (GMH)
    Grade 2: SEH with bleeding into the ventricles (IVH)
Hemorrhages with ventricular dilatation
    Grade 3: SEH + IVH + hydrocephalus
    Grade 4: SEH + IVH + hydrocephalus + parenchymal hemorrhage

This classification by extent of hemorrhage and by the presence or absence of ventricular dilatation (or hydrocephalus) is helpful and is used extensively. It does, however, have limitations as it tends to imply progression. The pathogenesis of hydrocephalus is usually on the basis of an obliterative arachnoiditis, which is certainly not a matter of degree, nor do grade 4 lesions necessarily represent the extension of SEH, GMH, or IVH; they may occur by a completely different mechanism. The more destructive parenchymal hemorrhages also tend to have a more serious long-term prognosis, while the outlook of the other three grades do not seem to differ too much from each other.

Hambleton and Wigglesworth have developed an hypothesis to explain the possible pathogenetic mechanism for IVH.[30] They take into consideration the loose supporting tissue in the germinal matrix, the thin-walled capillaries that course through this tissue, and the metabolic and hemodynamic factors that affect blood pressure and cerebral blood flow. The various factors differ in nature and degree and depend on the infant's gestational age, which is inversely related to vulnerability (Figure 7-3). The importance in identifying these factors provides some idea as to how these lesions can be prevented; the

use of bicarbonate has been demonstrated to increase the risk of development of IVH.[32]

Comprehensive long-term studies are scarce at present. Schechner put together data from a small number of studies (Table 7-2) showing that infants with grades 1, 2, and 3 have a similar outcome: 47–83 percent are free of neurologic impairment, and 53–82 percent are free of intellectual impairment, with those in grade 1 doing only slightly better.[33] Those infants with a grade 4 IVH had a much more serious outcome, with only 5 percent having a normal intelligence quotient (IQ) and all having some degree of neurologic impairment. In the light of these data, it is worth considering whether an alternative classification system should be devised in order to take into account the different nature and outcome for the parenchymal hemorrhages. This is still a new area of clinical awareness, and it requires further study and investigation.

Other Hemorrhages

Subarachnoid

Subarachnoid hemorrhage is probably the most common intracranial hemorrhage but is usually clinically quite insignificant. It is found in full-term infants, particularly where there has been some history of difficult delivery, and in preterm infants where there has been some history of hypoxia. It can also be found in association with other hemorrhages or as part of a generalized bleeding diathesis. The clinical picture and long-term outcome are variable and generally reflect associated pathologic conditions. Hydrocephalus is also a possible consequence.

Subdural

Subdural hemorrhages in the neonatal period are almost exclusively traumatic lesions of the full-term infant. They most commonly occur in situations where there is cephalopelvic disproportion or abnormal deliveries, e.g., breech or other presentations requiring forceps extraction.

Lacerations in the tentorium or falx are associated with large bleeds and appear early in the neonatal period; they usually have a serious, and often a fatal, outcome.

The clinical picture with rupture of superficial vessels is determined by the extent and progression of the bleed. The development of seizures and increased intracranial pressure are possible consequences. Not uncommonly, small or self limiting lesions may manifest much later as chronic subdural

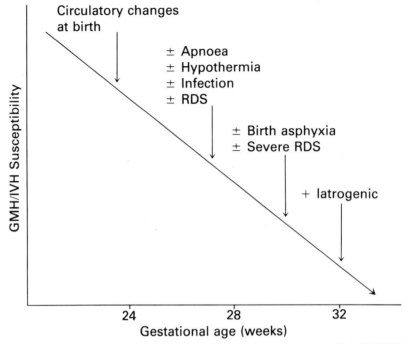

Figure 7-3. Hypothetical scheme to explain increasing stress required to elicit GMH-IVH with advancing brain maturation. (Reprinted with permission from Pape KE, Wigglesworth JS: Hemorrhage, ischemia, and the perinatal brain. Clinics in Developmental Medicine, 69/70. Philadelphia, Lippincott, 1979, p. 146.)

Table 7-2

Outcome of Infants with IVH

Grades	1(%)	2(%)	3(%)	4(%)
Neurologic				
Normal	83	76	47	0
Suspect	8	18	41	15
Abnormal	8	6	12	85
Psychologic				
Normal IQ	67	53	82	5
IQ 71–85	17	44	12	25
IQ 51–70	8	0	0	40
IQ 50	8	3	6	30
Total no. of cases 83	12	34	17	20

Reprinted with permission from Schechner S: Intraventricular hemorrhage in the premature infant. Presented at the March of Dimes Symposium on Prenatal Hypoxia and Brain Damage, New York, November 1981.

effussions. Of infants with these lesions, 50–80 percent do well on follow-up study.[34]

Intracerebellar

Intracerebellar lesions are not uncommonly found at autopsy in small premature infants. They may represent an extension of an IVH and have also been allegedly linked with the use of positive-pressure ventilation applied by face mask with a tight band around the occiput. Not much is known of this lesion, but it has been suggested that cerebellar function be thoughtfully assessed in the child who was premature.[34]

CNS Infections

Bacterial meningitis is responsible for 1–4 percent of neonatal deaths. It is more common in premature than in term infants. *E. Coli* is the most common infecting organism, followed closely by group B hemolytic streptococcus. Almost all organisms that cause sepsis in the newborn can cause meningitis, and this is the usual route of infection. Mortality and morbidity are high, particularly in the premature infant. Cerebral palsy, mental retardation, seizures, deafness, blindness, and hydrocephalus are all possible consequences. Sequelae of bacterial meningitis in older age groups are not as common nor as severe as those occurring in the neonatal period.

Nonbacterial meningitides are most commonly represented by the TORCH infections, i.e., toxoplasmosis, rubella, cytomegalovirus (CMV), herpes, and syphilis. They have a greater significance as intrauterine infections and are discussed in Chapter 5. Herpes simplex infections deserve specific mention, since they can occur during birth and result in high mortality and morbidity.

Kernicterus

Kernicterus represents the deposition of bilirubin in the basal ganglia. The incidence of this condition in full-term infants has been dramatically reduced by the prevention of Rh incompatability and the treatment of hyperbilirubinemia with exchange transfusions. Although the lesion is now uncommon in its full expression, some deposition of bilirubin is seen in low-birthweight infants at autopsy, particularly in those who had significant metabolic disturbances. The determining factors are felt to be those that increase the permeability of the blood-brain barrier to free bilirubin.[35]

Metabolic Factors

The major metabolic disturbances involving hypoxia and acidosis have been alluded to in the role they play in the pathogenesis of hypoxic–ischemic insults and IVH. The other metabolic factor that should be mentioned is hypoglycemia. This was more of a problem when the feeding of newborn infants was delayed. It remains a problem in low birthweight and SGA infants who have poor glycogen stores. There is some question whether hypoglycemia per se or some associated pathologic condition is the cause of morbidity. Haworth et al. demonstrated that the long-term outcome of infants of diabetic mothers was not related to the presence of symptomatic hypoglycemia in the neonatal period.[36]

Psychosocial and Economic Factors

No discussion of the perinatal factors that affect development can ignore the importance of healthy mother–infant relationships.[37] This applies particu-

larly to the sick premature infant who is surrounded by technology and must remain in the hospital for a prolonged period. This aspect of perinatal care requires as much attention as the treatment of medical problems and the maintainance of homeostasis.

The broader issues of prenatal and even preconceptual factors also deserve special mention. Hagberg et al. comment that these factors do not necessarily act as a cause of brain damage but as a predisposing factor, altering the vulnerability of the fetus to perinatal events that would otherwise be of minor significance.[38] Although they were discussing adverse medical factors during pregnancy, the concept can be expanded to include psychosocial phenomena. Knobloch et al. evaluated the factors that affected the outcome of infants with a birthweight of less than 1501 g.[39] They found that significantly more mothers of infants with major handicaps had less than a 12th-grade education (40 percent versus 18 percent) and that significantly more families received Medicaid (75 percent versus 29 percent). In a follow-up study of low birthweight infants, Neligan et al. found that the outcome of the infants was strongly associated with measures of mother's care of the child.[40]

Moser stresses the importance of intervention in the prevention of psychosocial mental retardation and applies this principle to children who are at risk for developing cerebral palsy (see Chap. 9). Perkins et al. applied the principle of prevention to the management of adolescent pregnancies and found that the outcome of these pregnancies did not differ significantly from those of the general population.[41]

These findings point strongly to the issues of prevention at many levels, particularly to the need for thoughtful scientific investigation of etiology and application of the knowledge to health education and the improvement of standards of living through public health policies.

PERINATAL FACTORS IN DEVELOPING COUNTRIES

The discussion of etiological factors has dealt only with data from developed or industrialized centers. Data from developing countries is scarce. Health care as reflected in high infant and neonatal mortality can be compared to levels in the U.S. before the 1940s. Stein and Rosen report an infant mortality of 41.73 for 1977 in Soweto, South Africa.[6] This corresponds to the infant mortality in the U.S. in 1940.[3] Stein and Mouton reviewed 103 autopsies on newborn infants and found that 30 of 84 singletons were born at term and 19 of those died from perinatal hypoxia. Perinatal hypoxia accounted for 36 percent of all causes of death.[42] In the newborn population surveyed, the incidence of low-birthweight infants was 20 percent and in the autopsy study 72 percent of the infants were of low birthweight. Contrast these figures to the ones for developed countries mentioned above where the figures are 10 percent and 90 percent, respectively. One can then readily see that there is a higher rate of low birthweight infants, but there is a proportionally higher mortality of term infants. Analysis of their data also reveals a high incidence of SGA infants at 15 percent.

The combination of low socioeconomic circumstance and limited antenatal care and perinatal services accounts for this situation. The data mentioned above reflect a population that has seen a dramatic improvement in services, however. In 1950 the infant mortality was a bleak 232 to every 1,000 live births. This latter figure may well represent what exists in even less-developed parts of the world.

It must be remembered that Little's original paper in 1862 reflected a population that was undergoing the process of industrialization.[1] In the group of children he presented, 40 percent were born at term with some adverse perinatal problem. In a group of African children with mental handicaps in Rhodesia (now Zimbabwe), Axton and Levy found that 60 percent of children with birth related problems had birth trauma as an etiological factor while only 20 percent were premature.[43] In a survey of etiological factors responsible for developmental delays in 725 children in a Soweto Clinic, Rubin and Davis found that 40 percent had perinatal problems with 70 percent of these being related to birth asphyxia and trauma.[44]

Therefore while the post-industrial states are wrestling with the problems of very low-birthweight infants, the populations that are undergoing the process of industrialization are trying to come to terms with providing adequate antenatal and perinatal services. The common denominator should be seen in the identification of etiological factors with a view towards prevention. The large discrepancy beween the contrasting population groups represents an anachronism, ideally what is needed worldwide is a sharing of information and services.

REFERENCES

1. Little WJ: On the influence of abnormal parturition, difficult labours, premature birth and asphyxia neonatorum, on the mental and physical condition of the child, especially in relation to deformities. Trans Obstet Soc Lond 3:293, 1862

2. Hagberg B, Hagberg G, Olow I: Gains and hazards of neonatal care: An analysis from Swedish cerebral palsy epidemiology. Dev Med Child Neurol 24:13, 1982

3. Wegman ME: Annual summary of vital statistics—1979: With some 1930 comparisons. Pediatrics 66:823, 1980

4. Wegman ME: Annual summary of vital statistics—1980. Pediatrics 67:755, 1981

5. Kiely JL, Paneth N, Stein Z, et al: Cerebral palsy and newborn care. II. Mortality and neurological impairment in low birthweight infants. Dev Med Child Neurol 23:650, 1981

6. Stein H, Rosen EU: Changing trends in child health in Soweto. South Afr Med J 58:1030, 1980

7. Hagberg B: Epidemiological and preventive aspects of cerebral palsy and severe mental retardation in Sweden. Eur J Pediatr 130:71, 1979

8. Stanley FJ: An epidemiological study of cerebral palsy in western Australia (1956–1975). 1. Changes in the total incidence of cerebral palsy and associated factors. Dev Med Child Neurol 21:701, 1979

9. Kiely JL, Paneth N, Stein Z, et al: Cerebral palsy and newborn care. I. Secular trends in cerebral palsy. Dev Med Child Neurol 23:533, 1981

10. Paneth N, Kiely JL, Stein Z, et al: Cerebral palsy and newborn care. III. Estimated prevalence rates of cerebral palsy under differing rates of mortality and impairment of low birthweight infants. Dev Med Child Neurol 23:801, 1981

11. Philip AGS, Little GA, et al: Neonatal mortality risks for the eighties: the importance of birthweight/gestational age groups. Pediatrics 68:122, 1981

12. Lee K, Paneth N, Gartner LM, et al: The very low birthweight rate: Principal predictor of neonatal mortality in industrialised populations. J Pediatr 95:759, 1980

13. Britton SB, Fitzhardinge PM, Ashby S: Is intensive care justified in infants weighing less than 801 gm at birth? J Pediatr 99:937, 1981

14. Pape KE, Buncic RJ, Ashby S, et al: The status at 2 years of low birthweight infants with birthweight of less than 1001 gms. J Pediatr 92:253, 1978.

15. Hack M, Fanaroff AA, Merkatz IR: The low birthweight infant—evolution of a changing outlook. N Engl J Med 301:1162, 1979.

16. Kumar SP, Anday EK, Sacks LM, et al: Follow up studies of very low birthweight infants (1,250 gms or less) born and treated within a perinatal center. Pediatrics 66:438, 1980

17. O'Reilly DE, Walentynowicsz JE: Etiological factors in cerebral palsy: An Historical review. Dev Med Child Neurol 23:633, 1981

18. Dale A, Stanley FJ: An epidemiological study of cerebral palsy in western Australia 1956–1975. II. Spastic cerebral palsy and perinatal factors. Dev Med Child Neurol 22:13, 1980

19. Myers RE: Experimental models of brain damage: Relevance to human pathology, in Gluck L (ed): Intrauterine Asphyxia and the Developing Fetal Brain. Chicago, Year Book Medical Publishers, 1977

20. Myers RE: Lactic acid accumulation as a cause of brain edema and cerebral necrosis, resulting from oxygen deprivation. Adv Perinatol 1:85, 1979

21. Banker BQ, Larroche JG: Periventricular leukomalacia of infancy: A form of neonatal anoxic encephalopathy. Arch Neurol 7:386, 1962

22. Davies PA, Tizard JPM: Very low birthweight and subsequent neurological defect. Dev Med Child Neurol 17:3, 1975

23. Volpe JJ: Observing the infant in the early hours after asphyxia, in Gluck L (ed): Intrauterine Asphyxia and the Developing Fetal Brain. Chicago, Year Book Medical Publishers, 1977

24. Dubowitz L, Dubowitz V: The Neurological Assessment of the Preterm and Full Term Infant. Clinics in Developmental Medicine, no. 79. Philadelphia, Lippincott, 1981

25. Nelson KB, Ellenberg JH: Apgar scores as predictors of chronic neurologic disability. Pediatrics 68:36, 1981

26. Minkowski A, Amiel–Tison C, Cukier F, et al: Long term follow up and sequelae of asphyxiated infants, in Gluck L (ed): Intrauterine Asphyxia and the Developing Fetal Brain. Chicago, Year Book Medical Publishers, 1977

27. Krishnamoorthy KS, Fernandez RA, Momrose KJ, et al: Evaluation of neonatal intracranial hemorrhage by computerized tomography. Pediatrics 59:165, 1977

28. Papile L–A, Burstein J, Burstein R, et al: Incidence and evolution of subependymal hemorrhage: A study of infants with birthweight of less than 1,500 gms. J Pediatr 92:529, 1978

29. Volpe JJ, Pasternak JP, Allan WC: Ventricular dilation preceding rapid head growth following neonatal intracranial hemorrhage. Am J Dis Child 131:1212, 1977

30. Hambleton G, Wigglesworth JS: Origin of intraventricular hemorrhage in the preterm infant. Arch Dis Child 51:651, 1975

31. Pape KE, Wigglesworth JS: Hemorrhage, ischemia and the perinatal brain. Clinics in Developmental Medicine, no. 69/70. Philadelphia, Lippincott, 1979

32. Wigglesworth JS, Keith IH, Girling DJ, et al: Hyaline membrane disease, alkali and intraventricular hemorrhage. Arch Dis Child 51:755, 1976

33. Schechner S: Intraventricular hemorrhage in the premature infant. Presented at The March of Dimes Symposium on Fetal Hypoxia and Brain Damage. New York, November 1981

34. Volpe JJ: Neonatal intracranial hemorrhage. Clin Perinatol 4:77, 1977

35. Ritter DA, Kenny JD, Norton HJ, et al: A prospective study of free bilirubin and other risk factors in the development of kernicterus in premature infants. Pediatrics 69:260, 1982

36. Haworth JC, McRae KN, Dilling LA: Prognosis of infants of diabetic mothers in relation to neonatal hypoglycemia. Dev Med Child Neurol 18:471, 1976

37. Klaus MH, Kennell JH: Maternal–Infant Bonding. St. Louis, C.V. Mosby, 1976

38. Hagberg G, Hagberg B, Olow I: The changing panorama of cerebral palsy in Sweden (1954–1970). III. The importance of fetal deprivation of supply. Acta Paediatr Scand 65:403, 1976

39. Knobloch H, Malone A, Ellison PH, et al: Considerations in evaluating changes in outcome for infants weighing less than 1,501 grams. Pediatrics 69:285, 1982

40. Neligan GA, Kolvin I, Scott DMcI, et al: Born too soon or born too small (A follow-up study to seven years of age). Clinics in Developmental Medicine, no. 61. Philadelphia, Lippincott, 1976

41. Perkins RP, Nakashima II, Mullin M et al: Intensive care in adolescent pregnancy. Obstet Gynecol 52:179, 1978

42. Stein H, Mouton SCE: Neonatal mortality in a black urban community. South African Medical Journal 55:413, 1979

43. Axton JHM, Levy LF: Mental handicap in Rhodesian African children. Developmental Medicine and Child Neurology 16:350, 1974

44. Rubin IL, Davis M: Developmental disabilities in a population undergoing the process of industrialization. Presented at the Academy of Cerebral Palsy and Developmental Medicine, Detroit, Michigan, 1981

Irwin A. Schafer

8

Genetics of Mental Retardation

Physicians in a variety of specialities participate in the management of infants, children, and adults with developmental disabilities such as cerebral palsy or mental retardation. Parents, siblings, and other family members will often question the provider about the cause of the patient's problem and whether there is a genetic component. These are important questions, since if a genetic etiology is established, genetic counseling, antenatal diagnoses, and, in a few instances, early treatment can be offered to the family to prevent or ameliorate the problem in subsequent offspring. It is equally important to the family if a nongenetic etiology can be established as the cause of the patient's disability, since this would imply that the parents do not have a high recurrence risk for subsequent pregnancies. The problem is defining an etiologic basis for the patient's retardation. In some patients the diagnosis is straightforward; in others it will tax the acumen of the most astute clinician. Physicians who manage developmentally disabled or retarded patients, regardless of their specialities, must be aware of the role that genetics may play in the etiology of their patients' problems. This chapter will provide a framework for genetic evaluation of the patient with mental retardation.

MENTAL RETARDATION

Mental retardation is a symptom and not a medical diagnosis. It may be defined as slower than normal rates of psychomotor development in childhood

with significantly subaverage intellectual function in adulthood. In practice, an individual is classified as retarded if the intelligence quotient (IQ) measures less than 70, regardless of cause or pathogenesis. This is an arbitrary definition based on the gaussian distribution of intelligence in the population. Analyses of published IQ curves provide a basis for segregating retarded individuals into two large groups (Fig. 8-1).[30,38] Curve A is the conventional representation of the distribution of intelligence. Individuals that deviate by −2 standard deviations from the mean IQ of 100 are classified as retarded. Based on a normal distribution approximately 2.27 percent of the population would have an IQ less than 70 and only 1.2 children per 1000 will score below 50. Curve C shows the actual distribution of measured intelligence, with 2.6–3.0 percent of the population falling into the retarded range. This deviation from the expected distribution may be explained by curve B. Superimposed on curve A is a second curve with a mean IQ 35 and a range from 0–70, representing the organic causes of mental retardation. The 3–4:1000 who score below 50 on the IQ testing reflect the additive effects of mendelian genetic and environmental (organic) causes of severe mental retardation.[1] Based on these data, the mentally retarded individual can be broadly classified as mildly affected if the IQ is 51–69 and severely affected if the IQ is below 50.

The distinction between mild and severe retardation is biologically meaningful to the clinician, since it is in the latter group that organic etiologies are frequently established as the basis of the patient's

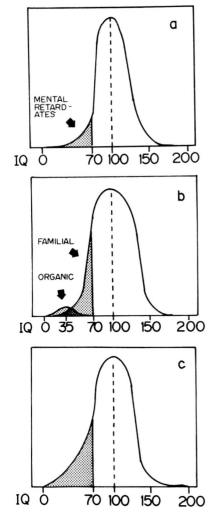

Figure 8-1. (a) Conventional representation of the distribution of intelligence. (b) Distribution of intelligence as represented in the two-group approach. (c) Actual distribution of intelligence. (From Zigler, E: Familial retardation: A continuing dilemma. Science 155:292, 1967. Copyright 1967 by the American Association for the Advancement of Science.)

disability. This classification must be tempered with common sense because of the limitation in the tests currently in use to assess intelligence. A number of factors must be evaluated before a diagnosis of mental retardation can be made. The guideline the physician must follow is that all chidren, even those with severe anatomic deformities, must be assumed to be capable of normal mental development until proved otherwise. In all instances children must be helped to reach their full potential.

Mild

Mild mental retardation is seven to eight times as common as severe mental retardation. The mildly retarded individual usually shows normal head size, height, and weight. There may be retarded siblings, and the parents may also be mildly retarded. The degree of retardation in relatives tends to shade into normality. This group as a whole appears normal on physical examination. Laboratory tests carried out to detect cytogenetic or biochemical genetic defects are usually normal. The mildly retarded group has been called familial, cultural–familial, simple, or physiologic retardation.

The evidence is strong that the determinants of intelligence are polygenic.[2] Polygenic inheritance involves the additive effects of several genes of small effect that interact with other genes and the environment to produce a continuous variation of a trait with a gaussian distribution, as shown in Figure 8-1.[6] Most individuals in the mildly retarded range represent a perfectly normal expression of the population gene pool. They do not differ physiologically from individuals of greater intellect but represent the lower portion of the IQ curve, reflecting normal intellectual variability. The polygenic model fits emperic data gathered from several studies.[31] In familial retardation, approximately 28 percent of first-degree relatives (parents, siblings), 7.8 percent of second-degree relatives (aunts, uncles, grandparents), and 3.1 percent of third-degree relatives (cousins) may also be retarded (see Table 8-3 for the proportion of genes shared in common). Clinical experience confirms these data that mild mental retardation without other associated problems is frequently familial. Empiric-risk data that may be used to counsel couples considering reproduction are shown in Table 8-1.

The physician should be aware that the mildly retarded are fertile and that a normal child can be born into the family of retarded parents. Without adequate stimulation, however, this normal child may function in the retarded range. Environmentally caused defects in intellectual function may be indistinguishable from genetic problems on IQ testing. Conversely, a small minority of patients with definable mendelian single-gene mutations, cytogenetic defects, and malformation syndromes may fall into the mild retardation category by IQ testing.

Diagnosis and Management

Diagnosis and genetic counseling in mild mental retardation are often more challenging than in severe retardation. The key to management is early diagnosis

Table 8-1
Counseling Data

Normal or retarded persons who have had at least one retarded child	Risk of having another retarded child (%)
Retardate × retardate	42.1
Retardate × normal or unknown	19.9
Normal sibling of retardate × normal	12.9
Normal (no retarded siblings × normal)	5.7

Normal persons who have not had any children	Risk of having a retarded first child (%)
Normal sibling of a retardate × retardate	23.8
Normal sibling of a retardate × normal	1.8
Normal sibling of two or more retardates × normal	3.6
Normal (all siblings normal) × normal	0.53

Data from Reed EW, Reed SC: Mental Retardation: A Family Study. Philadelphia, Saunders, 1965. Reprinted with permission.

through regular assessments of psychomotor development. Physical examination is usually normal. Every evaluation should include a three-generation pedigree of the family. Biochemical screening of neonates for disorders of amino acid and carbohydrate metabolism and for hypothyroidism are routine practice in many areas and in part relieve the clinician of biochemical testing. These screening tests do not establish a diagnosis but identify infants at risk. Definitive diagnoses require additional biochemical studies and specific management of a diagnosis if an inborn error of metabolism is confirmed. Even in the absence of physical abnormalities in the patient, chromosome analysis may be indicated to rule out the fragile-X-chromosome syndrome (discussed below). Other extensive laboratory evaluations are usually not indicated, since most mildly retarded individuals grow normally and show adequate physical development.

Educators, social workers, and psychologists will play the major role in planning the educational program and in providing guidance to the parents. The child's well-being dictates that a collaborative effort be mounted between the parents and the professionals responsible for medical and educational components of a comprehensive management plan. Institutionalization should be avoided. Emotional and behavioral problems can be managed through counseling and proper care.

Severe

Individuals with severe mental retardation frequently have a definable organic cause for their disability. The reported prevalence of severe retardation (IQ less than 50) in population studies is 0.25–0.54 percent.[1] Many affected individuals have associated congenital malformations that produce high mortality in the first 10 yr of life.[10] This probably accounts for the reported prevalence of severe mental retardation in only 0.3 percent of the adult population (20–64 yr).

The family pattern of disability varies from that described for the mildly retarded. Most commonly, the severely retarded are single cases in their family, the parents are of normal intelligence, and, if other affected siblings are born, they are retarded to approximately the same degree as the index case. Although the severely retarded comprise a small proportion of the retarded population, they consume a disproportionally large share of medical and community resources because they show the least social competence and the most severe associated physical handicaps.

The importance of defining the etiologic basis of retardation in these patients becomes apparent in reviewing surveys of institutional and ambulatory populations. Schafer et al. recently surveyed the distribution of etiologic diagnoses in community and institutional populations in Northeastern Ohio and compared these data to other published surveys (Table 8-2).[13,17,32] In the published surveys, many individuals with seizures or neurologic problems were thought to have cerebral palsy and were classified as having a central nervous system (CNS) dysfunction due to a prenatal or perinatal cause. To compensate for differences in the proportion of those unclassified, based on the criteria employed for assigning an etiologic diagnosis, an alternative distribution was formed

Table 8-2
Etiology of Severe Mental Retardation: Comparison of Regional and Institutional Surveys to Northeastern Ohio Data (% Distribution)*

Study†	Genetic (chromosome)	Genetic (single Gene)	Multiple Congenital Anomalies	CNS Malformations	CNS Dysfunction§	Infectious Disease	Postnal (Excluding Infection)	Infantile Psychosis	Other	Unclassified
Regional 1	36	5	20	2	16	7	1	2		12
2	19	10	10	4	22(30)	4	2			20(12)
3	24	3	2	2	6(22)	4	3			53(37)
Institutional 4	12	7	16	15	32	9	4	1		4
5	4	3	16	25	18	17	5	0		1
6	7	4	3	1	19(37)	6	4	1	11	53(35)

Category‡

*Regional, Uppsala; institutional, Central Colony, Wisc., and Rinnekoti Institution, Finland.
†1, Uppsala; 122 patients.[13] 2, Cleveland Metropolitan General Hospital; 194 patients.[32] 3, 169 county programs, Northeastern Ohio; 842 patients.[32] 4, Central Colony; 1224 patients.[17] 5, Rinnekoti Institution; 338 patients.[16] 6, Institutional populations, Northeastern Ohio; 558 patients.[32]
‡Figures in parentheses show change in distribution of diagnoses after adjustment for unclassified patients.
§Perinatal or unknown prenatal causes. (Data presented as the percent distribution of the total study population.)

64

by reassigning individuals with seizures, spasticity, or paresis in the unclassified categories to the category of CNS dysfunction with perinatal or unknown prenatal cause (see Table 2). Depending on which classification is used, 12–50 percent of severely retarded persons in Northeastern Ohio fall into the unclassified category. It has been estimated that in institutionalized populations, 45 percent of cases can be attributed to genetic causes or predisposition, with 15 percent of the total representing high-risk segregating-chromosome or single-gene mutations.[17] In the retarded population living at home the proportion of high-risk segregating cases (15 percent) is probably similar to that found in the institutionalized population. The genetic causes of severe retardation were underrepresented in the survey population in Northeastern Ohio.

Would the numbers of unclassified individuals be reduced if diagnostic services were regionalized in clinics staffed with specialists in pediatrics, neurology, genetics, and laboratory diagnosis? The results of the survey in Northeastern Ohio suggest that this may indeed be the case, since the proportion of unclassified patients was lowest in the population served by a hospital-based clinic staffed by specialists.[32] Without a specific diagnosis, the application of preventive measures through genetic counseling, antenatal diagnosis, and treatment is not possible. If the prevalence of severe retardation is to be reduced by the application of genetics, families with a high risk of producing a retarded child must be identified and offered genetic counseling and other preventative services. Clinical recognition of single-gene defects and chromosome anomalies is essential, since these etiologies constitute a large proportion of families that fall into the high-recurrence risk group.

Genetic Transmission and Chromosome Behavior

In human beings the hereditary material deoxyribonucleic acid (DNA) is carried by chromosomes. Somatic cells contain 23 pairs of chromosomes for a total chromosome number of 46. Each chromosome can be accurately identified by its size, shape, and banding pattern. Twenty-two pairs are termed *autosomes*, while the 23rd pair consists of the sex chromosomes. Except for the sex chromosomes in males (XY), members of a chromosome pair are morphologically similar, or homologous.

Somatic cells increase in number by mitosis, a process by which each chromosome from the parental cell is replicated and represented in each of two daughter cells. The germ cells (egg and sperm) have a haploid number of chromosomes—23. This reduction in chromosome number is achieved by meiotic division, which separates each member of a chromosome pair so that the gamete receives half the parental genome. At the time of fertilization when the egg and sperm fuse, the diploid number (46) of chromosomes is restored. Gene segregation, assortment, and recombination occur during the process of meiosis and provide a mechanism to expand genetic variability. The number of genes coding for proteins in the human genome has been estimated at 100,000.[18] A sample definition of a gene is that portion of the DNA responsible for the primary structure of a polypeptide. Each amino acid in a polypeptide is designated by a triplet of nucleotides in the DNA (a codon). A peptide with 500 amino acids would be coded by 1500 nucleotide bases, or, stated differently, the gene for that polypeptide contains 1500 nucleotide bases. The term *locus* is used to designate the position of the gene on the chromosome. Since chromosomes are paired, a gene on chromosome no. 21 has a counterpart at the same locus of its partner chromosome. Exceptions are the sex chromosomes of the male, which do not constitute a homologous pair (XY).

The term *allele* is used to designate an alternate form of the same gene. A change in a single nucleotide base or group of bases may lead to an altered gene product. Any allele is subject to error and is apt to mutate to another form. Some mutations are trivial, while others seriously affect protein function, produce disease, and affect phenotype. Mutant alleles at different loci can produce similar characteristics or traits in a person. These observed characteristics are termed the patient's *phenotype*. The phenotype is far removed from the genes producing the change. Mental retardation as a phenotype is the best example of this principle. It is estimated that at least 300 mutant genes at different loci can alter brain function, producing the clinical phenotype of mental retardation.[25] With this as background, one can now examine the distribution of single gene traits in families that may be associated with mental retardation.

Distribution of Single Genes in Families

Dominant inheritance. Each autosomal locus has two alleles or genes (a,a). If one gene is altered (A) and produces in the patient a deviation from the normal, it is called *dominant*. In dominantly inherited traits, the gene is expressed in the heterozygote (Aa genotype). Autosomal dominant inheritance is characterized by vertical transmission of the trait through

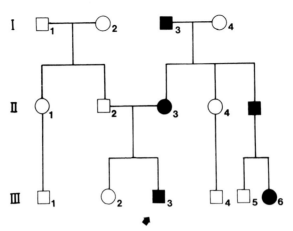

Figure 8-2. Transmission of a dominantly inherited mutant allele through a family. □, male: ○, female; → proband.

the family, with male and female offspring equally affected (Fig. 8-2). The usual mating types one encounters are Aa (affected) with aa (unaffected). On the average, 50 percent of the offspring from these parental genotypes will be affected. Individuals who do not manifest the trait usually have not inherited the mutant allele and cannot pass the trait to their offspring.

As with every generalization, there are exceptions. Dominant genes may show variable degrees of penetrance in which the gene is not fully expressed. This accounts for the so-called skipped generations in some pedigrees. Clinical assessments of "normal" family members will frequently reveal a trait indicating the presence of the gene, thus eliminating the gaps or skips in the pedigree. In some instances, heterozygotes for a mutant allele will mate (Aa × Aa). The genotype of offspring will be AA (25 percent), Aa (50 percent), and aa (25 percent). The homozygotes for the mutant allele (AA) are usually more severely affected than those in the more common Aa patient. The ratio of affected to normal offspring from this type of mating is 3:1. Most dominant genes code for structural genes rather than for enzymes. Severe mental retardation due to a mutant autosomal dominant gene occurs in 1–4.8 percent of institutionalized retarded populations.[29] Examples of dominantly inherited diseases associated with brain dysfunction include neurofibromatosis, tuberous sclerosis, and Huntington's chorea.

Note that new mutations are not an unusual observation in autosomal dominant disorders. When the affected patient reproduces, there is a 50 percent risk that the mutant gene will be transmitted to the off-

spring. The patient's parents, on the other hand, are at no greater risk than the general population of producing another affected child in subsequent pregnancies.

Recessive inheritance. In autosomal recessive inheritance the affected individual is homozygous for the mutant allele (aa). The parents are phenotypically normal but each must carry one mutant allele (Aa). Mating between heterozygotes (Aa × Aa) produces the following genotypes: AA, 25 percent; Aa, 50 percent; aa, 25 percent. The ratio of normal (AA,Aa) to affected offspring (aa) is 3:1. Relatives rather than nonrelatives are more likely to be carriers of the same mutant gene. Mating of relatives would increase the risk of producing infants affected with mental retardation due to rare mutant alleles. This is illustrated in Table 8-3.

If a recessive disease occurs with a frequency of 1:10,000 persons, the frequency of heterozygote carriers is about 1 in 50. The probability that two unrelated individuals would both carry the gene is 1 in 50 × 1 in 50, or 1 in 2500. If they married, the chance that they would produce a child with disease would be 1 in 10,000 (1 in 50 × 1 in 50 × 1 in 4 = 1 in 10,000). If one member of the couple was a carrier of the mutant allele and the genotype of the other unknown, the probability of their producing an affected child would be 1 in 2 (carrier) × 1 in 50 (heterozygote frequency) × 1 in 4 (probability of homozygote in offspring) = 1 in 400. If this couple were first cousins (i.e., they had 1 in 8 of their genome in common), the probability that they will produce an affected child is increased 1 in 2 (carrier) ×

Table 8-3

Proportion of Genes Shared by Relatives

Relatedness	Relationship to Affected Individual	Proportion of Genes in Common with Affected Individual
First degree	Parent, child, sibling,	1 in 2
	monozygotic twin,	1
	dizygotic twin	1 in 2
Second degree	Grandparent, grandchild,	1 in 4
	uncle, aunt, nephew, niece,	1 in 4
	half-sibling	1 in 4
Third degree	First cousin	1 in 8

1 in 8 (probability that mate inherited mutant allele from a common ancestor) × 1 in 4 (probability of homozygosity in offspring) = 1 in 64.

When dealing with rare autosomal recessive disorders it is important to determine if the parents of the proband are related. Approximately 1117 diseases inherited as autosomal recessive traits are now catalogued, and more will be discovered.[23] Recessive genes usually code for enzymes. Severe mental retardation due to mutant autosomal recessive genes occurs with an estimated prevalence of 1.5–4.18 percent in institutional populations.[29] Examples of recessively inherited disorders producing mental retardation include phenylketonuria (PKU), maple syrup urine disease, and other inborn errors of amino acid and carbohydrate metabolism. In many disorders transmitted in families as autosomal recessive traits, the biochemical basis of mental retardation is not defined. For example, microcephaly inherited as an autosomal recessive trait is thought to account for approximately 5 percent of severely retarded institutionalized individuals.[27] Congenital malformation syndromes associated with mental retardation may also show this pattern of inheritance, as in the Zellweger (cerebrohepatorenal) syndrome.[23]

X-linked recessive inheritance. Genes on the sex chromosomes are unequally distributed to males and females within families. Males receive their X chromosome from the mother, while females receive one X chromosome from the mother and the other from the father. If a female is a carrier of a mutant allele (A) on one X chromosome and a normal allele (a) on the other, the mutant allele will show a distribution in her offspring (Fig. 8-3). Fifty percent of the sons will inherit the mutant allele and be affected; 50 percent of the daughters will be carriers of the mutant allele and, in the great majority of instances,

will be phenotypically normal. In the female, only one X chromosome is active; thus, females are genetic mosaics. Chance appears to determine whether the X chromosomes inherited from the father or the mother are active in a cell. On average, in a given individual 50 percent of paternal X chromosomes and 50 percent of maternal X chromosomes are functioning.[21] As with any random distribution, there are extremes at either end. In rare instances a disproportionally large number of active chromosomes is derived from either paternal or maternal origin. If the female inherits a mutant allele on the X chromosome from her mother, and if in the process of random inactivation of the maternal and paternal X chromosome she is left with 95 percent active maternal X chromosomes, she may show the phenotypic manifestations of a disease that is usually restricted to males. If the male who inherits the mutant allele (A) from his mother reproduces with a female (aa) who does not carry the mutant allele, all their daughters will be heterozygote carriers, while the sons will be normal, (Fig. 8-4).

The daughters who are heterozygote carriers of the mutant allele will distribute it to their offspring with the pattern shown in Figure 8-3. The prevalence of X-linked recessive disorders causing severe retar-

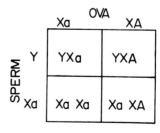

Figure 8-3. X-linked recessive mutation transmitted through carrier female. A, mutant allele.

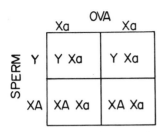

Figure 8-4. X-linked recessive mutation transmitted through affected male. A, mutant allele.

dation in institutional populations is estimated at 8–14 percent. Examples of X-linked recessive disorders that are associated with mental retardation are the Lesch-Nyhan syndrome and Hunter's syndrome (mucopolysaccharidosis).[23]

Fragile-X-chromosome syndrome. X-linked recessive inheritance has been demonstrated in many families by pedigree analysis. In most, a defined genetic defect had not been established. It has long been known that up to 30–50 percent more males than females are institutionalized because of mental retardation; it appears that social and institutional factors cannot account for this skewed sex ratio. This excess of males could indicate one or more unrecognized forms of X-linked mental retardation.

Recently, an abnormality in the X chromosome of mentally retarded males was described in cultured lymphocytes. It is characterized by a constriction near the end of the long arm of the X chromosome, resulting in a small knot separated by a thin stalk from the main portion of the chromosome. The thin stalk is often broken; hence the designation *fragile X*.[12,20,35]

This marker chromosome has now been reported in many families with mentally retarded male members. The fragile-X-chromosome marker has also been detected in some mildly retarded females (IQ 55 to 75).[12] In addition, some females who are obligate carriers, in whom pedigree evidence indicates that they possess the X mutation, do not show a fragile-X-chromosome marker on cytogenetic analysis. Information on this syndrome is rapidly evolving, but many questions remain unanswered. Why are some females with this marker retarded and others completely normal? Is the mechanism underlying these observations based on the random inactivation of the X chromosome discussed in the preceding section? Antenatal diagnosis is not now possible, since the fragile X marker cannot be reproducibly detected in

cultured fibroblasts but should be possible in the future, when this technical problem is solved.

The major clinical points to emphasize are that the fragile-X-chromosome syndrome, next to trisomy 21, is probably the most common cause of mental retardation that can be specifically diagnosed and may represent 2.5 percent of mental retardation in males. Mentally retarded individuals may be normal in phenotype and show no associated malformations. Although affected males predominate, the marker can also be detected in a small proportion of mildly retarded females.

In the past, chromosome analyses were seldom carried out in mentally retarded individuals who showed no associated congenital malformations, since the yield of positive results was low. The recognition of the fragile-X-chromosome marker and the familial nature of the mental retardation associated with this marker alter the clinical indications for chromosome studies. Cytogenetic analyses for the fragile-X-chromosome marker should be considered in mentally retarded individuals who are phenotypically normal and in whom an etiology has not been established.

Chromosome Errors

Medical cytogenetics deals with numerical and structural abnormalities of the human chromosome complement. Each of the 46 chromosomes can be accurately identified by special staining techniques. Abnormalities in chromosome structure or number can affect both the autosomes and the sex chromosomes. Down's syndrome may be associated with an increase in the normal chromosome number from 46 to 47. It may also be seen in individuals with 46 chromosomes who show an aberration in chromosome structure due to translocation of the long arm of chromosome no. 21. The chromosomes in these patients show an extra piece of chromosome no. 21, which is attached to another chromosome, usually one of the G group (chromosome no. 14). These persons are genetically trisomic for the long arms of chromosome no. 21 but show a normal chromosome count of 46.

Most clinicians have little difficulty in diagnosing the Down's syndrome phenotype. Chromosome analysis is carried out to determine whether the phenotype reflects an abnormality in chromosome number (47 trisomy) or an abnormality in chromsomes structure (46 translocation). Down's syndrome due to trisomy of chromosome no. 21 has a low recurrence risk (1 percent or less). Its frequency in the general population is related to parental age. Translocation

Down's syndrome in 50 percent of affected children results from a balanced translocation in either the mother or father. The carrier parent is phenotypically normal but has 45 chromosomes, including the translocated one (14q21q). The carrier parent theoretically produces gametes in equal proportion. Assuming union with a normal gamete from the noncarrier parent, there is a 2 in 6 risk that the zygote will be monosomic for chromosome no. 21 or 14 and a 1 in 6 risk that the zygote will be trisomic for chromosome no. 14. These gamete combinations are not usually viable and result in abortion.

The three remaining types of gametes can produce viable offspring. Theoretically, 1 in 6 offspring should have a balanced translocation like their normal carrier parent, 1 in 6 will be chromosomally normal, and 1 in 6 will show translocation Down's syndrome. The actual probabilities for a translocation carrier to produce a live-born infant with Down's syndrome differ from the theoretical expectations. Counting just live-born infants, the expected distribution would be 1 in 3 with a normal chromosome complement, 1 in 3 with a balanced translocation like their phenotypically normal carrier parent, and 1 in 3 with translocation Down's syndrome.[15,34] If the mother is the carrier, the risk is 10–15 percent that an affected infant will be produced, while if the father is a carrier, the risk is approximately 2 percent. The reasons for this deviation from the expected sex ratios are yet to be explained.

Variation in normal chromosome number and structure usually occurs as the result of errors that take place during the meiotic division of the gametes. Minor variations in structure may be of no clinical consequence and represent familial markers. Other errors in which there are segmental deletions or additions of genetic material result in abortion of the fetus or the birth of the infant with congenital malformations, mental retardation, or both. Examples of clinically recognized chromosomal errors include cri du chat syndrome, trisomy 13, and trisomy 18.[11]

Although this chapter has focused on variations in the number and structure of autosomes, the same abnormalities can occur with sex chromosomes. Turner's syndrome, characterized by deletion of an X chromosome, has a 45 XO chromosome karyotype. This error occurs in about 1:3000 live births.[22] Multiple X and Y karyotypes are also well documented. Turner's syndrome can be used to introduce the concept of mosaicism. Increases or decreases in chromosomes number in the gametes occur as a result of unequal division of the chromosomes during meiotic division. If this nondisjunction occurs after fertilization during an early cleavage division of the zygote, an individual with two or more cell lines with different chromosome numbers is produced. In the example of a Turner mosaic, some cells will have a normal XX karyotype with 46 chromosomes, while others will show 45 chromosomes with a deleted X (XO). The proportion of normal to abnormal cells may vary from tissue to tissue, and this will determine the patient's phenotype. On the average, mosaics are less severely affected than their nonmosaic counterparts.[9]

Human chromosome abnormalities are periodically catalogued, and several excellent texts on human cytogenetics are available.[3,11] It is estimated that 10–35 percent of severely retarded individuals in institutional populations show a chromosome defect.[29] By far the largest group is composed of individuals with the diagnosis of Down's syndrome. Chromosome abnormalities associated with severe mental retardation probably occur with an even higher prevalence in populations living at home, since these individuals are younger than retarded individuals living in institutions and effects of differential mortality due to associated congenital malformations would not yet be a selective factor.

Carrier detection. For recessively inherited and X-linked recessive disorders, specialized tests for the detection of heterozygotes may be available. This is especially important in sisters of boys affected with X-linked recessive disorders, since, regardless of the father's genome, there is a 50 percent risk that the sons of female heterozygotes will be affected with the disease. Chemical or cytogenetic examination of parents and siblings may provide a diagnosis in both recessive and X-linked recessive disorders even after the proband has died. For example, medical records of a patient with Lesch-Nyhan syndrome (X-linked recessive) may record cerebral palsy, self-mutilation, choreoathetosis, and hyperuricemia. A suspected diagnosis could be confirmed if cell strains from the mother were found to be deficient for hypoxanthine–guanine phosphoribosyl transferase activity. Carrier detection by screening population groups is applicable to selected genetic disorders that produce mental retardation.[19] Because of the low frequency of most mutant alleles that produce mental retardation and the technologic problems in laboratory detection of carriers, carrier detection is most productive when applied to specific pedigrees in which the information will be used for making future reproductive decisions.

Diagnosis and Management

The analysis of the symptoms of mental retardation requires an adequate data base coupled with a thorough physical examination. Events in the prenatal and perinatal periods which could adversely affect brain function require documentation, as do details of the patient's postnatal psychomotor development and health history. A three-generation pedigree should be obtained on every patient to evaluate possible genetic components. These initial steps in assessment can establish an etiologic diagnosis for retardation in many patients without extensive additional laboratory tests.

Pertinent information related to events in the prenatal period that may damage the brain include CNS infections (rubella, cytomegalovirus [CMV], toxoplasmosis), therapeutic x-irradiation of the mother, maternal alcoholism or diphenylhydantion (Dilantin) treatment, maternal exposure to toxins (lead and mercury) or endocrine metabolic problems in the mother (diabetes).

Is the patient retarded because of perinatal injury? The presence or absence of severe anoxia, traumatic delivery, early onset of seizures, prolonged metabolic acidosis, prematurity, and intrauterine growth retardation are a few of the factors that need evaluation.

Postnatal data should include details of the individual's developmental history. Was psychomotor development deviant from birth or did developmental arrest follow a postnatal CNS infection or trauma? At least 2 percent of the severely retarded individuals in the survey of Northeastern Ohio were disabled as a result of trauma to the head, which included accidents and the battering found in child abuse. If the child developed normally for a period, leveled off, and then began to lose previously possessed functions, a genetic degenerative CNS disease is a diagnostic possibility.

Genetic disorders producing mental retardation, although they may begin prenatally, often do not become manifest until well after birth. The family pedigree will provide clues to genetic etiologies, especially if first-degree relatives are also retarded or if there is a history of consanguinity. The data base may show that the etiology of the patient's disability is environmental and not genetic in origin.

Physical examination provides additional information to direct the diagnostic assessment. The mentally retarded individual who has other congenital malformations may represent a chromosome defect or a multiple malformation syndrome inherited as a single-gene defect or a polygenic trait or may reflect fetal exposure to an environmental teratogen. Cytogenetic analyses would be indicated in many of these individuals. Computed axial tomography (CAT) scans should be considered in all patients with microcephaly, macrocephaly, other suspected CNS malformations, or focal neurologic findings.

In the absence of associated malformations, the possibility of an inborn error of metabolism should be eliminated by appropriate metabolic screening tests. If the history of physical examinations suggests a degenerative process of the brain, enzyme analysis using serum, leukocytes, or cultured dermal fibroblasts may be indicated to rule out or establish a diagnosis of genetic sphingolipidoses.[33]

Cerebral palsy, mostly spastic tetraplegia, is commonly associated with severe mental retardation and, in many instances, reflects gross perinatal complications.[8] A significant number of individuals with severe mental retardation and cerebral palsy have an unremarkable perinatal history. These patients represent a diagnostic enigma. If the pedigree analysis shows no family trends, the overall empiric recurrence risk is low (approximately 2 percent).[14]

Patients with primary seizure disorders not due to inborn errors of metabolism represent a heterogenous group. Some represent clear genetic etiologies, such as tuberous sclerosis (autosomal dominant). Most are currently classified as idiopathic and include children with infantile spasms. In individuals with severe mental retardation associated with seizures, there is a familial occurrence in approximately 1 in 3. The familial recurrence risks based on age of onset and type of seizure varies from approximately 5 percent in infants with onset of seizure under 2 mo to 19 percent in those with infantile spasms.[28] It is obvious that diagnostic sorting in this group of patients is difficult because so little is known about their basic difficulty.

The majority of individuals without obvious malformations will fall into the category of environmental brain damage, which includes prenatal and postnatal infection and trauma to the head. Brain damage unfortunately occurs during the medical management of metabolic derangements that complicate burn therapy, diabetes mellitus, diarrhea, and other problems where it could be avoided.

Of particular interest from a genetic point of view are those infants with primary CNS malformations. Hydrocephalus not associated with spina bifida, infection, perinatal hemorrhage, hydrocephaly, or porencephaly may show family aggregation. Most familial cases occur in males with stenosis of the aqueduct of Sylvius and are transmitted in families as X-linked recessive traits.[4] The anencephaly–spina bifida–hydrocephalus group of neural tube defects is presumably a polygenic disorder, with a recurrence risk of 5 percent after the birth of one affected first-degree relative and of 10 percent after the birth of two.[5] Microcephaly not secondary to prenatal infection or associated with other malformations may be inherited as an autosomal recessive trait. These patients at birth have a head circumference three standard deviations below the mean; CAT scans show a small brain with no malformations. Females predominate, and the recurrence risk in subsequent offspring is high.[28] Each of these disorders may be diagnosed antenatally by sonography before the 20th wk of gestation. Measurement of α-fetoprotein in maternal serum and amniotic fluid is an important diagnostic adjunct in the antenatal detection of neural tube defects. Other CNS malformations that may show single gene transmission in families include lobar holoprosencephaly (autosomal recessive and dominant), Dandy–Walker defect (recessive), and agenesis of the corpus callosum (X-linked).[36]

In approximately 20 percent of individuals a specific etiologic diagnosis will not be established.[13,16,17,26,32] Before consigning the patient to the diagnostic category of unknown or "pure" mental retardation, the clinician must assess the social and environmental factors that may have contributed to the patient's functional deficiencies. The psychotic patient who is classified as severely retarded is perplexing. Is the psychotic behavior the result or the cause of the patient's retarded mental function? There is little question that emotional or sensory deprivation can produce functional mental retardation. In some instances the functional disability the patient exhibits can be reversed by placing the patient in a stimulating environment that provides for emotional needs. In dealing with infants and young children, this may require the child's removal from the home. Retarded function due to sensory deprivation may be completely reversed in deaf individuals if this defect is recognized early and adequately treated.

Infants with multiple malformations and potentially severe mental retardation have a high mortality. A causal diagnosis should therefore be made as close to birth as possible to obtain information that will permit prognostic and genetic counseling for the family. All fetal, stillborn, and neonatal deaths should be thoroughly examined in an effort to establish a diagnosis. Genetic etiologies with high recurrence can be identified by thorough autopsies including cytogenetic and biochemical analyses of tissues when appropriate. The central focus of all diagnostic efforts is the delineation of nongenetic causes for severe mental retardation that carry low recurrence risks from genetic causes that may place the family in a high-risk category. The high-recurrence risk group, which is estimated to comprise 15 percent of the total, includes single-gene mutations and segregating-chromosome errors.

The identification of genetic etiologies for severe mental retardation is frequently a demanding and expensive clinical exercise but, for the family and society, the potential benefits are large. It is in this high-risk group of families that genetics can be applied to the prevention of severe mental disability. Prevention of brain damage can be effected by early initiation of dietary therapy in PKU and galactosemia. In some forms of propionic acidemia, methylmalonic aciduria, and multiple decarboxylase deficiency, the mutation affects the cofactor binding site of the apoenzyme and the problem can be treated by the administration of pharmacologic amounts of the appropriate vitamin.[7] The number of biochemical genetic diseases that can be treated effectively is small at present. For most high-risk families, prevention is focused on genetic counseling, which provides the parents with the information required to make informed decisions about future reproduction. Detection of selected genetic diseases can now be made early enough in pregnancy to permit parents the option of abortion. Many parents elect this course, since it ensures them the birth of unaffected children in subsequent pregnancies[24]

The severely damaged infants who survive the neonatal period present a difficult problem in long-term management. The patient's potential for development and the severity of associated malformations are the major determinants in planning health care and educational programs. Parents should participate in the care plan from the onset. The goals of management should be directed toward providing a better life for the patient through health maintenance and the creation of an environment that provides social contact and sensory stimulation. The physician usually thinks that medical management is effective when a patients' disease is cured or symptoms are significantly ameliorated. By contrast, health care professionals working with the severely retarded patient may equate effective management with making life bearable for the patient, the family, and themselves. Obviously, prevention of severe brain damage offers

the best hope for the future. Continued efforts to understand the genetic and environmental factors that facilitate normal brain development may provide additional diagnostic methods and therapies to attain this goal.

REFERENCES

1. Abramowicz HK, Richardson SR: Epidemiology of severe mental retardation in children: Community studies. Am J Ment Defic 80, 18, 1975
2. Bodmer WF, Cavalli-Sforza LL: Genetics, Evolution and Man, San Francisco, W.H. Freeman, 1977
3. Borgaonkar DS: Chromosomal Variation in Man. A Catalogue of Chromosome Variants and Anomalies (ed 3). New York, Alan R. Liss, 1980
4. Burton BK: Recurrence risks for congenital hydrocephalous. Clin Genet 16:47, 1979
5. Carter CO, Roberts JA: The risk of recurrence after two children with central nervous system malformations. Lancet 1:306, 1967
6. Carter CO: Genetics of common disorders. Br Med Bull 25:52, 1969
7. Desnick RJ (ed): Enzyme Therapy in Genetic Diseases: 2 Birth Defects. Original Art Series 16. New York, Alan R. Liss, 1980
8. Durkin MV, Kaveggia EG, Pendleton E, et al: Analysis of etiologic factors in cerebral palsy with severe mental retardation. Eur J Pediatr 123:67, 1976
9. Ford CE: Mosaics and chimeras. Br Med Bull 25:104, 1969
10. Forssman H, Akesson HO: Mortality of the mentally deficient: A study of 12,903 institutionalized subjects. J Ment Defic Res 14:276, 1970
11. deGrouchy J, Turleau C: Clinical Atlas of Human Chromosomes. New York, Wiley, 1977
12. Turner G, Brookwell R, Selikowitz M, et al: Heterozygous expression of X-linked mental retardation and the marker X: fra (X) (q27). N Engl J Med 303:662, 1980
13. Gustavson KH, Hagberg B, Hagberg G and Sars K: Severe mental retardation in a Swedish county. II. Etiologic and pathogenic aspects of children born 1959–1970. Neuropädiatrie 8:293, 1977
14. Hagberg B, Habgerg C, Olow I: The changing panorama of cerebral palsy in Sweden, 1954–1970. Acta Paediatr Scand 64:193, 1975
15. Hamerton JL, Human Cytogenetics, vol. 2. New York, Academic Press, 1971
16. Iivanainen MM: A study in the origins of mental retardation in clinics, in Developmental Medicine no. 51, Spastics International Medical Publications. London, William Heineman, 1974
17. Kaveggia EG, Durkin MV, Pendleton E, et al: Diagnostic/genetic studies on 1,224 patients with severe

mental retardation. Proceedings of the Third Congress of the International Association for the Scientific Study of Mental Deficiency. Polish Medical Publishers, Warsaw 1972
18. Krome W, Wolfe U: Chromosomes and protein variation in the biochemical genetics of man, in Brock DJH, Mayo O (eds): New York, Academic Press, 1978
19. Levy HL: Genetic screening. Adv Hum Genet 4:1, 1974
20. Lubs HA: A marker X chromosome. Am J Hum Genet 21:231, 1969
21. Lyon MF: Sex chromatin and gene action in the mammalian X chromosome. Am J Hum Genet 14:135, 1964
22. Maclean N, Harnden D, Court-Brown W, et al: Sex chromosome abnormalities in newborn babies. Lancet 1:286, 1964
23. McKusick VA: Mendelian Inheritance in Man (ed 5). Baltimore, Johns Hopkins University Press, 1978
24. Milunsky A (ed): Genetic Disorders of the Fetus. New York, Plenum Press, 1979
25. Morton NE, Rao DC, Lang-Brown H, et al: A genetic study of mental defect. J Med Genet 14:1, 1977
26. Moser HW, Wolfe PA: The nosology of mental retardation including the report of a survey of 1378 mentally retarded individuals at the Walter A. Fernald State School. Birth Defects 7:117, 1971
27. Opitz JM: Diagnostic/genetic studies in severe mental retardation, in Lubs AA, de la Cruz F (eds): Genetic Counseling. New York, Raven Press, 1977
28. Opitz J: Diagnostic/genetic studies in mental retardation. Post grad Med 66:205, 1979
29. Opitz JM: Mental retardation: Biological aspects of concern to pediatricians. Pediatr Rev 2:41, 1980
30. Penrose LS: The Biology of Mental Defect. New York, Grune & Stratton, 1963
31. Reed EW, Reed SC: Mental Retardation: A Family Study. Philadelphia, Saunders, 1965
32. Schafer IA, Ross JL, Schafer MW, et al: The Demography of the Mental Retardation in Six Northeastern Ohio Counties. Report to the Commissioner. Columbus, Ohio Department of Mental Retardation, 1981
33. Stanbury JB, Wyngaarden JB, Fredrickson DS: The Metabolic Bases of Inherited Disease (ed 4). New York, McGraw-Hill, 1978

34. Stene J: A statistical segregation analysis of (21q21q) translocation. Hum Hered 20:465, 1970
35. Sutherland GR: Heritable fragile sites on human chromosomes. II. Distribution, phenotypic effects and cytogenetics. Am J Hum Genet 31:136, 1979
36. Warkany J, Lemire RJ, Cohen Jr MM: Mental Retardation and Congenital Malformations of the Central Nervous System. Chicago, Year Book Medical Publishers, 1981
37. Yunis JJ (ed): New Chromosomal Syndromes. New York, Academic Press, 1977
38. Zigler E: Familial retardation: A continuing dilemma. Science 155:292, 1967

Hugo W. Moser

9

Prevention of Psychosocial Mental Retardation

It is a truism that social and environmental factors profoundly influence physical health. Physicians in virtually every branch of medicine each day attempt to modify these influences to enhance their patients' physical health, and examples of successful individual approaches are provided throughout this book. The purpose of this chapter is to summarize data that indicate that social and environmental factors, in the aggregate, appear to have a specially significant role for the development of children at risk, including those with cerebral palsy. The role of these environmental factors appears greater than had been recognized previously and, unless it is taken into account, may confound studies that attempt to evaluate effects of biologic factors, e.g., follow-up studies of very low birth weight infants. Finally, and most important, there is recent evidence that with the assignment of resources and a broadly based approach, the ill effects of an adverse environment can be overcome to an astounding degree. Major research questions remain on what are the key components of such intervention, when to apply them, and how to do this in an economically feasible way.

ENVIRONMENTAL FACTORS

The Child with Handicaps

Low Birth Weight and Socioeconomic Status

Drillien's classic clinical follow-up studies in Edinburgh provide an example of additive effects of low socioeconomic status (SES) and very low birth

weight (Table 9-1).[5,6] In these studies, intellectual function was tested serially in 3- to 5-year-old children in order to evaluate the effects of prematurity and SES. In families with superior SES, birth weight had only a slight effect on intellectual performance. For the lowest SES children, moderately reduced birth weight had no or slight effect on intellectual performance. A major reduction of average intellectual function, however, was observed in children with very low birth weight born to low SES families. Figure 9-1 shows the changes in developmental quotients (DQ) between 6 and 24 mo as a function of birth weight and SES. Note that the average DQ of high SES, very low birth weight children increases with age but that this is not true for the low SES, very low birth weight children. Oski has commented that "if you are going to be born small, it is better to be born rich."[15]

The reasons for these observations are complex. It is unlikely that they reflect "simply" inherited low intellectual function; if that were the case, similar degrees of impairment would be expected at all birth weights. The apparent increase of DQ with age for high SES, low birth weight children suggests that the high SES environment provides something that helps to alleviate handicaps. Whatever this is, it does not seem to be a function of biologic maturation alone, since then one would not expect it to depend on SES. Nutritional factors appear not to have had a major role, since physical growth did not differ to the same extent.[4]

To summarize, it is the combination of severe reduction in birth weight and low SES that appears to produce significant reduction in average intellectual function, suggesting that biologic and environ-

75

Table 9-1
Mean Scores on Intelligence Testing at Different Ages by Birth Weight and Maternal Grade

Maternal Grade	Age (yr)	Birth Weight*			
		3 lb 8oz and under	3 lb 9oz–4 lb 8oz	4 lb 9oz–5 lb 8oz	5 lb 9oz and over
1 and 2: Middle class and superior working class	3	98	101	102	108
	4	100	102	104	110
	5+	104	112	110	118
3: Average working class	3	80	92	99	103
	4	73	93	101	103
	5+	74	93	104	106
4: Poor working class	3	66	80	93	97
	4	64	84	88	98
	5+	59	87	93	95

From Drillien CM: A longitudinal study of the growth and development of prematurely and maturely born children. II. Mental development, 2–5 years. Arch Dis Child 36:233, 1961. Reprinted with permission.
*Note that significant impairment was observed only in children with very low birth weight and low SES.

mental risks have aggravated each other. The mechanism of this interaction is exceedingly complex and will be discussed in the following sections, which deal with the effects of environmental factors on the cognitive development of children who have no known biologic handicaps. Again, adverse environmental factors may potentiate the effects of biological handicaps on child development, and for this reason the study and remediation of these adverse factors has relevance for the child with cerebral palsy.

The Child Who Is Biologically Intact

Genetic Determinants of Intelligence

There is strong documentation that parents who are retarded or who have a low intelligence quotient (IQ) are at increased risk of having children who function in the retarded range. When the father and mother are both retarded, there is an eight-times normal risk that their children will be retarded, and there are intermediate levels of increased risk if one parent or other relatives are retarded.[19]

Other strong evidence for genetic determinants of intelligence come from studies of twins and of adopted children. The combined data for studies of 6000 sets of twins reared together showed an 0.85 intraclass correlation for intelligence for identical twins and 0.59 for fraternal twins.[12] Studies of 122 sets of

identical twins reared apart showed the correlation for intelligence to be 0.82.[9] Although these studies have technical limitations that may tend to exaggerate the degree of correlation, there is no doubt that significant correlations do exist.[14] Similar conclusions have been derived from the studies of adopted children. Comparisons were made between the IQs of adopted children, their biologic parents, and their adopted parents. The correlation between the IQ of the biologic parent and the adopted child (living apart) was 0.48; for the foster parent and adopted child (living together), 0.19; and for control biologic parents and children (living together), 0.58.[13]

Attempts have been made to derive from these and related stuides quantitative estimates of the relative importance of genetic and environmental factors, but this is not possible because of unavoidable deviations from ideal experimental design in studies that involve human beings.[14]

Psychosocial Mental Retardation

Although many persons are mentally retarded because of recognized abnormalities of brain structure and function, there is a still larger group of persons who function in the mildly retarded range (IQ 50–70) but who have no demonstrable physical or physiologic abnormality.[11,21]

The first group is clearly heterogenous and comprises many distinct entities. The second group, i.e., mental retardation without demonstrable abnormalities, represents a "continuing dilemma."[21] The group

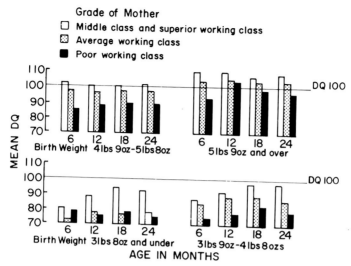

Figure 9-1. Mean DQ by age, birth weight, and mother's SES of children included in the Drillien follow-up studies. Note particularly the changes in DQ for the children with birth weight of 3 lb 8 oz and under. The high SES children experienced gains, while the low SES group failed to do so. (From Drillien CM: A longitudinal study of the growth and development of prematurely and maturely born children. II. Mental development, 2–5 years. Arch Dis Child 36:233, 1961. Reproduced with permission.)

is large; it comprises up to 2–3 percent of the general population, is more than 5 times as common as mental retardation due to known organic causes, and is a characteristic feature that occurs more commonly among families of lower SES.[2] Finally, it commonly affects more than one family member. Does this group represent the consequence of the observation that human intelligence appears to be distributed along a normal gaussian curve and hence must have a lower end? Is it a consequence of assortive breeding of people with relatively low intelligence? Is it the result of disadvantaged and impoverished environment? Or is it a combination of all three factors? The uncertainty about the nature of this category is reflected in its name, which has shifted from *familial* to *cultural-familial* to *sociocultural* and currently to *psychosocial* mental retardation.[1]

In the early part of this century, genetic factors were considered the major and possibly exclusive cause of this entity, and this conclusion had profound effects.[8] These included the segregation of retarded people in large institutions and sterilization laws, embodied in Chief Justice Oliver Wendell Holmes's statement that "three generations of imbeciles are enough." A major new development is the strong suggestion from recent studies, described below, that what appeared to be an inevitable cycle of retardation in successive generations can be interrupted, at least in part, by intensive environmental intervention. These new findings have important implications for national policy.

Identification of the Child at Risk for Psychosocial Retardation

Psychosocial retardation is more common among those of lower SES and in families where one or both parents function in the mentally retarded range. The pernicious effect of the combination of these two factors is demonstrated by the studies of Garber and Heber in a black and disadvantaged section of Milwaukee, a section which had the lowest median income and educational level and the highest level of population density and condemned housing.[7] Twenty-two percent of the population had an IQ of 75 or less. Although low SES status applied to nearly all persons in this area, it was found that the mother's IQ had a profound influence on her children's intellectual development (Fig. 9-2). When the mother's IQ was less than 80, the children's average IQ fell progressively,

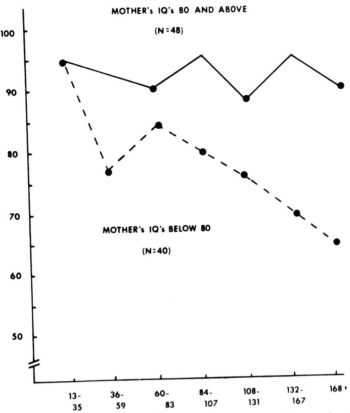

Figure 9-2. Mean IQ with increasing age in children in a disadvantaged section of Milwaukee, according to IQ of mother. None of the children received intervention. (From Garber HL, Heber R: The efficacy of early intervention with family rehabilitation, in Begab MJ, Haywood HC, Garber HL (eds): Psychosocial Influences in Retarded Performance, vol. 2. Strategies for Improving Competence. Baltimore, University Park Press, 1981. Reproduced with permission.)

a pattern characteristic of the child with psychosocial mental retardation, while this fall did not occur in the children of the higher IQ mothers.

Ramey et al. have developed a set of criteria for the identification of children at high risk for psychosocial retardation.[16] A great advantage of these criteria is that they can be applied at the time of the child's birth on the basis of information available routinely on birth certificates. The most predictive factors were race and the mother's educational level. Other factors that increased risk were mother's age, birth order (third or later), time of initiation of prenatal care, low birth weight, and a previous live birth now dead. A subsequent follow-up study has shown that application of these criteria identified correctly

80 percent of the children who functioned poorly in first grade.[18]

RESULTS OF ENVIRONMENTAL INTERVENTION

It has been pointed out that parents who function in the retarded range are at higher risk of having children who are retarded and that intelligence is genetically determined to a considerable extent. As noted, these two observations provided plausibility to the "nature" side of the "nature versus nurture" argument and formed the basis of national policies that are now

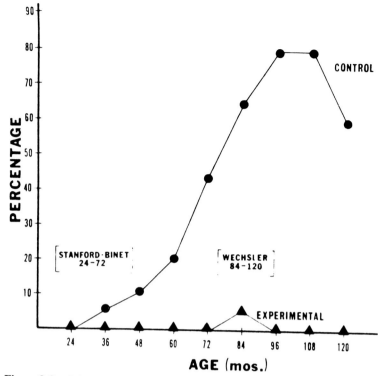

Figure 9-3. Effect of intervention on IQ of children included in the Milwaukee project. The chart lists the percentage of children whose IQ is more than one standard deviation below norm for age. Intervention was discontinued at 72 mo. Note that difference between the experimental and control groups still is readily demonstrable 3½ yr later. (From Garber HL, Heber R: The efficacy of early intervention with family rehabilitation, in Begab MJ, Haywood HC, Garber HL (eds): Psychosocial Influences in Retarded Performance, vol. 2. Strategies for Improving Competence. Baltimore, University Park Press, 1981. Reproduced with permission.)

considered inappropriate. It is evident that parents who are disadvantaged and who function in the retarded range may not be able to provide an optimal environment for their children's development and that the familial cycle of psychosocial mental retardation may be due, at least in part, to environmental factors. Three studies (two recent and one older) provide evidence that this is indeed the case.

Milwaukee Project

The Milwaukee project involved 40 children and families from the particularly disadvantaged section of Milwaukee already referred to.[7] All children were in a very high risk category for psychosocial retar-

dation (see Fig. 2). They were divided randomly into an experimental and a control group. Intervention for the experimental group was extremely intensive: the children received educational programs seven hours a day, five days a week, from age three to six months until entrance into first grade at six years. Concurrently the mothers received a rehabilitation program including vocational training, counseling, adult education, and group sessions. The children's development was assessed by independent evaluators. Figure 9-3 shows dramatic differences between the mean IQs of the experimental and the control group. Analogous differences were observed in language and social development, mother–child interaction, and problem-solving skills. The experimental group's su-

Table 9-2

Cognitive Development of Children (aged 42 mo) Enrolled in the Abecedarian Project

Subscale*	Experimental Group (23 children)		Control Group (24 children)			
	X	SD	X	SD	F	P <
Verbal	50.07	6.96	46.00	7.60	4.14	0.05
Perceptual performance	46.26	7.49	41.92	8.72	4.39	0.04
Quantitative	51.74	7.31	43.83	9.54	13.99	0.001
Memory	51.74	5.07	48.58	6.94	4.24	0.05
Motor	50.00	6.96	47.33	7.24	1.75	

From Ramey CT, Haskins R: The Causes and Treatment of School Failure: Insight from the Caroline Abecedarian project, in Begab MJ, Haywood HC, Garber HL (eds): Psychosocial Influences in Retarded Performance, vol. 2. Strategies for Improving Competence. Baltimore, University Park Press, 1981. Reprinted with permission.
*McCarthy subscale scores.

perior performance was still demonstrable at age 10, four years after cessation of the program.

Abecedarian Project

The Abecedarian project is a preschool and school-age program for black children from a rural community in North Carolina who are known to be at high risk for psychosocial mental retardation on the basis of the criteria developed by Ramey and associates.[16-18] The intervention was as intensive as in the Milwaukee project, but differed from it in specifics of curriculum and did not include a formal rehabilitation program for the mothers. Care was taken to provide excellent general health care and nutrition for both the experimental and the control groups. The project has now been in progress for six years. Clear improvements in IQ and social interactions have been

Table 9-3.

Contrast Group (N = 12)

		EXPERIMENTAL PERIOD						FOLLOW-UP STUDY				
	Before Transfer			After Transfer				Follow-up Test*		Length of Post-experimental Period, Months	Change in IQ During Post-experimental Period	Total Change in IQ from Initial to Follow-up Test
	Initial Test[b]		Chrono-logical Age, Months, at Transfer	Last Test[b]		Length of Experi-mental Period, Months	Change in IQ, Initial to Last Test					
CASE NUMBER* SEX	Chrono-logical Age, Months	IQ		Chrono-logical Age, Months	IQ			Chrono-logical Age, Months	IQ			
14........ F	11.9	91	....	55.0	62	43.1	−29	81	64	26.0	+ 2	−27
15........ F	13.0	92	....	38.3	56	25.3	−36	81	52	42.7	− 4	−40
16........ F	13.6	71	....	40.9	56	27.3	−15	75	80	34.1	+ 9	−45
17........ M	13.8	96	....	53.2	54	39.4	−42	82	51	28.8	− 3	−45
18........ M	14.5	99	....	41.9	54	27.4	−45	62	35[b]	20.1	−19	−64
19........ M	15.2	87	....	44.5	67	29.3	−20	101	89	56.5	+22	+ 2
20........ M	17.3	81	....	52.9	83*	35.6	+ 2	77	91	24.1	+ 8	+10
21........ M	17.5	103	....	50.3	60	32.8	−43	73	49	22.7	−11	−54
22........ M	18.3	98	....	39.7	61	21.4	−37	74	78	34.3	+17	−20
23........ F	20.2	89	....	48.4	71	28.2	−18	106	75	57.6	+ 4	−14
24........ M	21.5	50	....	51.6	42	30.1	− 8	91	68	39.4	+26	+18
25........ M	21.8	83	....	50.1	60	28.3	−23	96	61	45.9	+ 1	−22
Mean........	16.6	86.7	....	47.2	60.5	30.7	−26.2	83.3	66.1	36.0	+ 5.6	−20.6
Standard deviation....	3.2	13.9	....	5.6	9.7	5.8	14.1	12.3	16.5	12.2	13.8	25.6
Median........	16.3	90.0	....	49.3	60.0	28.8	−30.0	81.0	66.0	34.2	+ 6.0	−24.0

* Arranged according to age at time of initial test.
[b] Kuhlmann Binet (1922) IQ.
* Stanford Binet (1916) IQ.

From Skeels HM: Adult status of children with contrasting early life experiences: A follow-up study. Monogr Soc Res Ch Dev 105:1, 1966. Reprinted with permission.

Table 9-4.

Experimental and Contrast Groups: Occupations of
Subjects and Spouses

Case No.	Subject's Occupation	Spouse's Occupation	Female Subject's Occupation Previous to Marriage
Experimental Group:			
1[a]	Staff sergeant	Dental technician	. . . .
2	Housewife	Laborer	
3	Housewife	Mechanic	Nurses' aide
			Elementary school teacher
4	Nursing instructor.	Unemployed	Registered nurse
5	Housewife	Semi-skilled laborer	No work history
6	Waitress	Mechanic, semi-skilled	Beauty operator
7	Housewife	Flight engineer	Dining room hostess
8	Housewife	Foreman, construction	No work history
9	Domestic service	Unmarried	
10[a]	Real estate sales	Housewife	. . . .
11[a]	Vocational counselor	Advertising copy writer[b]	. . . .
12	Gift shop sales[c]	Unmarried	. . . .
13	Housewife	Pressman-printer	Office-clerical
Contrast Group:			
14	Institutional inmate	Unmarried	. . . .
15	Dishwasher	Unmarried	. . . .
16	Deceased	. . . .	. . . .
17[a]	Dishwasher	Unmarried	. . . .
18[a]	Institutional inmate	Unmarried	. . . .
19[a]	Compositor and typesetter	Housewife	. . . .
20[a]	Institutional inmate	Unmarried	. . . .
21[a]	Dishwasher	Unmarried	. . . .
22[a]	Floater	Divorced	. . . .
23	Cafeteria (part time)	Unmarried	. . . .
24[a]	Institutional gardener's assistant	Unmarried	. . . .
25[a]	Institutional inmate	Unmarried	. . . .

[a] Male.
[b] B.A. degree.
[c] Previously had worked as a licensed practical nurse.

From Skeels HM: Adult status of children with contrasting early life experiences: A follow-up study. Monogr Soc Res Child Dev 105:1, 1966. Reprinted with permission.

demonstrated (Table 9-2). It is particularly striking that in the experimental group there is no longer any correlation between the child's cognitive development and the mother's IQ.

Skeels Study

The Skeels study is unique in that it provides a 30-yr follow-up.[20] In 1932 Harold Skeels, a psychologist on the staff of the Iowa Child Welfare Research Station, State University of Iowa, became the first psychologist to be employed by the Iowa Board of Control of State Institutions. As part of his duties he examined a group of white orphans aged 6–24 mo. Table 9-3 lists the ages and IQ's of these children. Those children who were not adopted were assigned to an orphanage that provided adequate physical care

but, as described in the Skeels monograph, was hopelessly devoid of the opportunities for social interaction, play, and intellectual stimulation that are now recognized as vital. Skeels noted that only a few of the children who had their entire elementary-school experience in the orphanage school were able to make the transition to the public junior high school, and, as the subsequent follow-up study showed, very few made satisfactory vocational or marital adjustments (Table 9-4).

The intervention technique employed by Skeels came about as the result of a serendipitous event: Skeels had examined two girls aged 13 and 16 mo who functioned at the 6- and 7-mo level, were considered unsuitable for adoption, and were transferred to an institution for the mentally retarded. He saw the girls again 6 mo later and was astounded to observe totally unexpected developmental gains. By chance, the two girls had not been assigned to the usual children's unit at the institution but had been placed in a ward with women aged 18–50 yr whose mental ages were estimated to be 6–9 yr. These women "adopted" the children, gave them love and affection, and competed with each other to stimulate the children's development. The children recouped all their intellectual deficit, continued normal gains, at ages 4 and 5 yr were able to qualify for adoption in normal households, and, as Skeels showed 30 yr later, became successful citizens.

Because of this totally unexpected and highly encouraging experience, this same plan was followed with 11 additional children, thus establishing the 13-member experimental group, and its progress was compared with that of 11 children who remained at the orphanage (the contrast group). At 50 months the cognitive development of the experimental group was far superior to that of the contrast group (see Table 9-3), somewhat analogous to the findings in the Milwaukee project (see Fig. 9-3). What makes this study unique is that 30 yr later Skeels was able to trace all 25 subjects. Table 9-4 lists their vocations and marital status. The contrast between the two groups speaks for itself.

Follow-up Study and Conclusions

All three studies concern children proved to be at high risk for psychosocial mental retardation. In the Milwaukee project and the Skeels study, respectively, intervention was proved to have prevented mental retardation, 4 and 30 yr after the intervention had been discontinued. Long-term follow-up is not yet available for the Abecedarian project.

The projects complement each other in that they involve both rural and urban populations and different races. Intervention techniques differed but in each instance were intensive and longterm. The Skeels study is unique in that much of the stimulation was provided by women who were thought to be mentally retarded.

It is cautioned that in the aggregate these three studies involve no more than 150 children and must be replicated. Furthermore, the specific approaches were intensive and too costly for general application. The investigators are fully aware of this. They took the position that the important initial question was to determine whether massive environmental intervention would have *any* effect, and they elected at that time not to approach the issue of cost-effectiveness.[7a]

Several excellent articles have reviewed the methodology and implications of these three related studies.[1,3,18] It seems likely that the greatest and most persistent effects are achieved when intervention is aimed at both the mother and the child and even at the "ecology" of the whole family. It was at first thought that the effects of many structured but less intensive programs aimed at the child only would "wash out" a year after the program had ceased, but a recent 10-yr collaborative follow-up study of children who participated in the Head Start program showed a significant reduction in the percentage of children who were placed in special education classes and who were school dropouts, even though no differences in IQ were demonstrable.[3,10] Thus, although these less intensive interventions fail to show the dramatic differences associated with the three studies cited above, it now seems likely that they do have favorable long-term effects.

IMPLICATIONS FOR THE CHILD WITH CEREBRAL PALSY

The studies with physically intact children cited above strongly suggest that environmental intervention can significantly improve the intellectual performance of children at high risk for psychosocial mental retardation. Despite the convincing evidence for the importance of genetic determinants of intelligence, it appears that remedying environmental deficiencies offers significant hope. The challenge is to define those elements of the interventions that are most decisive and to develop means to deliver them at acceptable cost. The potential benefits to the individual and to society are very large indeed, and educational and behaviorist professionals require the support of the medical community to accomplish this task. In my view, children with cerebral palsy and their families have a special stake in this endeavor. Cerebral palsy is more common in the premature child, the child of an adolescent mother, or in low SES families, all of them at risk for psychosocial mental retardation. Furthermore, the results of Drillien cited earlier suggest that the effects of biologic and environmental risk may be additive.[5,6] In any case, the achievement of optimum cognitive and social growth will increase the capacity of persons with cerebral palsy to help themselves, and this, in many ways, is the main aim of all efforts.

REFERENCES

1. Begab MJ: Issues in the prevention of psychosocial retardation, in Begab MJ, Haywood HC, Garber HL (Eds): Psychosocial Influences in Retarded Performance, vol. 1. Issues and Theories in Development. Baltimore, University Park Press, 1981, pp 7–27
2. Birch HG, Gussow JD: Disadvantaged Children: Health, Nutrition, and School Failure. New York, Grune & Stratton, 1970
3. Bronfenbrenner U: Is early intervention effective? A report on longitudinal evaluations of preschool programs. DHEW Pub. no. (OHD) 75-25, Washington, DC, U.S. Government Printing Office, 1975
4. Drillien CM: A longitudinal study of the growth and development of prematurely and maturely born children. II. Physical development. Arch Dis Child 33:423, 1958
5. Drillien CM: A longitudinal study of the growth and development of prematurely and maturely born children. VII. Mental development, 2–5 years. Arch Dis Child 36:233, 1961
6. Drillien CM, Thomson AJM, Burgoyne K: Low birthweight children at early school-age; a longitudinal study. Dev Med Child Neurol 22:26, 1980
7. Garber HL, Heber R: The efficacy of early intervention with family rehabilitation, in Begab MJ, Haywood HC, Garber HL (eds): Psychosocial Influences in Retarded Performance, vol. 2. Strategies for Improving Competence. Baltimore, University Park Press, 1981, pp 71–87
7a. Garber HL: Personal communication
8. Goddard HH: The menace of mental deficiency from the standpoint of heredity. Boston Med Surg J 175:1, 1916
9. Jensen AR: IQ's of identical twins reared apart. Behav Genet 1:133, 1970
10. Lazar I, Snipper AS, Royce J, et al: Policy implications of preschool intervention research, in Begab MJ, Haywood HC, Garber HL (eds): Psychosocial Influences in Retarded Performance, vol. 2. Strategies for Improving Competence. Baltimore, University Park Press, 1981, pp 275–291
11. Lewis EO: Types of mental deficiency and their social significance. J Ment Sci 79:298, 1933
12. Loehlin JC, Nichols RC: Heredity, Environment and Personality: A Study of 850 Sets of Twins. Austin, University of Texas Press, 1976
13. Munsinger H: The adopted child's IQ: A critical review. Psychol Bull 82:623, 1975
14. Nichols RC: Origins, nature, and determinants of intellectual development, in Begab MJ, Haywood HC, Garber HL (eds): Psychosocial Influences in Retarded Performance, vol. 1. Issues and Theories of Development. Baltimore, University Park Press, 1981, pp 127–154
15. Oski FA, Stockman JA: The Year Book of Pediatrics. Chicago, Year Book Medical Publishers, 1981, p 48
16. Ramey CT, Stedman DJ, Border S, et al: Predicting school failure from information available at birth. Am J Ment Def 82:525, 1978
17. Ramey CT, Finkelstein NW: Psychosocial mental retardation: A biological and social coalescence, in Begab MJ, Haywood HC, Garber HL (eds): Psychosocial Influences in Retarded Performance, vol. 1. Issues and Theories in Development. Baltimore, University Park Press, 1981, pp 65–92
18. Ramey CT, Haskins R: The causes and treatment of school failure: Insight from the Carolina Abecedarian project, in Begab MJ, Haywood HC, Garber HL (eds): Psychosocial Influences in Retarded Performance, vol. 2. Strategies for Improving Competence. Baltimore, University Park Press, 1981, pp 89–112
19. Reed EW, Reed SC: Mental Retardation: A Family Study. Philadelphia, Saunders, 1965, pp 51–69
20. Skeels HM: Adult status of children with contrasting early life experiences: A follow-up study. Monogr Soc Res Child Dev 105:1, 1966
21. Zigler E: Familial mental retardation. A continuing dilemma. Science 155:292, 1967

PART III

Assessment of Associated Dysfunctions

Bruce K. Shapiro   Renee C. Wachtel
Frederick B. Palmer   Arnold J. Capute

10

Associated Dysfunctions

In 1964, cerebral palsy was defined as a disorder of movement and posture due to a defect or lesion of the immature brain.[2] This definition was useful from a diagnostic standpoint because (1) the site of the defect was placed in the central nervous system (CNS) and (2) progressive (degenerative) processes were excluded. Although useful from the diagnostic viewpoint, this definition is limited by its exclusive motor focus. Motor deficiency may not be the most devastating handicap for the person with cerebral palsy. Since the insults producing the motor deficits in the developing brain are not discrete, additional or associated neurologic dysfunctions are common. An alternative definition for cerebral palsy recognizing these associated dysfunctions is *a chronic neurologic disorder of movement and posture due to a defect or lesion of the immature brain. The motor disability serves as a neurodevelopmental marker indicative of associated cerebral dysfunctions such as mental retardation, learning disability, seizures, deafness, sensory loss, and other dysfunctions.* The rationale for highlighting the associated dysfunctions rests on two premises: (1) associated deficits are common and (2) knowledge of the associated deficits is necessary to ensure full habilitation.

The incidence of specific dysfunctions can be debated, but the high frequency of additional neurologic deficits in children with cerebral palsy is well established. Tablan, as cited by Jones, reported that 88 percent of the patients with cerebral palsy have three or more disabilities (Table 10-1).[8] Among the disorders noted were cognitive dysfunction, hearing loss, language disorders, visual defects, behavioral disturbances, and perceptual deficiencies. Others have found significant degrees of sensory loss, seizures, and orthopaedic problems.

Studies of the outcome of adults with cerebral palsy show that 7–60 percent of people with cerebral palsy are gainfully employed.[3,6,15] The differences among these studies preclude direct comparisons, but even the most optimistic study reports that 40 percent of involved adults will *not* be gainfully employed. Although motor disabilities are a factor, cognition, personality factors, and other associated dysfunctions seem to be important variables. Full habilitation sets independence as the long-term goal, but most individuals with cerebral palsy do not reach this goal. Locomotion is but a single consideration. Communication, activities of daily living, and transportation are probably more important to the outcome.

The more frequently associated deficits are listed in Table 10-2. The interactions of the associated dysfunctions negate the idea of "straight forward" cerebral palsy. Present knowledge is limited only to assessing the relationship of single associated deficits to outcome of cerebral palsy. For complete understanding, however, it will be necessary to identify and appreciate not only the effect of isolated additional dysfunctions but also the interaction of multiple dysfunctions and their effects on outcome.

Table 10-1

Frequency of Disability in 333 Cerebral
Palsy Patients

Number of Disabilities	Percentage
2	11.7
3	40.0
4	32.0
5	11.7
6	3.0
7 or more	1.6

Data from Jones M: Differential diagnosis and
natural history of the cerebral palsied child, in
Samilson R (ed): Orthopedic Aspects of Cerebral
Palsy. Philadelphia, Lippincott, 1975.

ASSOCIATED DYSFUNCTIONS

Cognitive Dysfunction

Because the brain insult is seldom discrete, cognitive dysfunction is probably the most common associated deficit of cerebral palsy. Although professionals working with young children with cerebral palsy are most concerned about mental retardation, it should be remembered that more subtle dysfunctions exist in those children and are manifested clinically by learning disabilities. These subtle dysfunctions in central processing are difficult to assess in the young child who may also have associated dysfunctions in speech and language, vision, and hand use. Differentiating between limited motor and limited intellectual abilities requires an experienced evaluator. Although it is not possible to measure the cognitive potential in every child with cerebral palsy, it is possible to assess the vast majority of children. Just as the topographical diagnosis of cerebral palsy often requires several examinations, so does the cognitive examination need to be repeated several times for a satisfactory assessment of language and problem-solving abilities. Repeated assessment of cognitive abilities is necessary to permit readjustment of habilitation goals.

One may question whether this emphasis on cognitive assessment is justified. Does it matter whether a child with a profound motor handicap, no expressive language, and little hand function is mildly or profoundly mentally retarded? The answer is yes. Much time and effort may be expended to implement techniques that compensate for the lack of expressive language, but failure results because the child lacks the cognitive ability to benefit from the circumven-

Table 10-2

Associated Deficits

Cognitive dysfunction
Communication disorders
Visual dysfunction
Seizures
Emotional and behavioral disorders
Sensory impairments
Orthopaedic deformities

tion. In order to develop appropriate expectations and avoid frustration for the therapist, family, and child, cognitive level must be determined.

The association of mental retardation with cerebral palsy is well-established. "Significant subaverage general intellectual functioning existing concurrently with deficits in adaptive behavior and manifested during the developmental period" has been reported in 30–70 percent of the population with cerebral palsy. Generally, the more limbs involved, the more significant the retardation. Previously, the athetoid cerebral palsied patient was felt to be an exception, having overall intelligence higher than the general population of cerebral palsy despite the four-limb involvement. More recently, the picture of the child with extrapyramidal cerebral palsy has changed. As a result, physicians are seeing fewer of the "bright" children who had kernicterus and more with significant intellectual impairment due to hypoxic–ischemic insults.

Suggestive data exist relating outcome of motor therapy and employability to intellectual ability. Several studies have suggested that increased degrees of cognitive limitation adversely affect the child's ability to benefit from motor therapy. Intellectual potential has also been related to later employability. Of adults with cerebral palsy who have similar degrees of motor handicap and constellations of associated dysfunctions, those with intellectual quotients (IQs) greater than 70 are more likely to be successfully employed.

An IQ over 70 is, however, no guarantee of success for the child with cerebral palsy. As noted above, subtle deficiencies in central processing manifest themselves as *an uneven profile* or *scatter* on psychologic testing and as learning dysfunction in the school-age child. In cerebral palsy, scatter is simply a marker of disordered neurologic functioning. In our experience, children who "scatter" seldom do as well as would be predicted by the summary score. Educational habilitation programs must recognize the relative strengths and weaknesses. The question whether to remedy weaknesses or capitalize on strengths by circumvention remains unanswered. The prevalence of learning dysfunction in cerebral palsy is unknown but appears high.

These problems and others of cognitive and intellectual impairment are discussed in Chapters 8, 9, 15, and 31.

Communication Disorders

The inability to communicate is a major handicap of the individual with cerebral palsy. (Chap. 16). Far more handicapping than the inability to walk is the inability to speak. Disorders of communication in cerebral palsy may be divided into three groups: speech disorders (oromotor dysfunction), language disorders (central processing dysfunction), and hearing loss (auditory dysfunction). These groups are not independent and may coexist in the same child. When the habilitation of one of the disorders of communication (e.g., hearing loss) is not progressing as expected, the presence of an additional communication disorder (e.g., language disorder) should be excluded.

Speech Disorders

Oromotor function remains the most neglected and poorly understood aspect of cerebral palsy. Although a good deal of attention has been paid to the topographic and physiologic classification of cerebral palsy, little attention has been focused on the associated oromotor dysfunction. Presently there is an ill-defined base for describing the neuropathophysiology of oromotor dysfunction. Despite this, occupational therapists and speech pathologists have become involved in the therapy of oromotor dysfunction without the ability to properly classify the oromotor problems. The present state of the art is trial and error. Even though the possibility of aiding certain types of dysfunction exists, there is a lack of well-designed experimental studies that delineate distinctive clinical syndromes and document therapeutic efficacy.

Language Disorders

Although it was previously thought that the communication disorders seen in cerebral palsy were only on a speech basis (peripheral oromotor mechanism), later findings tend to support the concept of language dysfunction as a coexisting handicap. Deficits in central processing are the rule in cerebral palsy. This fact is of significant importance in the treatment of the speech and language disorders of cerebral palsy. It is unlikely that simple speech (articulation) therapy will be effective in treating language disorders. The

efficacy of language therapy is unproved. If the inability to communicate is on the basis of peripheral oral dysfunction, then children should do well with alternative methods of communication. If, however, the dysfunction is more central, then these children may indeed have difficulty communicating by alternative means.

Hearing Loss

The child with cerebral palsy is at greater risk than the general population for auditory dysfunction. Deafness has been reported in 6–16 percent of the population with cerebral palsy. Kernicteric athetoid children have the highest incidence of hearing loss—approximately 60 percent; however, it is not infrequent to see children with cerebral palsy still not diagnosed as having significant hearing impairment as late as 4 yr of age. It is frequently difficult to assess the degree of hearing loss because of the cognitive disability. The assessment of acoustic reflex threshold with impedance audiometry and the availability of brainstem auditory-evoked responses promise to improve the identification of communicatively handicapping, sensorineural hearing loss.

The acoustic reflex threshold measures the decrease in compliance (increase in impedance) of the middle ear system, resulting from the contraction of the stapedius muscle's reacting to a sound stimulus. If the sound is loud enough, muscles in both the probe and stimulus ears contract, yielding bilateral reflexes. Minimal cooperation is required for eliciting this response. The acoustic impedance bridge easily measures this reflex threshold as well as determines tympanic membrane mobility. Inability to determine acoustic reflex thresholds may result from middle ear dysfunction in the probe ear (including cranial nerve VII, which supplies the stapedius muscle), a severe cochlear loss in the stimulus ear, moderate conductive loss in the stimulus ear, or interruption in the brain stem acoustic reflex pathways. If acoustic reflex thresholds cannot be elicited, one can usually determine the reason by ipsilateral stimulation and monitoring in addition to the usual contralateral elicitation.[7] Availability of equipment, ease of administration, and reliability of results make determination of acoustic reflex thresholds a valuable assessment tool.

Assessment of brain stem auditory-evoked potentials is not a screening technique but may be necessary in situations where behavioral audiometry and impedance testing are unreliable, inconclusive, or technically difficult. Evoked potential audiometry is based on the finding of a consistent series of electroencephalographic (EEG) responses occurring within

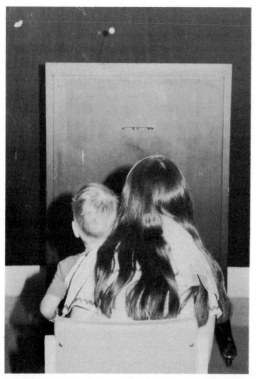

Figure 10-1. The STYCAR method for determining visual acuity. A white ball is presented from behind a dark screen, and the child's response is noted by the examiner (observing through the slit). It is possible to derive an estimate of visual acuity by using a ball of known size that is presented at a known distance.

10 msec of an auditory stimulus. These responses are of low amplitude; hence, computer averaging is needed. The latency phase of these peaks is proportional to the intensity of the auditory stimulus. As a result, it is possible to draw a latency-intensity of stimulus curve and infer hearing abilities.[13] Although normal-evoked potential audiometry results cannot ensure the presence of perfect hearing, this test may nevertheless be useful in a battery to exclude a communicatively handicapping hearing loss.

Visual Dysfunction

Strabismus is the most common visual disturbance associated with cerebral palsy (approximately 50 percent) and is readily recognizable. (See Chap. 14) Refractive errors and visual field cuts are more difficult to assess in young children. Traditional methods—assessing refractive errors by Snellen chart testing and visual field function by visual tangent screen testing (perimetry)—are based on higher cognitive functions and therefore cannot be used until a mental age of seven or eight. It is possible, however, to clinically document refractive errors and visual field cuts before this age.

The testing of vision in the child with cerebral palsy might prove difficult because of the movement disorder, cognitive limitations, attentional aberrations, language problems, and central visual processing dysfunction. The Sheridan Test for Young Children and Retardates (STYCAR) mounted balls test is ideal for the child with significant motor impairment, since it requires only a minimum of cooperation and may obviate the need for retinoscopy under anesthesia. The test relies on the child's ability to move the eyes to fix on a novel object (white ball against a black background) and requires a cognitive level of approximately 6 months (Fig. 10-1). Balls ranging from 2.5–0.125 in diameter are presented from behind a screen. The child's visual response is noted by the examiner through a slit in the screen. Although generally presented from a distance of 10 ft, distractibility may necessitate presenting material at 5 ft. The child who cannot sit alone may be supported on a friendly lap. Standard visual acuity measures (Snellen equivalents) have been published for this method.[19]

Infants with cerebral palsy are often diagnosed as cortically blind, since they demonstrate pupillary reactions but do not visually respond to a threatening gesture. Visual abilities are developmental; pupillary reactions develop during intrauterine gestation, whereas a response to visual threat does not occur until 3 months of age. Therefore, children whose central visual processing abilities are less than a 3-month level may be thought to be cortically blind. The ability to visually follow horizontally may help resolve the question of cortical blindness, since this ability occurs by two months and usually precedes the development of a response to threatening gesture.

Homonymous hemianopsia has been noted in 25 percent of patients with hemiplegia.[20] When present, it is usually (85 percent) associated with sensory deficit on the affected side. Asymmetric somatic undergrowth should alert one to the possibility of a visual field cut in the child who is unable to participate in formal perimetry. To document this, the child can be seated on the parent's lap and a stimulus presented to draw the child's attention forward while the examiner brings a red ring or other bright object in a circular fashion from behind to directly in front of the child (Fig. 10-2). A consistently diminished unilateral response suggests a visual field cut. The disability resulting from hemianopsia is usually slight, but it must be recognized when designing communication boards and planning educational strategies.

Just as the child with cerebral palsy may have peripheral and central communication dysfunction, so may he or she have peripheral *and* central visual dysfunction. The child with cerebral palsy frequently demonstrates an inability to interpret visual symbols. Visual processing dysfunction may be responsible for an inability to identify letters, making assessment of visual acuity and reading more difficult.

Ophthalmologic problems, assessment, and treatment are discussed in detail in Chapter 14.

Seizures

Seizures occur more frequently in children with cerebral palsy than in the general population; 25–35 percent of children with cerebral palsy have seizures, and those with spastic hemiparesis and quadriparesis have the highest frequency.

The long-term effects on learning and behavior from medications given to control seizures are unknown. Perlstein and Hood reported a series of 173 hemiplegic children.[17] The mean IQ of the 76 children with seizures was 70.2, while the mean IQ of those without seizures was 83. This is consistent with the results of Crothers and Paine.[3] Whether the relative lowering of intellectual function is caused by the same neurologic dysfunction as that which caused the seizures and cerebral palsy or is related to the treatment of the seizures remains to be shown.

Seizure disorders are discussed in Chapter 13.

Emotional and Behavioral Disorders

Children with brain damage are four to five times more likely to have behavioral disorders than children without brain damage.[18] The primary behavioral disturbances seen in the child with cerebral palsy are the same as those seen in the hyperkinetic syndrome of childhood (Strauss syndrome): attentional abberrations, impulsivity, and distractability. Hyperactivity may also be noted, although this is not infrequently masked by motor deficiency.

As the child grows, cerebral palsy takes on a different significance for the child, family, and society. When considering the behavior of the child with cerebral palsy, the role of the family cannot be overstressed. MacKeith recognized the central role that parents play in the treatment and called parents

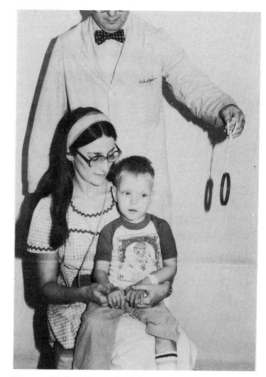

Figure 10-2. A method for assessing the presence of a visual field cut (homonymous hemianopsia) in the young child (see text for explanation).

"the keystone of the therapeutic arch."[11] Transitional points are times when family stress can be expected. Time of diagnosis, school entrance, school change, puberty, graduation, moving away of a sibling, and death or infirmity of a parent are such points.[10] Guidance at these times may diminish the secondary emotional disturbances resulting from such stresses.

Secondary behavioral disorders are common in the adolescent with a handicap. Normal adolescent concerns of socialization, sexuality, independence, and future vocation are compounded by continued dependence because of motor and other handicaps and parental overprotectiveness. This is further intensified by the parents' concerns about their own mortality and the ultimate achievement of their child. Little formal research has addressed methods to prevent and treat the secondary problems noted in adolescence.

Adolescence is not the only emotionally troubled time. The social life for adults also has limitations. Klapper and Birch reported that fewer than 10 percent of people with cerebral palsy marry and as many as 25 percent are described as social isolates.[9] Multiple factors responsible for social failure include poor communication abilities, poor hand function, immobility, lack of transportation, mental retardation, and behavioral disorders (see Chapter 33).

Pseudodegeneration

It is not uncommon to see a number of adolescents with cerebral palsy stop walking. Not infrequently, these individuals are referred for evaluation of a progressive neurologic disorder. Generally, they may have been marginal walkers, requiring assistive devices, who have gone through a growth phase. Whether the work of walking becomes excessive because of change in body habitus or whether the individual decides that trying to walk is too inefficient and ungainly is unclear. A further consideration may be an increase in dystonia and a corresponding decrease in choreoathetoid movements, commonly seen in adolescence. Similar regression in speech performance has been noted.

Sensory Impairments

Sensory impairments are thought to be more prevalent in hemiplegia and are postulated to be secondary to parietal lobe dysfunction. Although most investigations have focused on hemiplegia, any child demonstrating significant left–right asymmetry is at risk for sensory impairment. Dysfunctions have been noted (in decreasing order) in stereognosis, two-point discrimination, position sense, sharp–dull discrimination, pain, light touch, and temperature sense.[20] The severity of sensory involvement is not necessarily related to the degree of motor impairment. Children with the most severe sensory impairment, the so-called blind limb, show diminished arm usage out of proportion to the degree of motor handicap.

As is true for many of the associated dysfunctions, age and cognition are limiting factors in determining the presence of sensory impairments. In addition to unilateral functional neglect, skeletal undergrowth serves as a marker of sensory impairment. The association of even mild asymmetric somatic undergrowth is very closely associated with sensory impairment. Mild degrees of somatic undergrowth may be detected by comparing the nail beds of corresponding fingers and eliciting Allis' sign.

In addition to somatic undergrowth and functional neglect, visual neglect (visual field cut) is also a marker of sensory dysfunction. It is possible to develop a clinical impression of visual field cut earlier

than one can formally assess sensory impairment. The presence of a visual field cut should alert clinicians to the possibility of sensory impairment, since 85 percent of children with homonymous hemianopsia have associated sensory loss.

Upper-extremity function has been directly related to outcome in cerebral palsy. Good hand function allows the child to circumvent the limitations imposed by the motor (e.g., wheelchair usage, adaptive devices for activities of daily living) and speech (e.g., sign language, typewriters, and other supplemental methods of communication) deficits. As a result, upper-extremity function has been the focus of multiple treatment approaches—surgery, splinting, various forms of peripheral manipulation, and pharmacologic therapy. Although motor function may be improved, the optimal habilitation of the sensory-impaired limb remains unknown.

Orthopaedics

When discussing the associated dyfunctions, one must not neglect the resultant orthopaedic deformities. Although the brain lesion is static, the peripheral manifestations are dynamic. The orthopaedist approaches the direct effects of the neurophysiologic dysfunction—contracture, imbalance, instability, and malalignment—with the goals of (1) correcting deformity, (2) preserving function, and (3) relieving pain.

Orthopaedic deformities are common. Of 108 cerebral palsied children admitted to The John F. Kennedy Institute for Handicapped Children in 1977, significant contractures were noted in 45.3 percent, previous orthopaedic surgery in 21.3 percent, scoliosis in 13.9 percent, and hip dislocation in 4.6 percent.[12] Positional orthopaedic deformities occurred in patients with extrapyramidal lesions despite involuntary movements and variability of tone. Habilitation goals frequently had to be readjusted because of an intervening orthopaedic deformity adversely affecting posture and locomotion.

One of the most common orthopaedic handicaps is hip dislocation (see Chap. 23). Spastic diplegia and quadriplegia have approximately a 4-percent incidence of hip dislocation if ambulatory and a 25-percent incidence if nonambulatory.[14] Patients with extrapyramidal cerebral palsy with obligatory asymmetric tonic neck reflexes (ATNR) are at risk for scoliosis and dislocating the hip on the occiput side. With dislocation, gait balance and the ability to sit are impaired, thus limiting the child's musculoskeletal development. Scoliosis and fixed pelvic obliquity are frequent concomitants of hip dislocation.[4]

CLASSIFICATION OF CEREBRAL PALSY

Although cerebral palsy was initially classified to allow for specific therapies, the classifications remain useful because associated deficits tend to cluster, forming specific subclasses of cerebral palsy. The topographic and physiologic classifications remain useful in predicting associated deficits.

Spastic hemiplegia remains the most common type of cerebral palsy. Hemiplegias have the lowest rates of mental retardation. The tetrad of hemiplegia—somatic undergrowth, sensory impairment, homonymous hemianopsia and seizures—must be recognized and addressed for full habilitation to occur. Spastic quadriplegia tends to have an increased incidence of mental retardation. These children are at greater risk for opthopaedic deformity and require close monitoring of the status of the hips and careful positioning to prevent hip dislocation and scoliosis. Seizures occur at approximately the same rate as in hemiplegia. Children with asymmetric quadriplegia should also be assessed for sensory dysfunction and visual field cuts. Children with spastic diplegia tend to have mild cognitive impairment. Hand function and speech are usually minimally affected, but, as is true of quadriplegia, close monitoring for orthopaedic complications is needed. Seizures are relatively infrequent in spastic diplegia.

The most common etiology of extrapyramidal cerebral palsy used to be kernicterus, resulting from erythroblastosis fetalis. The syndrome of kernicterus was associated with choreoathetosis, high-frequency hearing loss coupled with central auditory imperception, supraversion gaze palsy, and poor dentition.[16] This association is rarely seen today. Prematurity and hypoxia are responsible for the etiology of extrapyramidal cerebral palsy to an increasing degree. More severe cognitive disturbance, complex seizures, severe oromotor dysfunction, and orthopaedic handicaps are now being seen with these lesions.

The clustering of associated dysfunctions is in a dynamic state. Improved obstetric and neonatal care are resulting in better outcomes. Although the rate of cerebral palsy is felt to be decreasing as a result of these interventions, it is unclear whether the child who develops cerebral palsy, despite improved care, is likely to be more handicapped than previously.

Even though the classification of cerebral palsy is useful to focus attention on the associated dysfunctions, the term cerebral palsy does not encompass the entire spectrum of central motor disability. As motor therapists strive to improve the "quality" of movement, the point at which *clumsiness* becomes *motor impairment* is obscured. Specific motor therapy may not be required in the minimal or mild forms of motor dysfunction. Minimal or mild motor dysfunction may not be disabling; however, it serves as a marker for associated deficits in other areas of neurologic function. The associated deficits may prove more handicapping than the motor dysfunction. This is particularly true in the behavioral and cognitive areas, where gross motor delay is a frequent presenting sign in mental retardation and clumsiness or soft neuromotor signs are prevalent in children with learning disabilities. Some workers have suggested reclassifying central motor dysfunctions to include the minimal and mild forms of motor dysfunction as well as cerebral palsy.[2]

PERSPECTIVE

Cerebral palsy is but one of a heterogeneous group of disorders known as the *developmental disabilities*. These disorders have varied manifestations but are appropriate to group because they are the result of chronic nonprogressive, neurologic dysfunction commencing in the pediatric age group. Disorders are classified by the most obvious presenting symptom; hence, children with motor disability are diagnosed as having cerebral palsy, children with cognitive disability are diagnosed as having mental retardation or learning disability; and children with speech and language disorders fall into the category known as communication disorders (central communicative disorders, autism, deafness).

To reflect not only the most obvious manifestations, and consequently fully describe the child, complete diagnosis is necessary before habilitation. The child with *language delay* may be hearing impaired, have poor oromotor abilities or a central communication disorder, be mentally retarded, or choose not to speak. It is imperative that the reason for the language delay be discerned before the nonspecific institution of *language therapy*. If children are to be specifically treated, then the concept of developmental delay must be replaced by a comprehensive diagnosis.

The diagnosis of cerebral palsy is insufficient;

it should make the clinician think of the other associated deficits that might prevent the long-term achievement of independent function. It should be remembered that the etiologies responsible for cerebral palsy do not exert discrete influences but are responsible for diffuse dysfunction. As such, it is not unusual to find multiple handicaps. Attempts to treat cerebral palsy without cognizance of the associated deficits can result in incomplete habilitation. To enable a child to ambulate yet miss his or her mental retardation is unacceptable.

The treatment of the associated dysfunctions commonly becomes an end unto itself, however, and the effects of the underlying brain dysfunction are dealt with by having more therapists involved as new symptoms are noted. The pediatrician, neurologist, orthopaedist, ophthalmologist, audiologist, speech pathologist, psychologist, teacher, occupational therapist, and physical therapist may all be involved in the treatment of the child with cerebral palsy. The potential for chaos exists, and, left unchecked, the treatment of the cerebral palsied child may become overbearing to the family. A coordinated, interdisciplinary approach to the cerebral palsied child enables all those who treat the child to share their perspectives. Treatment priorities or habilitation plans must be ordered to prevent the parents from trying to do everything at once. By setting achievable goals, more realistic impressions are transmitted to the family. The progress made by the child can be more objectively assessed within the context of full habilitation when the primary therapist is not solely responsible for the assessment of efficacy.

Most therapies employed to treat cerebral palsy are based on the belief that peripheral manipulation is able to repair or bypass CNS dysfunction. This premise remains unproved. Those who employ a particular therapy are obligated to demonstrate that it is more effective than doing nothing. Workers are still at the point where therapeutic endeavors are justified because they "work for some children." If the therapy of cerebral palsy is to progress, then clinicians must scientifically distinguish groups of children for whom therapy is effective. Researching therapeutic efficacy requires a homogeneous population. The number and varied expression of associated deficits makes this a formidable task, yet to use a heterogeneous population carries the risk of not being able to answer the question of efficacy.

In cerebral palsy, motor dysfunctions and associated deficits are manifestations of diffuse brain dysfunction. An understanding of the interactions of the motor components and the associated deficits is requisite for establishing realistic habilitation goals. It is only by appreciating the full spectrum of the dysfunctions that new and more effective methods of treatment can be developed.

REFERENCES

1. Bax M: Terminology and classification of cerebral palsy. Dev Med Child Neurol 6:295, 1964
2. Capute A, Shapiro B, Palmer F: Spectrum of developmental disabilities: Continuum of motor dysfunction. Orthoped Clin North Am 12:3, 1981
3. Crothers B, Paine R: The Natural History of Cerebral Palsy. Cambridge, Harvard University Press, 1959
4. Drummond DS, Rogala EJ, Cruess R, et al: The paralytic hip and pelvic obliquity in cerebral palsy and myelomeningocele, in American Academy of Orthopaedic Surgeons: Instructional Course Lectures, vol. 30. St. Louis, Mosby, 1980, p 7–36
5. Grossman H (ed): Manual on Terminology and Classification in Mental Retardation. Baltimore, Garamond/Pridemark Press, 1973
6. Hansen E: Cerebral palsy in Denmark. Acta Psychiatr Neurol Scand (suppl) 146: 1960
7. Hayes D, Jerger J: Impedance audiometry in otologic diagnosis. Otolaryngol Clin North Am 11:759, 1978
8. Jones M: Differential diagnosis and natural history of the cerebral palsied child, in Samilson R (ed): Orthopedic Aspects of Cerebral Palsy. Philadelphia, Lippincott, 1975
9. Klapper Z, Birch H: The relation of childhood characteristics to outcome in young adults with cerebral palsy. Dev Med Child Neurol 8:645, 1966
10. MacKeith R: The feelings and behavior of parents of handicapped children. Dev Med Child Neurol 15:524, 1973
11. MacKeith R: The restoration of the parents as the keystone of the therapeutic arch. Dev Med Child Neurol 18:285, 1976
12. Marquis P: Personal communication, 1979
13. Mizrahi E, Dorfman L: Sensory evoked potentials: Clinical applications in pediatrics. J Pediatr 97:1, 1980
14. Phelps WM: Prevention of acquired dislocation of the hip in cerebral palsy. J Bone Joint Surg 41A:440, 1959
15. Pollock G, Stark G: Long-term results in the management of 67 children with cerebral palsy. Dev Med Child Neurol 11:17, 1969

16. Perlstein M: The clinical significance of kernicterus, in Swinyard C (ed): Kernicterus And Its Importance in Cerebral Palsy. Springfield, Ill. Charles C Thomas, 1957

17. Perlstein M, Hood P: Infantile spastic hemiplegia: Intelligence, oral language and motor development. Courrier 6:567, 1956

18. Rutter M, Graham P, Yule W: A Neuropsychiatric Study in Childhood. London, Heinemann, 1970

19. Sheridan MD: The STYCAR graded balls vision test. Dev Med Child Neurol 15:423, 1973

20. Tizard J, Paine R, Crothers B: Disturbances of sensation in children with hemiplegia. JAMA 155:628, 1954

Norberto Alvarez

11

Neurologic Examination

It is the responsibility of the pediatrician (or general practitioner) to detect early signs of developmental delay. Early detection will allow for early identification and appropriate management of problems and, hence, improved outcome. The role of the pediatrician is enhanced, since there is a greater need for medical services in infancy (see Chap. 2). As the child grows, less medical and more social, education, and vocational needs must be satisfied. In addition, it is desirable that the pediatrician play an important role in the long-term management of children with cerebral palsy.

DEVELOPMENTAL SCREENING

Developmental screening identifies those infants and children who will need a more extensive assessment. It should not be a difficult and time-consuming task. There are several standardized tests from which one can choose.[1-4] Simple tests for hearing screening should be included in addition to the test for motor, social, and linguistic performance. Table 11-1 represents a progression of milestones that covers the important developmental stages of babies and children. The items included have been drawn from well-established scales. Each developmental level, or epoch, represents a span of two months. As a rule of thumb, any child at least one epoch behind chronologic age deserves a more extensive evaluation.

HISTORY

A complete personal and family history as well as a detailed history of pregnancy, delivery, and neonatal course are important. The presence of a positive family history is suggestive of a familial disorder, but a negative family history does not exclude this possibility.

Information should be obtained about maternal illnesses, diet, medications, and the use of socially accepted toxins such as alcohol and cigarette smoking, since these are all known to cause problems in the fetus (see Chap. 5). A negative history during pregnancy does not exclude an acquired congenital infection, since these can be asymptomatic. A history of an abnormal delivery, e.g., face, breech, or transverse presentation, may indicate prior fetal disorders, as the fetus with a central nervous system (CNS) malformation or motor disorder is likely to present in an abnormal position. Information such as "prolonged labor," "did not cry right away," and "was blue at birth," are vague terms and do not necessarily reflect the cause of handicap. In many obstetric services, intensive monitoring of high-risk pregnancies can provide relevant information (see Chaps. 5 and 6).

A detailed developmental history is essential. Developmental milestones that parents most frequently remember with some accuracy are smiling, sitting, standing, walking, first words, feeding alone,

Table 11-1
Progression of Developmental Milestones

Age	Fine Motor	Gross Motor	Personal and Socialization	Language	Vision	Hearing
1 mo	Opens hand randomly	Turns head to either side when in prone position Holds head erect for 2 or more sec when upright	Regards face	Cries	Focuses briefly on objects Blinks at bright light Optical blink reflex with habituation After several trials, turns to a diffuse light	Startles and blink change sucking and respiration patterns in response to noise Acoustic blink reflex with habituation after several trials
2 mo	Hands mostly fisted	Keeps head up when upright In prone position, raises head up and maintains it at 45° for few seconds	Smiles in response to friendly sounds	Make different cries Some open vowel sounds	Follows moving object at 90° horizon Watches mother's face at feeding time	Shifts eyes to voice Alerting reaction to voice or sound
4 mo	Looks at hands Brings hand to mouth Begins to show ulnar-palmar prehension Plays with fingers at midline	Maintains head up and chest up to 90° Rolls to supine from prone	Smiles spontaneously	Begins to babble	Follows in all directions Watches own hands Converges eyes on ball	Turns head to voice in horizontal plane
6 mo	Reaches accurately for a toy with either hand Transfers toys from hand to hand Radial palmer prehension	Turns head to side of noise Pulls to sit Has no head lag from supine position Rolls to prone position when supine Sits with support	Begins to self-feed a cracker	Laughs and squeals	Displays visually directed reach	Turns head to side of noise, although may not localize the source of the sound

Age	Fine Motor	Gross Motor	Social	Language	Vision	Hearing
8 mo	Holds one cube in one hand and reaches for second. Thumb opposition for cube. Begins inferior pincer grasp	Sits without support for 2–3 min. Assume quadruped position when prone	Responds to name. Withdrawal with strangers	Repeats two-syllable words. Laughs. Uses single-and double-syllable words	Visual axes are parallel. Squints are no longer observed. Quick response to testing or peripheral vision. Watches a rolling ball	Localized sound by a compound visual maneuver consisting of horizontal followed by a vertical component
10 mo	Pokes with index finger	Can assume sitting position alone. Crawls. Begins to stand using furniture and cruises	Uses language to attract attention. Plays peek-a-boo. Initiates hand clapping	Says one word. Understands "no" and "bye-bye"	Fixes on small objects. Maintains interest for minutes	Localized hearing test at three feet above and below ear level with a single head movement
12 mo	Thumb finger grasp and, in many cases, neat pincer grasp	Stands alone. Walk few steps alone. Walks with one hand held	Follows simple orders. Helps with dressing. Waves goodbye	Jargon plus three or four words. Recognizes names of a few common objects	Looks for and finds toys that rolled out of sight	Immediate response to hearing tests. Comprehends simple commands
18 mo	Scribbles spontaneously. Tower of three cubes	Walks alone without difficulty	Removes socks, pulling from toes. Points to two or three body parts and some common objects on request	Commands 10 words. Combines two words. Names common object. Uses gestures to communicate	Searches for hidden objects	See language

(continued)

Table 11-1
Progression of Developmental Milestones (*continued*)

Age	Fine Motor	Gross Motor	Personal and Socialization	Language	Vision	Hearing
24 mo	Tower of four cubes Dumps raisin from a bottle	Kicks ball forward Throws ball over head Walks backwards Walks up steps Jumps in place	Uses spoon Helps in simple tasks in house Follows simple commands Removes shoes	Makes two- to three-word sentences Begins use of pronouns A 200-word vocabulary	Anticipates trajectory of a moving object	
3 yr	Tower of 8–10 cubes Imitates vertical line Copies a circle	Walk up stairs, changing feet Pedals tricycle	Washes and dries hands Puts on clothing	Uses plurals Vocabulary of 1000 words	Can be tested for visual activity with small pictures Has 20/40 vision	
4 yr	Copies a cross Laces shoes Buttons clothes Identifies longer line	Balances on 1 foot for at least 5 sec	Dresses with supervision	Engages in long conversations	Recognizes colors Has 20/30 vision	
5 yr	Draws a man (three parts)	Skips Hops on one foot	Separates from mother easily Brushes teeth	Adult sentence structure	Can be tested with letters	
6 yr	Copies square	Balances on one foot for 20 sec	Follows three to four serial commands	Defines words	Has 20/20 vision	

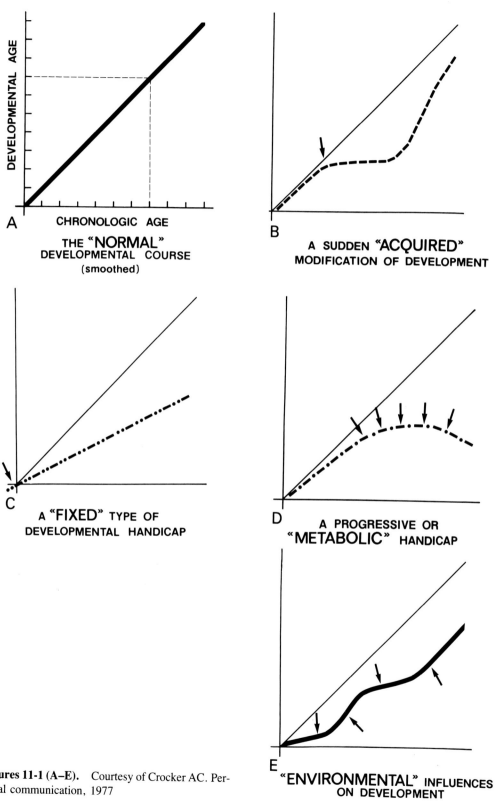

Figures 11-1 (A–E). Courtesy of Crocker AC. Personal communication, 1977

101

and sphincter control. In the case of older children, school records may be helpful.

After the personal history is completed, the examiner should be able to categorize the patients in one of the subgroups represented in Figures 11-1 (A–E). Categorization helps determine the approach to further investigation.

Physical and Neurologic Examination

Although in most cases a single examination may be adequate, in some situations two or three interviews may be needed for a complete evaluation. This is preferable to sedation, although it might be necessary for fundoscopy or special investigations.

General Physical Examination

A complete physical examination is mandatory. Clues on etiologic diagnoses may be found outside the CNS; e.g., eyes and skin have a common embryologic origin with the CNS. Tables 11-2 and 11-3 show skin and eye disorders associated with developmental delays. The spleen and liver are enlarged in several metabolic disorders, as seen in Table 11-4. Dysmorphic features are suggestive of congenital disorders.[5]

Anthropometric measures should include head circumference, height, and weight. Each should not be considered in isolation. Measurement of head circumference is an effective method for early detection of microcephaly and hydrocephalus. Head circumference beyond the 97th percentile or below the 3rd percentile for age and sex is always an indication for further evaluation. Rapid increases in head circumference, e.g., a jump from the 50th to the 75th percentile, are also an indication of further examination, even if the head circumference is still within the normal range. In a recent prospective study, Ellenberg and Nelson found that unusually small or large heads were both associated with an increased rate of cerebral palsy.[6]

Premature children tend to grow at a faster rate than term newborns, and at one point they may look "hydrocephalic." A similar situation may be seen in severely malnourished infants, whose normal heads may look too big for their small bodies.

NEUROLOGIC EXAMINATION

The classical neurologic examination is presented in Table 11-5. The order in which the examination is done can be changed, but it is advisable to do it in the same order each time to avoid omitting some items. A complete neurologic examination can be obtained in almost every patient, although some

Table 11-2

Skin Lesions Associated with Neurologic Disorders

Lesion	Description
Tuberous sclerosis	Adenoma sebaceum Subungual fibromas Depigmented skin lesions (ash leaf) Thickened skin areas (shagreen patch)
Neurofibromatosis	Cafe-au-lait spots Subcutaneous tumor (neurofibromas)
Sturge–Weber disease	Port wine hemangioma in the distribution of the trigeminal nerve, usually unilateral; mostly in the ophthalmic and maxillary division of the nerve
Ataxia telangiectasia	Telangiectasis (dilated venules) in the bulbar conjunctiva and malar areas of the face
Linear sebaceous nevus	Linear, hyperkeratotic, verrucous lesion in forehead and tip of the nose, with midline location
Nevus unis lateralis	Linear group of dark papules raised above normal skin; no specific distribution
Incontinentia pigmenti	Hyperpigmentation of skin lesions characterized by reddened vesicular and bullous eruptions that later become verrucous and hyperkeratotic

Table 11-3

Ocular Abnormalities Associated
with Developmental Delay

Clouding of cornea

Congenital syphilis
Mucopolysaccharidosis I, IV, VI, or VII
Mucolipidosis IV

Lens opacities

Galactosemia
Cretinism
Down's syndrome
Prenatal rubella

Dislocation of lens

Homocystinuria
Marfan's syndrome

Cherry red spot in macula

Tay–Sach's Disease (GM_2 gangliosidosis)
GM_1 gangliosidosis
Niemann–Pick disease

Chorioretinitis

Congenital syphilis
Toxoplasmosis
Cytomegalic inclusion disease
Prenatal rubella

tests require active cooperation and may be difficult
to perform and interpret. In this situation, the patient
may need to be reexamined at a later visit.

Posture and Gait

Since motor deficiency is the hallmark of cerebral palsy, gait abnormalities are common. Children with discrete lesions in the motor area may have
minimal motor disorders that can go unnoticed for
years. The children usually have a normal intelligence
quotient (IQ) and are brought to consultation at preschool or early school age because of a history of
"recent weakness in one leg" or problems with activities that require coordination or strength, e.g., ice
skating or dancing. More often than not, they have
a nonrelevant past medical history. Sometimes a history of wearing out one shoe more than the other or
intermittent tiptoeing may be the only suggestive clues.
The physical and neurologic examination may only

Table 11-4

Hepatosplenomegaly

Gaucher's disease

Mucopolysaccharidosis (most types)

Niemann–Pick disease

Glycogen storage disease types I and II

Generalized GM_1 gangliosidosis

Galactosemia

Mucolipidosis II

reveal minimal abnormal signs, e.g., some tiptoeing,
mild or no equinovarus, slight increase in deep tendon
reflexes, intermittent Babinski's sign, mild increase
in muscle tone, or unsustained clonus, and there may
be trophic changes in the affected limb (a small cortical lesion in the mesial prerolandic area may be
responsible for this disorder). Early recognition of
these gait disorders may save the child and the parents
unnecessary testing and anxiety. The evaluations of
gait disorders have been improved with the recent
development of gait laboratories where computerized
analysis of gait disorders can be performed (see Chap.
12).

Obvious abnormal gait disorders are easily recognized.

Spastic

In the spastic hemiplegic gait the patient walks
with equinus posture of the foot. This is circumduc-
tion of the legs with pelvic elevation and foot drag-
ging on the affected side. Normal associated movements are decreased on the paretic side. The patient
with spastic paraparesis walks with a stiff gait, ad-
ducting the lower extremities, which cross each other
in a characteristic "scissoring" pattern.

Choreoathetoid

Patients with dystonic–athetotic disorders have
markedly increased associated movements when
walking, e.g., grimacing, opening and closing of eyes,
throwing the head backward or from side to side, and
writhing contortions of the tongue and neck; the characteristic athetoid movements of the fingers and hands
become markedly exaggerated.

Cerebellar

Patients with cerebellar disorders walk with a
broad base, staggering and swaying from side to side,
and are very unsteady. Falls are not unusual.

Table 11-5
Neurologic Examination

Mental status

Gait and stance

Cranial nerves

   I. Olfactory
        Sense of smell

  II. Optic
        Sense of vision

  III. }
  IV. } Oculomotor
  VI. }   Eye position and motility; pupils

  V. Trigeminal
       Sensibility of face, including cornea
       and $\frac{2}{3}$ of scalp; motor innervation
       masseters and temporalis muscle

  VII. Facial
       Muscles of facial expression,
       lacrimation, salivation, and taste

  VIII. Acoustic
       Hearing; vestibular functions

  IX. } Glossopharyngeal
  X. } Vagus
       Swallowing, deglutition, voice,
       sucking, vomiting, cough, and
       salivary secretions

  XI. Spinal accessory
       SCM—trapezius muscle

  XII. Hypoglossal
       Tongue

Motor system

  Muscle
    Trophism (bulk of muscle)
    Tone
    Strength

  Deep tendon reflexes

  Spinal reflexes

  Motility
    Presence of normal range
    Lack of motility
    Presence of abnormal movements

Cerebellar testing

Sensory functions

Exteroceptive
  Touch, pain, temperature

Proprioceptive
  Pressure, position, vibration sense

Complex sensory functions
  Stereognosis
  Two-point discrimination
  Discrimination of weight, shape, and
  texture

Other Disorders

A gait disorder is also associated with damage to the posterior tract of the spinal cord or with peripheral nerve disorders. This sensory ataxia is exaggerated when the eyes are closed. Several other varieties of abnormal gaits do not conform any classic pattern.

Muscle Bulk

The bulk of the muscle, as observed or palpated by the examiner, gives an idea of the trophism of the muscle. There is no objective test to measure trophism. Measurement of the circumference of the limb may serve as a crude method to quantify muscle bulk; however, a certain degree of subjectivity will always be present. Muscle atrophy is frequently seen in patients with cerebral palsy, mostly as a consequence of disuse in paralyzed limbs or when malnutrition is superimposed. Since muscle atrophy may also be an expression of lower motor neuron disease, the recent development of localized muscle atrophy deserves further evaluation. Compression of the spinal cord by tumors, as seen in neurofibromatosis, or peripheral nerve compressions (e.g., the associated incidence of nerve root and peripheral nerve compressions observed in dystonic–athetotic patients)[7] are some of the possible causes. The potentially treatable conditions, if undiagnosed, will result in muscle atrophy, with consequent loss of function.

Muscle Tone

The extent of motion and the degree of the resistance encountered when a particular joint is moved through its maximal range of motion are the bases for the definition of the muscle tone.

Well-trained examiners may have a high degree of correlation when evaluating the same patient, but the lack of quantatitive, objective measurements of muscle tone is an important limiting factor. Attempts have been made to quantify muscle tone by computer analysis of the stretch reflex, but this is not available in the clinical setting.[8] Until bedside objective tests are developed, this aspect of neurologic examination will remain open to disagreement, mostly for the diagnosis of mild cases and notably for the evaluation of changes produced by any antispastic therapy.

Hypertonia

A high degree of resistance with limited range of motion is characteristic of hypertonicity. Two well-defined types of increased muscle tone have been described.

Spasticity. Spasticity represents increased resistance to fast stretching that suddenly gives way—the "clasp-knife" phenomenon. It is the most common abnormal muscle tone observed in cerebral palsy and is usually associated with increased deep tendon reflexes, clonus, Babinski sign, and certain spontaneous assumed postures. Associated joint contractures secondary to inadequately treated, long-standing hypertonicity can also be seen.

Rigidity. Rigidity represents continuous increased resistance to slow stretching and is observed during the whole range of motion—the "lead pipe" phenomenon. Poor facial mimic expression with drooling and a decrease in associated movements when walking are also observed.

The "cog wheel" phenomenon is the result of a concomitant tremor and is manifested by a series of jerks during passive stretching. Rigidity is frequently seen in association with the use of psychotropic medications.

Hypotonia

Decreased resistance with increased range of motion is characteristic of hypotonia. Approximately 20 percent of children with cerebral palsy will be hypotonic. Often, a phase of hypotonia, which may last variable periods, precedes the picture of hypertonic cerebral palsy. Hypotonia, particularly in infancy, can pose a diagnostic dilemma (Table 11-6).[9]

Muscle Strength

The evaluation of muscle strength is usually performed by comparing the patient's strength with that of the examiner. This can be limited because it requires cooperation. Simple tests like stepping on a bench or standing up from squatting or lying may be helpful. When quantitative measures of muscle strength

Table 11-6
Disease Associated with Hypotonia

Muscle disorders

  Congenital myopathies
  Metabolic myopathies
  Hypothyroidism
  Polymyositis

Neuromuscular junction

  Myasthenia gravis and myasthenic syndrome
  Neonatal myasthenia gravis

Peripheral neuropathies

Anterior horn cell disorders

  Werdnig–Hoffmann disease
  Arthrogryposis multiple congenita

CNS disorder

  Acute cerebral insult
  Chromosomal abnormalities—Down's syndrome
  Toxicity
  Metabolic–degenerative disorders

are needed, a dynamometer or myothenometer can be used.

Muscle weakness is a feature of both hypertonic and hypotonic cerebral palsy. Table 11-7 provides guidelines for the assessment of muscle strength.

Deep Tendon Reflexes

Deep tendon reflexes are usually reported on a scale from 0 (absent) to 4+ (very active). This is an extremely subjective measure and reflects the discretion of the examiner.

Deep tendon reflexes are increased in both hypotonic and hypertonic cerebral palsy and are usually associated with other signs of upper motor neuron involvement. An interesting situation is presented by the child, with the clinical diagnosis of cerebral palsy without deep tendon reflexes. If deep tendon reflexes have never been observed, the diagnosis of cerebral palsy should be reviewed. Slowly progressive polyneuropathies or other lower motor neuron disorders are possible. Diseases that affect the fetus, e.g., Werdnig–Hoffmann disease, render them prone to abnormal deliveries, with the likelihood or superimposed brain damage. Children born by breach presentation may sustain damage to the lumbosacral

Table 11-7
Assessment of Muscle Strength

Number	Description
0	No muscle contraction
1	A flicker, or trace, of concentrations without actual movement, or con tractions may be palpated in the absence of apparent movement; minimal or no motion of joints (0 percent to 10 percent of normal movement)
2	The muscle moves the part through partial arc of movements with gravity eliminated (11 percent to 25 percent of normal movement)
3	The muscle completes the whole arc of movement against gravity (26 percent to 50 percent of normal movement)
4	The muscle completes the whole arc of movement against gravity, together with variable amounts of resistance (51 percent to 75 percent of normal movement)
5	The muscle completes the whole arc of movement against gravity and maximal amount of resistance several times without signs of fatigue; this is normal muscular power (76 percent to 100 percent)

plexus. Children born with myelomeningoceles or other spinal cord malformations can also be included.

If a previously documented deep tendon reflex is no longer elicited, it may be the result of a fixed contracture or an intercurrent disease such as diabetes or uremia.

Abnormal Movements

Long-standing abnormal movements as expressions of brain damage are found in some forms of cerebral palsy. Dystonic–athetoid movement disorders, secondary to basal ganglia damage, are probably the most common. Ballismus, hemiballismus, and cerebellar tremors are also seen. Tics, either as an isolated phenomenon or as a component of Gilles de la Tourette's syndrome, can also occur in cerebral palsy. Repetitive stereotyped movements seen in children with mental retardation are not necessarily a consequence of acquired brain lesions. Movements

of this sort are classically observed in children with autism.

Because of lack of cortical inhibition of lower brain stem and spinal cord centers, severe spastic cerebral palsy can have generalized or localized tonic contractions. This massive reflex response can be mistaken for seizures. Quite frequently contractions can be precipitated by bladder or bowel distention. Myoclonus, seen as brief, sudden jerks in the limbs, might fall into the same category. Reflex rhythmic myoclonus can also be induced by exteroceptive stimulation, e.g., when the patient is changed, bathed, or having physical therapy. Myoclonus can also be the expression of a seizure disorder. A good evaluation of the surrounding circumstances might save unnecessary testing and inappropriate use of antiepileptic therapy. Diphenylhydantoin can induce paroxysmal choreoathetoid movements in the presence of brain damage. Lithium can induce tremors. Haloperidol may produce Parkinsonlike syndromes, and tardive dyskinesia is a complication usually associated with long-standing phenothiazine use. The recent development of movement disorders, therefore, requires further evaluation.

The use of videotapes and the Abnormal Involuntary Movement Scale are of great help in obtaining objective information needed for clinical follow-up study and evaluation of therapies.[10]

Sensory Evaluation

Unless there is a strong suspicions of sensory deficit, it is not necessary to test every senory modality. It is advisable to test all four extremities for changes in sensation to pinprick, touch, position sense, and vibration. This requires patient cooperation and therefore may be difficult to evaluate. Frequently the examiner must be satisfied with indirect responses, such as observations of wincing, mild postural changes, or changes in breathing pattern.

Some tests have been devised to quantitate sensory findings, such as cubes of different sizes, forms of different shapes, or instruments that apply measureable pressure, but since sensation is mostly a subjective phenomenon, its use in uncooperative patients is limited.

Cranial Nerves
Smell and Taste

The sense of smell is tested by the use of nonirritating aromatic substances such as tobacco, perfume, and coffee. The recognition of the aroma, even if not properly identified, is enough to certify the presence of smell. Taste requires the use of substances that are salty, bitter, sour, or sweet. In both cases a high degree of cooperation is needed. There are no bedside quantitative tests, and the results may be inconsistent in children. Deficits in smell and taste have never been fully evaluated in children with cerebral palsy. It is not clear whether deficiencies in smell or taste will further handicap the child.

Facial Nerve

Upper motor neuron disorders of the facial nerve (VII) result in decreased voluntary movements in the opposite lower half of the face (central facial palsy). In lower motor neuron lesions the whole face ipsilateral to the lesion is paralyzed (peripheral face palsy). Facial pareses are more common in hemisyndromes. Children with severe spastic quadriparesis as well as spastic diplegias and choreoathetosis may not show obvious facial involvement. Since the muscles innervated by cranial nerve VII participate in the mimic expression of the face, even uncooperative patients can be evaluated. Some maneuvers that stimulate emotional reactions such as laughing or crying will show asymmetric facial responses in peripheral facial palsy. In the case of central facial palsy, the voluntary performance of tasks, such as opening the mouth or closing the eyes, is needed to show facial asymmetry.

Mild facial asymmetries, although unnoticed in the young child, become more evident in older age. Hemisyndromes resulting from parietal lobe lesions affect the contralateral body growth. The motor component may not be as evident as the asymmetric body growth, which becomes more obvious as the child grows. At one point the facial asymmetry may be perceived as a new sign. Old pictures showing the presence of asymmetric facial movements, and findings such as ipsilateral hemiatrophy, may help to determine the chronic nature of the lesion.

For a discussion on cranial nerves II, III, IV, and VI, which are related to visual function and eye motility, see Chapter 14. Evaluation of cranial nerve VIII (hearing) is discussed in Chapter 16.

Eating and Swallowing

Watching a patient who is eating or drinking is a simple test to be included in the evaluation of every patient with cerebral palsy. Normal swallowing is a complex sensory motor function that requires several cranial nerves.[11]

Swallowing starts with an oral phase in which the food is moved from lips to pharynx, followed by a pharyngeal phase in which the food is passed through the pharynx. Simultaneously, the soft palate seals the nasopharynx to avoid nasal reflux, and the epiglottis closes to avoid aspiration. The esophageal phase, where contraction and relaxation of the upper esophageal spincter propels the bolus into the esophagus, is the last. It takes less than one second for the bolus to travel from the lips to the esophagus.

The motor supply of the oral phase, including sucking, is from the motor branches of cranial nerve VII. Cranial nerves IX and X supply the tensors of the palate, and cranial nerve XII supplies the tongue. The sensory innervation of the inner mucosae of the mouth is carried by nerve V; nerve IX carries the sensation from the palate and uvula. Cranial nerves VII, IX, and X are also responsible for taste. The motor branch of nerve V, which innervates the masseters and temporalis muscles, and of IX and X, which innervate the intrinsic muscle of the pharynx, supply the muscles involved in the pharyngeal phase. Nerve IX is responsible for the sensory innervation of the pharynx. The esophageal phase mostly depends on nerve X, with some contribution from nerve IX. This is the only phase in which the swallowing center is not essential. Thus it can be seen that the function of eating is a complex one involving a number of cranial nerves and their branches.

Poor sucking, nasopharyngeal regurgitation, coughing, and gagging at the time of feeding are the most common symptoms directly associated with swallowing disorders. Failure to thrive and the indirect consequences of recurrent aspiration are found clinically. Swallowing disorders are frequently seen in children with severe cerebral palsy and in almost all dystonic choreoathetotic patients. Bilateral cortical dysfunction in the frontal lobe, brain stem abnormalities (mostly in the pons–medulla areas), peripheral neuropathies, impairment at the neuromuscular junction, and intrinsic disease of muscles can all produce swallowing disorders.

Functional disorders, e.g., spontaneous gastroesophageal reflux or lack of esophageal peristalsis, may also simulate these symptoms. Disorders of swallowing may also be non-neurologic in origin, e.g., anatomic malformation such as cleft and lip palate, micrognathia, foreign bodies in the pharynx or esophagus, and vascular rings.

The presence of swallowing problems in patients with cerebral palsy deserves further evaluation with barium x-ray studies combined with esophageal manometry and endoscopy.[11] (See Chapter 18 for feeding team assessment and function.)

Articulation of words and phrases, as in the case of swallowing, is a function that depends on muscles innervated by nerves with centers in the pons and medulla. Some of the principles mentioned for swallowing also apply in articulation. More detail of disorders in articulation can be found in Chapter 16.

Neck

The muscles that turn the head (sternocleidomastoid) and shrug the shoulders (trapezius) are innervated by cranial nerve XI. In unilateral paralysis of the sternocleidomastoid, the chin is deviated to the opposite side (torticollis). In paralysis of the trapezius, the paralyzed shoulder is lower. In children with cerebral palsy, torticollis is often unrelated to lesions of nerve XI. Congenital hematomas in the sternocleidomastoid cause shortening of the muscle and turning of the head. Patients with cerebral palsy and diplopia may turn the head to one side to compensate for the visual defect. Patients bedridden with severe cerebral palsy and dystonic posturing may have a one-sided preference, and, if no corrective physical therapy is offered, the head will end up fixed in a torticollis posturing.

Acute torticollis may be seen secondary to cervical root compressions and unrelated nerve XI disorders; e.g., children with Down's syndrome have a tendency to subluxate (C1 on C2) and can present with acute torticollis that deserves further evaluation.

Tongue

Cranial nerve XII provides motor innervation of the tongue. Lesions of this nerve produce ipsilateral tongue paralysis with muscle atrophy. If the lesion is in the cerebral cortex or descending tracts, the impairment is contralateral to the lesions. It is unusual to have isolated damage to nerve XII with cerebral palsy. When problems in the movement of the tongue are observed, they are more often the result of central lesions, either in the cortex or in the efferent pathways. These lesions are often responsible for the dysarthria seen in patients with cerebral palsy.

NEURODEVELOPMENTAL EXAMINATION

The first objective of the neurologic examination is to establish a functional developmental level. The milestones reported by history must be confirmed—not only the level reached, but also the quality of the particular skill (See Chapter 19). Some aspects of spasticity may be misinterpreted by the patient or parent as a newly acquired developmental achievement, e.g., the development of pathologically in-

creased extensor neck muscle tone in a hypertonic infant may be misinterpreted as some degree of head control. The importance here is to match the infant's abilities with standardized norms.

The establishment of the neurodevelopmental level is important in order to (1) evaluate the extent of the pathology, (2) Develop the best therapeutic approach to achievement of optimal function, and (3) make a prognosis that will serve as a guideline for long-term management.

A paper by Ellenberg and Nelson discusses the predictive value of some developmental milestones obtained at 4 mo of age for the risk of cerebral palsy at age 7 yr.[6] Special attention was given to the following six milestones: support weight on legs, keep hands open, respond to red ring, support weight on forearm, sit with support, and respond to mirror image. Children who passed all six milestones were unlikely to have cerebral palsy, even in the presence of other abnormalities. Failure to pass any one item increased the risk of cerebral palsy, the last three being the ones with the highest predictive risk (12-fold to 17-fold).

The Special Case of the Newborn

The neurologic examination, as performed on all children, will not be sufficient for the newborn. Prenatal and perinatal damage very often produce a constellation of symptoms with very few or no focal signs. A neurologic examination that can assess the integrity of the nervous system is not necessarily optimal for the assessment of the maturity of the nervous system. Although interdependent, they need different evaluation techniques. To fill this gap, protocols have been developed and standardized[1,12,13] (see Table 11-8).

The screening test developed by Prechtl can help to detect newborns at risk,[3] although it does not lead to a neurologic diagnosis. The items with the most predictive values are body posture, observation of the eyes, spontaneous motor activity, resistance to passive movement, the tactile test, sucking, and motor response.

One of the most important variables is the behavioral state at the time of the examination. This in itself may be an important clinical sign. Responses present when the baby is awake may not be seen when he or she is sleeping. Different stages of sleep, i.e., rapid eye movement or quiet sleep, may affect the intensity of the responses. Factors that can affect the clinical assessment include (1) primary CNS pa-

Table 11-8

Some Expected Responses in Normal Appropriate-for-Gestational-Age Full-Term Infant

Habituation	
Light	Response to negative stimuli (blink or body movement) shut down within 10 stimuli
Sound	Startle reaction followed by decreased response after 5–10 stimuli
Movement and tone	
Posture (at rest)	Full flexion
Arm traction	Arm flexed at elbow at 140 degrees for 5 sec
Leg recoil	Flexion is completed instantaneously or after 5 sec
Leg traction	Knee flexion is maintained between 100–160°.
Head in prone position	Infant lifts head, nose, and chin off
Reflexes	
Walking	Two steps or some efforts with two legs
Sucking–palmar grasp	Present and strong
Neurobehavioral item	
Eyes	Centered, conjugate movements follow horizontally

Adapted from Dubowitz L, Dubowitz V: The Neurological Assessment of the Preterm and Full-Term Newborn Infant. Clinics in Developmental Medicine, no. 79. Philadelphia, Lippincott, 1981.

thology, (2) pathological conditions outside the CNS, e.g., septicemia and respiratory distress syndrome (RDS) and (3) other factors, e.g., maternal medication, jaundice, photo therapy, and hypothermia.

Some signs strongly suggestive of infants at risk are opisthotonic posture, constant head turning to one side, presence of nystagmus, constant strabismus, tremors not associated with crying when observed after the fourth day, asymmetries between right and left or differences between upper and lower extremities, absent or weak Moro reflex, hypotonia, and seizures.

Abnormal neonatal findings do not necessarily allow any prediction about neurologic outcome months or years later, but they are a strict indication for close follow-up study. In some infants the normal signs may disappear but reappear after a period. This silent period is, in itself, a justification for good neurologic screening in the newborn.[1]

The Special Case of the Child with Cerebral Palsy and Sensory Impairment

The presence of developmental delay does not necessarily imply a primary CNS deficiency. Sensory handicaps, either in the visual, hearing, or tactile

sphere, will be responsible for developmental delay even in the absence of CNS damage. The early recognition of sensory deficits improves the benefit of a specific therapy.

Vision

Visual handicap may be the only sensory deficiency, or it may be associated with other motor and sensory deficiencies.[15] A diagnosis of congenital blindness may be made at birth, but it may be difficult to make in some visually handicapped children; e.g., a visually handicapped child with normal intelligence will smile at six weeks of age.

The effect of visual handicaps vary according to associated deficits and the quality of education received. Of 100 children with visual handicaps reported by Zinkin, 68 functioned at three quarters of the level for their age, but Morris claimed that 66 blind children, with no other major handicap and with proper early education, reached the same level as their school-aged peers.[15,16]

Some aspects of development are strongly influenced by vision. Among them are the concepts of visual third dimension, which, in turn, conditions some motor milestones like pointing with the index finger, following falling objects, and transferring objects from hand to hand. Therefore, hand development could be delayed. A visually handicapped child will move the legs and feet more than the hands and arms. Pincer grasp may not be seen until the second year of life. All aspects of self-initiated motility, i.e., rolling, standing, crawling, and walking, will also be delayed. The parachute reaction is another example. Few severely impaired children develop it before 18 mo of age.

The poor visual–verbal link may be responsible for language delay. Expressions such as "no" and "give me," which are usually said in association with body gestures, require more time to be learned. Blind children also tend to be echolalic.

Hearing

In the case of hearing loss, language delay will be the main, if not the only, area affected. The diagnosis of hearing deficiency may be difficult at times in children with mild hearing deficits. Noise makers can not detect hearing loss limited to the middle to higher frequencies, and babies with residual hearing will respond normally.[17] Clapping hands, banging cubes, and stomping feet may create vibrations that can produce reactions in a hearing-impaired child. Normal children with a hearing impairment are invariably visually alert. Sound stimulations by bells in the peripheral visual field may produce pseudo-reaction. As happens with visual handicaps, hearing deficits are also frequent in children with cerebral palsy (see Chapter 16). Since language development

is most probably the best predictor of future cognitive functions, the presence of a hearing impairment should be evaluated as soon as possible.

Approximately 1:1000 neonates have a hearing impairment, but the incidence is 30–40 times higher in infants with certain risk conditions.[17]

SPECIAL INVESTIGATIONS

Metabolic Studies

Inborn errors in the metabolism of amino acids, lipids, carbohydrates, and organic acids almost always interfer with brain development.[18] They produce an array of neurologic signs that have developmental delay or mental retardation as a common denominator.

Useful screening tests are presented in Table 11-9. When positive, they should be followed by a more specific biochemical analysis and assay that require sophisticated laboratory tests. Some of these tests can also be used to identify carriers and diagnose affected fetuses in utero.

Electron microscopic (EM) examination of blood cells, skin, and conjunctival biopsies give nearly as much information as brain biopsy in the evaluation of lysosomal storage disorders.[18] Culture of the fibroblasts and amniotic fluid cells have shown diagnostic abnormalties of storage diseases, allowing a prenatal diagnosis (see Chapter 8).[19,20]

Table 11-9
Screening Test for Detection of Inborn Metabolic Disorders of the Nervous System

Test	Disease
Ferric chloride	Phenylketonuria (PKU)
Dinitrophenylhydrazine	Maple syrup urine disease
Cyanide nitroprusside	Homocystinuria
Blood ammonia	Urea cycle disorders
Benedict	Galactosemia; fructose intolerance
Berry spot and acid albumin turbidity	Mucopolysaccharides
Amino acids in blood and urine	In disorders involving overflow or transport defect, aminoacidopathies

Methods of Brain Imaging

Skull X-ray Study

With the introduction of computed tomography (CT) scanning, skull x-ray studies are no longer used in the routine evaluation of children with cerebral palsy. Their use is limited to document abnormalities of skull structures, e.g., fractures and craniosynostosis, or occasionally as an adjunct to the diagnosis of other diseases, e.g., Gaucher's disease, Niemann–Pick disease, or to document intracranial calcification as occurs with congenital infections.

Pneumoencephalogram

Pneumoencephalogram (PEG) was once the most commonly performed procedure. It has been reduced to almost total obsolescence by the advent of the CT scan.

Angiography

The visualization of the cerebral vasculature can be obtained by the intra-arterial injection of contrast material. In competent hands it is a complex but safe technique. In general, sedation is needed, but in some patients general anesthesia is necessary.

Cerebral angiography is particularly useful for the diagnosis or localization of intracranial vascular lesions, arteriovenous malformations, aneurysms, or chronic arthritis. For these lesions it is superior to CT scan, but its use in children with cerebral palsy is limited.

Echoencephalography

The technique for echoencephalography is simple. Sedation is usually not necessary, and it is a relatively quick procedure, lasting 30 min at the most. In contrast to CT scans, the equipment is small enough for bedside examination, and no radiation is involved. This makes it suitable for obstetric and fetal diagnosis.[21] It is also useful in newborn and children up to 4 or 5 yr of age while the skull is still unilaminar. After this age, the skull structure becomes diploic and acts as a shield, deflecting sound waves and limiting its use.[22]

Intrauterine ultrasonic cephalometry is used to measure the growth of the fetus in utero.[21,23] Prenatal diagnosis of fetal CNS malformations have been achieved by Hobbins in cases of anencephaly, hydrocephalus, porencephalic cysts, and meningocele.[24] Harvey et al used biparietal diameter measurements serially before and after delivery and were able to predict, at birth, which small-for-gestational-age (SGA) babies were more likely to have problems with perceptual performance and motor ability.[25]

Ultrasound is also accurate in the diagnosis of intraventricular bleeding and hydrocephalus and is used extensively in premature infants for the diagnosis and monitoring of these conditions.[26,27]

CT Scanning

The introduction of CT scanning in the last few years has had a profound impact on the practice of neurology. The CT scan is 100-times more sensitive than conventional radiography. The amount of radiation needed for a complete study is approximately one third of the dose of a single lateral skull x-ray film.[22,28] Contrast enhancement can be obtained with intravenous (IV) injections of radiopaque material.

CT scans are invaluable in the diagnosis of disorders that affect the ventricular system or produce distortion in the anatomic structure of the brain.[29]

They are indicated for the diagnosis of brain or brain stem tumors, progressive degeneration diseases of the CNS, presence of epileptic disorder, severe head trauma, acute and chronic infections of the CNS, comas of unknown origin, and suspicion of cerebrovascular accidents. They are not indicated following minor head trauma, and the scan has a low diagnostic yield for simple headaches, syncopal attacks, or dizziness without other neurologic signs.[30]

In children with cerebral palsy, the CT scan shows a high degree of accuracy in the diagnosis of developmental anomalies of the brain, the presence of generalized or localized brain atrophy, the evaluation of sequelae of cerebrovascular accidents, and the detection of intracranial calcifications. In the presence of hydrocephalus, the CT scan provides measurements of ventricular size as well as the thickness of the cerebral mantle. In obstructive hydrocephalus, the localization of the lesion can be determined. In patients with intraventricular shunts, the reduction of the ventricular size that follows the shunt placement and potential complications can be readily recognized.

Normal CT scans are not unusual in children with cerebral palsy. Some forms of cerebral dysgenesis, such as micropolygyria or neuronal heterotropias (see Chap. 2), and some of the causes leading to cerebral palsy, e.g., hypoxic–ischemic encephalopathies, produce changes at microscopical levels that will not be visible on CT scan. Structural lesions smaller than 1 cm may not be seen either.

New advances in technology have extended the use of the CT scan to the whole body. In the case of children with cerebral palsy, this will be of great help in the delineation of malformations of the lower spinal cord, e.g., small myelomeningoceles and syringomyelic cavitations.

Myelography

In children with cerebral palsy, myelography is indicated for the evaluation of spinal dysraphism or in cases of severe kyphoscoliosis when spinal cord compression is suspected.

Neurophysiologic Studies

Electroencephalogram

The electroencephalogram (EEG) is the most widely accepted technique for the evaluation of the neurophysiologic status of the brain. It is extremely useful in the diagnosis of epilepsy and is also a helpful adjunct in the evaluation of other CNS disorders.

Although the American EEG Society has set standards for EEG recordings, the wording of an EEG report is a matter of personal style.[31] The report usually has one of the three conclusions: normal, borderline, or abnormal.

Normal.   A normal EEG does not exclude the possibility of an epileptic disorder. Usually an EEG recording lasts 40–60 min, hence, any epileptiform activity that is less frequent than 1 an hour may not be seen in the first EEG. Besides, some epileptiform patterns are activated during sleep; therefore, an EEG that does not include drowsy and sleep states should be considered incomplete. If epilepsy is suspected, it is worthwhile to repeat the EEG with sleep deprivation or special procedures such as nasopharyngeal leads, sphenoidal leads, or, more rarely, chemical activation.

Repeated normal awake and sleep recordings reduce the likelihood of epilepsy. Furthermore, if a behavior suspected of being epileptic is observed with simultaneous normal EEG recordings, it is most probably not epileptiform in origin. Normal repeated EEGs can be found in patients in whom epilepsy is strongly suspected, however. In those cases, clinical judgment should prevail.

Normal EEGs are not unusual in children with cerebral palsy, particularly in the absence of epileptic disorders or structural lesions in the brain.

Borderline.   Borderline EEGs can be reported as borderline–normal or borderline–abnormal. The term is justifiable in the presence of (1) patterns of uncertain significance; after 40 yr of clinical experience, controversies still remain on the interpretation of certain patterns, e.g., positive spikes at 14–6 cps,[32] (2) artifacts, i.e., extracerebral activity recorded on the EEG that may occasionally be very difficult to differentiate from real cerebral activity, (3) other factors, e.g., medications (phenobarbital produces an increase in fast activities while diphenylhydantoin produces slowing), normal variations (old age produces a generalized slowing), and subtle deviations from normality (mild interhemispheric asymmetries, and poorly developed sleep patterns).[33]

In any event, any EEG reported as borderline should be followed by a personal discussion with an electroencephalographer to place it in the proper clinical context.

Abnormal.   Abnormal EEGs are found in a wide spectrum of CNS disturbances, which will not be discussed extensively in this chapter. It should be appreciated that EEG characteristics are the result of a combination of external and internal factors interacting with genetic factors. An EEG that shows abnormal patterns, even epileptiform abnormalities, may therefore be an expression of a genetic trait. Metrakos and Metrakos found spikes and wave discharges of 3 cps, with classic EEG patterns of the so-called centrencephalic or petit mal seizure in asymptomatic relatives of epileptic patients.[34] Olofson et al. showed the presence of paroxysmal activity, some resembling epileptiform patterns, in 2.7 percent of normal awake children and in more than 8 percent of children during drowsiness and light sleep.[35]

In view of these possibilities, an EEG referral should elaborate all the clinical symptoms and the reason for this request. Statements such as "Please do EEG. Patient has cerebral palsy" are technically unsatisfactory and do not fully use the skills of the clinical electroencephalographer.

Long-Term Monitoring

Radiotelemetry.   Recent technologic advances have increased the scope of EEGs. The use of EEG transmitted by radiotelemetry, combined with visual television recordings, provides a composite image of the patient with simultaneous EEG.[36] The patient can be observed in an unrestricted environment, and the EEGs can be several hours long. This technique allows correlation between abnormal behaviors and EEG changes and is particularly useful in the differential diagnosis between seizures and pseudoseizures.[37]

Portable cassette recordings.   Another useful method for long-term EEG recording is through the use of a portable cassette recording system.[38] The EEG is collected by amplifiers small enough to be hidden under normal hair and is recorded on a standard C-120 audio-cassette that is carried by the patient. This system is ideal for long-term EEG recording at home, work, and school without disruption of normal activities and without drawing the attention of classmates or friends. As with radiotelemetry, this is useful in the differential diagnosis of epilepsy and related disorders. In contrast with radiotelemetry, the clinical correlation of behaviors and EEG is obtained from descriptions by relatives, peers, or the patient. This is a limitation in that the temporal correlation might not be accurate.

EEG of the Newborn

The EEG of the newborn deserves special mention. Besides being of help as a diagnostic tool, certain EEG patterns during the newborn period are statistically reliable in predicting neurologic outcome.[39]

Rose and Lambroso in 1970, found a normal neurologic outcome in almost 90 percent of newborns with normal EEGs when examined at age 4–7 yr.[40] Even in the presence of clinical seizures, a normal EEG was associated with normal neurologic development in 75 percent of the children by age 5 yr. When the EEG was abnormal, the chance of normal neurologic examinations by age 5 was as low as 10 percent in some subgroups.

The use of serial EEG–polygraphic recordings might improve the determination of the prognostic profile of babies "at risk," e.g., hypoxic–ischemic insults, and might also prove to be a useful tool in evaluating the effect of therapies.[14] The EEG in newborn infants has also been found to be reliable in assessment of gestational age.[41]

BRAIN-EVOKED POTENTIALS

The advent of computer averaging of brain activity has made possible the evaluation of minute response to volleys of sensory stimulation. These tests are recognized as *evoked potentials* or *event-related potentials*. This technique is nonpainful, requires minimal cooperation, and can be done in infants and in patients with severe mental retardation.[42]

Evoked potentials should be considered in the evaluation of visual and hearing deficits when conventional methods fail.

Visual-Evoked Potentials

Normal visual-evoked potentials (VEPs) suggest that the visual system is most probably intact. It does not, however, guarantee that the information is appropriately used, since deficits in other structures may render the input nonfunctional.[43] Children with damage to the occipital cortex may show the presence of early components of VEPs with absence of late components. These children are behaviorally blind, even though the eye examination, including pupillary reflexes, can be normal.[44]

Although most often abnormal VEPs are the result of damage in the neural pathway, abnormalities can result from impaired vision, cataracts, refractory defects, visual field defects, and glaucoma.

Auditory-Evoked Potentials

In a clinical setting, auditory evoked potentials (AEPs) can be used to estimate hearing acuity and also as a diagnostic method to detect lesions in the auditory pathway.

Cortical electrical response audiometry can be used to determine, within a few decibels, the subjective hearing threshold.[45,46] This requires some cooperation and therefore may be difficult in young infants or children with brain damage.[47] The use of sedation can also affect the responses.[48]

AEP is useful when behavioral audiometry fails to elicit consistent responses. In this situation, the presence of cortical auditory-evoked responses indicates that the anatomic pathway is intact. This response does not imply that the patient can use the information in any meaningful way. In uncooperative patients, the benefit of a hearing aid can be assessed by AEP.[49]

A special situation is presented by children with cerebral palsy who are not deaf but are unable to speak. These patients may have normal responses to behavioral or impedance audiometry, which is a reflex activity based on brain stem centers. In these patients, the early components of the AEP, which reflects eighth nerve and brain stem activity, are normal, but the late components, which reflect cortical activity, may be abnormal, implying some form of dysfunction. It is suggested that this type of expressive language disorder may not respond to therapy, since it probably represents damage to the receptive areas of speech.

ELECTROMYOGRAPHY

Electromyography (EMG) can be performed with either surface (skin) or deep needle electrodes.

Surface EMG

The surface EMG is a simple, nonpainful, noninvasive technique, especially useful for the evaluation of groups of muscles in action, but it does not provide information about intrinsic muscle disorders or about disorders of neuromuscular junction. It may be useful in the study of patients with cerebral palsy who have orthopaedic disorders or when muscle rehabilitation therapy is indicated. Gait disorders can also be evaluated with surface EMG (see Chap. 12).

Recent advances in the neurophysiology and neuropharmocology of movement disorders have opened a new field for surface EMG. Recently, Hallet and Alvarez, using surface EMGs through a flexion–extension task involving the arms, established different patterns of abnormalities in patients with athetoid dystonic movement disorders, some of them amenable to treatment with EMG biofeedback.[50]

Needle EMG

The needle EMG is more complex. An electrode must be inserted into the muscles, and this produces discomfort and, quite often, pain. The use of needle EMG in cerebral palsy is very limited, since there is no specific EMG pattern associated with upper motor neuron disease. It is most suitable for the evaluation of lower motor unit disorders (anterior horn cell neuron, peripheral roots and nerves, neuromuscular junction, and muscle).

In children with myelomeningoceles, EMG helps to recognize the extent of the lesion. It might also be useful in the evaluation of the anal and urethral sphincter function. This is important in the management of the neurogenic bladder. Sometimes, congenital myopathies developing in the fetus may be responsible for dystocic deliveries. In these cases, specific EMG patterns will help to delineate the pathology in these hypotonic infants.

NERVE CONDUCTION TIME

The use of nerve conduction time is limited, since the causes of cerebral palsy do not produce damage to the peripheral nervous system. Recently, however, Alvarez and colleagues[7] reported several cases of median nerve compressions (carpal tunnel syndrome) in patients with athetotic–dystonic cerebral palsy. Some patients were asymptomatic. Patients who are bedridden, confined to wheelchairs, or use crutches are susceptible to traumatic neuropathies. It is in this group of patients susceptible to traumatic or compressive neuropathies that nerve conduction time can be of help in the management of cerebral palsy.

REFERENCES

1. Prechtl H: The Neurological Examination of the Full Term Newborn Infant (ed 2). no. 63. Philadelphia, Lippincott, 1977
2. Kenburg FW, Dodds JB: Denver Developmental Screening Test. Boulder, University of Colorado, 1969
3. Bayley N: Bayley Scale of Infant Development. New York, The Psychological Corporation, 1969
4. Touwen B: Neurological Development in Infancy. Clinics in Developmental Medicine, no. 58. Philadelphia, Lippincott, 1976
5. Smith D: Recognizable Patterns of Human Malformations, vol. VII. Major Problems in Clinical Pediatrics (ed 2). Philadelphia, Saunders, 1976
6. Ellenberg J, Nelson K: Early recognition of infants at high risk for cerebral palsy: Examination at four months. Dev Med Child Neurol 23:703, 1981
7. Alvarez N, Larkin C, Roxborough J: Carpel tunnel syndrome in dystonic athetoid cerebral palsy. Arch Neurol 11:311, 1982
8. Hallet M: Unpublished data
9. Dubowitz V: The Floppy Infant. Clinics in Developmental Medicine, no. 76 (ed 2). Philadelphia, Lippincott Co. 1980
10. Sandoz Pharmaceutical: A simple method to determine tardive dyskinesia symptoms. Aims examination procedure, East Hanover, NJ 1981
11. Fisher S, Painter M, Milmoe E: Swallowing disorders in infancy. Pediatr Clin North Am 28:845, 1981
12. Brazelton TB: Neonatal Behavior Assessment Scales. Clinic in Developmental Medicine, no 50. London, Heinemann, 1973
13. Dubowitz V, Dubowitz L: The Neurological Assessment of the Preterm and Full-Term Newborn Infant. Clinic in Developmental Medicine, no. 79. Philadelphia, Lippincott, 1981
14. Lombroso CT: Neurophysiological observations in diseased newborns. Biol Psychiatr 527, 1975
15. Zinkin PM: The Effect of Visual Handicapped in Early Development. Clinics in Developmental Medicine, no. 73. Philadelphia, Lippincott, 1979
16. Morris M: What affects blinds children's development? New Outlook Blind 50:258, 1956
17. Froa TJ: Assessment of hearing. Pediatr Clin North Am 28:757, 1981
18. Kolodny E, Cable WSL: Inborn errors of metabolism. Ann Neurol 11:221, 1982
19. Ornoy A, Sekeces B, Cohen R, et al: Electromicroscopy of cultured fibroblasts in amniotic fluid cells in the diagnosis of hereditary storage diseases. Monogr Hum Genet 10:32, 1978
20. Laboratory Report: Mayo Clin Proc 57:192, 1982
21. Campbell S: An improved method of fetal cephalometry by ultrasound. J Obstet Gynecol Br Commonw 75:586, 1968
22. Phelps ME, Hoffman EJ, Terporgosian MM: Attenuation coefficient of various body tissues, fluids and lesions at photo energies of 18 to 136 Kev. Radiology 117:573, 1975
23. Campbell S, Newman GB: Growth of the fetal biparietal diameter during normal pregnancy. J Obstet Gynecol Br Commonw 78:513, 1971
24. Hobbins J: Ultrasound in the diagnosis of congenital anomalies, Am J Obstet Gynecol 134:331, 1979
25. Harbey D, Prince S, Bunton J, et al: Abilities of children who were small for gestational age babies. Pediatrics 69:296, 1982
26. Pape KE, Wigglesworth JS: Haemorrhage, Ischemia and the Perinatal Brain. Clinics in Developmental Medicine, no. 69/70. Philadelphia, Lippincott, 1979
27. Levine MI, Wiggelsworth JS, Dubowitz V: Cerebral structure and intraventricular hemorrhage in the neonate: A real-time ultrasound study. Arch Dis Child 56:416, 1981

28. Perry BJ, Bridges C: Computarized transverse axial scanning (tomography). IV. Radiation dose considerations. Br J Radiol 46:1048, 1973

29. Baker Jr HL, Campbell JK, Houser OW: et al: Early experience with the EMI scanner for the study of the brain. Radiology 116:327, 1975

30. CT Scan Consensus Panel: Office for Medical Application of Research, Bethesda, MD

31. Klass DW, Daly DD (eds): Current Practice of Clinical Electroencephalography. New York, Raven Press, 1979

32. Mavsby RL: EEG patterns of uncertain significance, in Klass DW, Daly DD (eds): Current Practice of Clinical Electroencephalography. New York, Raven Press, 1979

33. Low M: Evaluation of psychiatric disorders and the effects of psychotherapeutic and psychotomimetic agents, in Klass DW, Daly DD (eds): Current Practice of Clinical Electroencephalography. New York, Raven Press, 1979

34. Metrakos K, Metrakos JH: Genetics of epilepsy, in Vinken PJ, Bruyn GW (eds): Handbook of Clinical Neurology, vol. 15. The Epilepsies. New York, American Elsevier, 1974

35. Olofsson O, Petersen J, Seldon U: The development of the electroencephalogram in normal children from the age of one through fifteen years. Paroxysmal activity. Neuropadiatrie 2:375, 1971

36. Porter RJ: Methodology of continuing monitoring with videotape recording and electroencephalography, in Wada JA, Penry JK (eds): Advances in Epileptology. The Tenth Epilepsy International Symposium. New York, Raven Press, 1980

37. Neill J, Alvarez N, Courcelle R: Differential diagnosis between seizures and pseudoseizures in mentally retarded. Paper presented at the 53rd Annual Meeting of the EPA, Baltimore, April 16, 1982

38. Sato S, Penry KF, Dreifus FE: Electroencephalographic monitoring of generalized spike wave paroxysm in the hospital and at home, in Kellaway, Petersen I (eds): Quantitative Analytic Studies in Epilepsy. New York, Raven Press, 1976

39. Obrecht R, Pollock MA, Evans S, et al: Predictions of outcome in neonates using EEG. Clin Electroenceph 13:46, 1982

40. Rose AL, Lombroso CT: Neonatal seizure states: A study of clinical pathological and electroencephalographic features in 137 full-term babies with long term follow up. Pediatrics 45:404, 1970

41. Lombroso CT: Quantified encephalographic scales on 10 preterm healthy newborns followed to 40–43 weeks CA by serial polygraphic recordings. Electroencephalographic clinic. Neurophysiology 46:460, 1979

42. Bickford R: Newer methods of recording and analyzing EEGs, in Klass DW, Daly DD (eds): Current Practice of Clinical Electroencephalography. New York, Raven Press, 1979

43. Goodn D, Squires K, Starr A: Long latency event related components of the auditory evoked potentials in dementia. Brain 101:635, 1979

44. Bodis–Wallner R: Visual association control and vision in man: Pattern evoked occipital potentials in a blind boy. Science 198:629, 1977

45. Gibson WPR: Essentials of Clinical Electrical Response Audiometry. Edinburgh, Churchill & Livingstone 1978

46. Davis H, Hirsch SK, Shelnutt J, et al: Further validation of evoked response audiometry (ERA). J Speech Hearing Res 10:717, 1967

47. Beagley HA, Gibson WPR: ERA in the diagnosis and treatment of hearing impaired children. Paper read at VIII Curso Monografico Y I Curso-Symposium International Sobre Nuevas Technicas de Exploracion Auditivas, Seville, Spain, 1974

48. Davis, H: Sedation of young children for electric response audiometry (ERA). Audiology 12:55, 1973

49. Rapin I, Graziannil S: Auditory evoked responses in normal brain damage and deaf infants. Neurology 17:881, 1967

50. Hallet M, Alvarez N: Derangement of voluntary movement in athetosis. Presented at the 105th annual meeting of the American Neurological Association, Boston, September 7–10, 1980

Ronald R. Riso,
E. Byron Marsolais

12

Electromyography and Gait Analysis

The use of instrumented gait analysis is among the most promising and productive developments for guiding the management of gait abnormalities in cerebral palsy patients. The principal application of electromyography (EMG) and gait analysis is to provide accurate timing information so that the investigator can determine when particular muscles are active during the walking cycle. This investigation into the coordination and orchestration of the various muscles demands that the electrical activity of the muscles be recorded while the person is actually walking with his or her characteristic gait and is properly referred to as "dynamic electromyography".

Such studies are particularly important to the understanding of cerebral palsy gait because the primary deficiencies are ones of neuromuscular control rather than muscle paralysis or weakness. Single muscles rarely operate in isolation. Through the stretch reflexes, an individual muscle can affect the activity of itself, its synergists, and its antagonists. Through the mechanism of the mass limb reflexes, the joint positions of the hip and knee can influence the activity of the muscles of the foot and ankle by purely neurophysiologic means. The vestibular system, too, has its influence and exerts changes in muscle tone whenever postural adjustments are made, such as in standing versus lying. This hierarchy of control is disrupted by damage to the brain and results in the diversity of gait disorders seen with cerebral palsy.[48]

Physicians' inability to describe and localize precisely the brain lesions present in each patient makes it difficult t predict how the damaged locomotor control system will operate when various surgical interventions are suggested. Furthermore, the enormous capacity for one muscle to be influenced by other muscles, joint positions, and postural changes makes static, isolated muscle testing frequently inaccurate. Dynamic EMG and gait analysis is now making it possible to produce a profile of each patient's muscle activity and limb motion during walking.

EQUIPMENT

EMG is the electrical registration of the ionic events that take place along the muscle fiber membranes during their excitation and contraction. The essential items required to perform dynamic EMG are (1) suitable electrodes to sense the electrical muscle activity, (2) a preamplifier to boost the weak electrical signals (usually only a few hundred microvolts) so that they can be transmitted without interference from environmental electrical noise and from lead wire motion artifact, (3) recording, analysis, and display apparatus such as oscilloscopes, audio monitors, tape recorders, and computer graphics, and (4) a foot-switch system capable of recording foot-to-floor contact patterns for each leg to provide an accurate record of the stance and swing events of the gait cycle against which the EMG data can be evaluated.

Differential Amplification

The most satisfactory EMG recordings are obtained with high-impedance differential amplifiers. This requires that at least two spatially distinct "active

117

electrode" sites be provided for each muscle being recorded and that a third (generally remote) location be employed for the attachments of a *ground* or *reference* electrode.

The reference electrode enables the differential amplifier to record only those signals that are specific to the active electrodes and that presumably originate in the muscle mass between them. Extraneous signals produced by remote sources such as the heart beat (electrocardiographic [ECG] signals) influence the reference electrode in combination with each of the active electrodes about equally and are excluded by the mechanism of differential amplification from the amplifier output.

Electrodes

EMGs are recorded with a variety of electrode types, each of which is best suited to a particular application. The major types used are surface-mounted electrodes and indwelling, fine wire, or needle electrodes. The number of muscle fibers whose electrical activity is recorded between the two active electrodes largely depends on the distance between them and on the surface area of the active electrodes. The recording tips of indwelling-type electrodes are very small in comparison to the gross contact area of the EMG surface-type electrodes. The major distinction between surface and indwelling electrode types is thus their ability to isolate the activity of a specific region of the muscle being studied.

Surface Electrodes

Surface electrodes (Fig. 12-1) are primarily suited to record the gross, massed activity of large muscles or muscle groups such as the gastrocnemius or the quadriceps femoris.[18,54] This characteristic renders them inappropriate for the study of small or deep muscles.

Indwelling Needle and Fine Wire Electrodes

For the study of deep muscles, such as the tibialis posterior, or when the individual activity of each of a group of small muscles, such as the peroneals, must be isolated, indwelling electrodes must be employed.

Very discreet regions of a particular muscle are typically studied using coaxial needle electrode arrangements (see Fig. 12-1). These are capable of registering single motor unit and isolated muscle fiber activity and are popularly used in electrodiagnostic laboratories.[10] Because of their rigid shaft, however, they are mainly used when studying restricted or isometric contractions and are not suitable for gait EMG studies, where the muscles may undergo large excursions beneath the surface of the overlying skin.

This difficulty is overcome by using extremely flexible, fine wire electrodes that are inserted percutaneously into the specific muscles under study with the aid of a hypodermic needle (see Fig. 12-1).[2] During insertion, the location of the electrode tips can be verified by stimulating the muscle through these electrodes. After confirming that the electrode tips

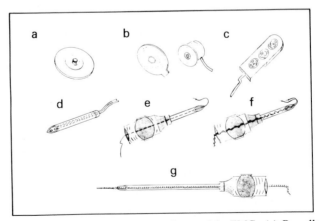

Figure 12-1.   Various types of electrodes used in EMG. (a) Pregelled disposable surface electrode; (b) reusable surface electrode with adhesive collar; (c) surface electrode with built-in preamplifier; (d) bipolar coaxial needle electrode; (e) monopolar indwelling electrode; (f) bifilar indwelling electrode; (g) special coiled wire indwelling electrode for chronic recording.

are, in fact, within the intended muscle, the hypodermic needle is withdrawn, leaving the fine wire electrodes behind. Discomfort upon insertion can be minimized by using sharp needles of small caliber (no. 23–26 gauge depending on the diameter of wire used).

Once installed, the fine wire electrodes are not felt, and the electrodes are practically innocuous. When it is time to remove the electrodes, a steady gentle pull straightens the hook at the tip and brings the wires out intact. A small possibility exists that an electrode tip could break off and remain behind in the tissue. The experience of many investigators has shown this to be an extremely rare occurrence when wire of at least 50 μ in diameter is employed; if this does happen, the small fragment of wire will cause no harm.[1] Because of its biologically inert properties, stainless steel wire is recommended. Silver and copper should be avoided because of their toxicity.[16,20] The material used to insulate the wire is also important. Insulation that consists of polyurethane and other plastics has been shown to have toxic properties.[5]

A special coiled wire electrode has been designed for use in truly "chronic" recording situations (see Fig. 12-1), in which percutaneous electrodes remain in place and function for months or even years.[13,47] These coiled wire electrodes exist in either single-filament or bifilar designs.

PROCESSING OF SIGNALS AND DISPLAY

The processing of EMG signals has been the subject of considerable research.[31] For purposes of this discussion, simple on-off information (phasing) about muscle activity is all that is determined from the EMG records. Data are filtered to improve the signal-to-noise ratio. The filter settings must be carefully chosen, however, to avoid removing substantial components of the EMG signal.[21,25,38] Automated evaluation of EMG data in gait studies is being developed to aid in interpreting the results.[3]

The amplitude of the recorded EMG signal is a function of many elements, including recording parameters such as electrode geometry, interelectrode spacing, position over or within the muscle, electrode impedance, and amplifier gain and bandpass (filter) characteristics.[34,76] The relationship between the force output of the muscle and the amplitude of the EMG signal depends not only on these details of the recording apparatus but also on certain physiologic conditions of the patient's neuromuscular system, e.g., fatigue, temperature, velocity of the movement, and the effects of any drugs that the patient may be using. For these reasons, care must be observed when comparing EMG data recorded from different patients or even from the same patient at different times. Reference to a number of studies on EMG and on the recording of bioelectrical events will be of assistance.[9,17,19,22–24,33,42]

FOOTSWITCH SYSTEM

A footswitch system capable of recording foot-to-floor contact patterns for each leg provides an accurate record of the stance and swing events of the gait cycle against which the EMG data can be evaluated. A simple trielectrode arrangement can be made with three separate strips of aluminum tape, each fixed to the medial, lateral, and heel portions, respectively, of each of the patient's shoes. With the shoes prepared in this fashion, the patient walks along an electrically conductive walkway while appropriate electronic circuitry records the contact events of the shoes with the floor.

DYNAMIC EMG OF A NORMAL CHILD'S GAIT

EMG data about gait function in normal and abnormal children and adults has been made available through many investigators.[7,11,12,15,28,40,44–46,50,64,68–70,73,75] In normal gait, the walk cycle is divided into the *stance* phase, in which the foot is in contact with the ground, and the *swing* phase, in which the foot is swung forward through the air in preparation for the next step. The stance phase accounts for approximately the first 60 percent of the cycle; the swing phase, for the remaining 40 percent.[50] Okamoto and Kumamoto found the length of the stance phase to be age related.[46] It represents approximately 50 percent of the gait cycle when measured about 3 mo after the onset of independent ambulation, but by 2 yr of age, stance duration begins to gradually increase until it plateaus at 62 percent at about 7 yr of age. In the cerebral palsy gait, Bleck has noted that a shortened stance phase relative to swing and a higher cadence are frequent findings.[7]

In normal gait the muscles of the posterior calf (posterior tibialis, triceps surae, and flexors of the toes) as well as the peroneals are active just after heel-strike to just before toe-off.[44,63,69] The dorsi-flexors of the foot are active primarily during the swing phase beginning just before toe-off but continue on until heel-strike is ended and foot-flat is achieved (from 50 percent of one gait cycle on into about 10 percent of the next). The hip extensors and the muscles of the thigh (gluteals, quadriceps, and hamstrings) are active from late swing through early stance (from 90 percent of 1 cycle through 10 percent of the succeeding gait cycle). One component of the quadriceps group, the rectus femoris, shows an additional activation period, from about 50–70 percent of the gait cycle. The hip adductors are active in late stance, from about 40–60 percent of the cycle, while the flexors of the hip (iliopsoas and sartorius) show activity at early swing, from about 60–80 percent of the gait cycle.[50]

SOME PROPERTIES OF ABNORMAL MUSCLES IN CEREBRAL PALSY

Studies employing dynamic electromyography have revealed some surprising results about the nature of spasticity and the properties of abnormal muscles in cerebral palsy.

Holt has shown that although stretch applied to a spastic muscle may increase that muscle's activity and hence intensify its spasticity (the classic expectation), in the same patient other hyperactive muscles may show markedly decreased activity when stretched.[32] As illustrated in Figure 12-2, the gastrocnemius, when at rest, showed considerable hyperactivity. When stretch was applied, however, activity was drastically reduced. Finally, release of the stretched muscle resulted in a rebound of activity in not only the gastrocnemius but also in the tibialis anterior.

Additional observations about the EMG responses of muscles to passive stretch and voluntary effort in cerebral palsy patients have been reported by Milner-Brown and Penn.[43] They have found in

many patients that voluntary movement of the knee joint is not necessarily impaired if either the flexor (hamstrings) or extensor (quadriceps) muscle groups retains the ability to contract upon activation and relax upon lengthening, even though the antagonist muscle group may exhibit continuous activity irrespective of the position of the joint or direction of the movement. According to these investigators, another frequently encountered situation in the lower limb of still other cerebral palsy patients was that both the knee flexors and the knee extensors showed reflexive activity in response to stretch applied to the flexors.

Holt also demonstrated that the functional activity of a muscle during locomotion may not be predicted from, and in fact may be actually reversed from, what is observed during isolated voluntary activity.[32] Figure 12-3 illustrates a situation in which a cerebral palsy patient with a drop-foot gait was found to possess good voluntary dorsiflexion when tested manually, and a strong dorsiflexor EMG was obtained. Yet during gait, the dorsiflexors were electrically silent. The opposite situation, in which EMG activity is present during gait but no activity is present during volitional effort, may also be encountered.

From the above observations, it is apparent that physical examination alone may not always reliably predict muscular activity during locomotion.

USE OF EMG STUDIES IN PLANNING SURGICAL TREATMENT

Muscle Release or Recessions

The value of dynamic EMG studies in planning surgery has been documented by many authors.[6,7,14,48–51,53,60,71] Perry initially investigated the validity of the traditional Silfverskiöld stretch test (Fig. 12-4) in determining whether there is a fixed contracture in the gastrocnemius or soleus muscle or in both.[53] The test is based on the anatomic fact that since the gastrocnemius is a two-jointed muscle, it

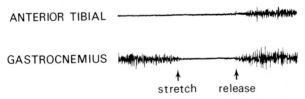

Figure 12-2. Stretch applied to hyperactive gastrocnemius muscle caused a reduction in hyperactivity. Release of stretch resulted in rebound activity in both the gastrocnemius and anterior tibial muscles.

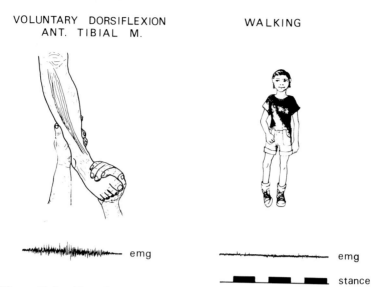

Figure 12-3. Manual muscle test results may not predict activity of muscle during walking. At left, patient successfully produces a voluntary contraction of anterior tibial muscle. (Note strong EMG activity.) At right, patient walks with drop-foot gait, and no activation of dorsiflexors occurs.

will be stretched when the knee is extended, but the soleus, which operates only across the ankle joint, will not be thus affected. If the ankle can be passively brought into dorsiflexion when the knee is flexed but not when the knee is extended (the positive test result), it is concluded that there is a contracture in the gastrocnemius but not in the soleus. Of 17 cerebral palsy patients with persistent equinus gait who underwent evaluation, 8 tested positively using the Silfverskiöld test. Yet under general anesthesia (which eliminates all neurologic input to the muscles), none of

these patients showed any significant differences in range of dorsiflexion with a change in knee position. None of the eight positive tests was therefore due to contracture per se but only to changes in neurologic tone due to knee position.

This finding alone would not seem to invalidate wholly the slow stretch test, since muscle tightness induced by extension of the leg (presumably attributable to the gastrocnemius), whether due to contractures or to spasticity, would still be a positive indication for surgical recession of the gastrocnemius

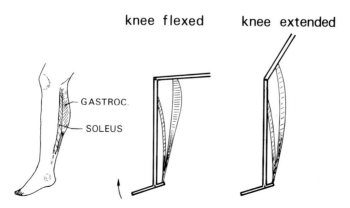

Figure 12-4. Silfverskiöld test.

to correct the functional equinus.[65] The important discrepancy, however, was the discovery from the EMG data that when the knee was extended, both the gastrocnemius and the soleus showed spastic activity on application of slow stretch. This spastic activity is apparently produced by the presence of a primitive extensor synergy, which acts to increase tone in both these muscles when the knee is extended. Since the surgical procedure of choice with spastic involvement of both the soleus and gastrocnemius muscles is to lengthen the heel cord (recession of the gastrocnemius while leaving the spastic soleus intact will be ineffective), reliance on the traditional muscle stretch test would have led to inappropriate treatment.

A considerable amount of study has also been directed to the muscles about the hip and knee. Eight clinical stretch tests were applied to 23 ambulatory children with spastic diplegic cerebral palsy.[51] Through the use of EMG, it was found that none of the clinical stretch tests was specific for any single muscle. For most of the stretch tests, marked EMG activity was elicited from muscles that the tests were designed to exclude from the stretching. A child with markedly positive "gracilis" clinical tests, for example, was found to have intense EMG activity in all the hamstring muscles during the testing. Another child, who showed a positive prone rectus test clinically, was demonstrated to have equally strong activation of the iliopsoas with EMG studies. These data corroborate prior criticisms on the lack of specificity of the tests.[58,71]

Sutherland and associates used the procedure of rectus femoris release to produce improvements in knee flexion during early swing in selected cerebral palsy patients who previously had stiff-knee gait due to rectus femoris spasticity.[71] The authors stressed the importance of objective or instrumented motion analysis in conjunction with EMG studies in establishing the indications for this surgery, which they caution are "narrow, precise and relatively infrequent." These include "prolonged stance phase, slow, labored and inadequate knee flexion" and EMG recordings showing hyperactivity of the rectus femoris. The EMG analysis must always include all the quadriceps muscles, since if the entire quadriceps group is active during swing phase, then isolated rectus release alone would be useless, and such patients should be excluded from this surgical treatment.

Several investigators have observed the most salient feature of spastic hip and knee muscles in cerebral palsy patients to be a prolongation of phasic response rather than a totally dysphasic response, although dysphasic activity is not uncommon. For example, among diplegics, Csongradi et al. have found

that in a study of 32 children with spastic cerebral palsy, rectus femoris activity was on the average present over 78 percent of the gait cycle, versus 31 percent for normal children.[15] Vastus medialis activity averaged 62 percent of the gait cycle, whereas this muscle's activity is only about 32 percent in normal children. This tendency toward prolonged activity was exhibited in these same patients in recordings of the medial hamstrings as well, where the average duration of activity was 71 percent as compared to 39 percent for normal children. The investigators further noted that the presence of spasticity in quadriceps was usually accompanied by hamstring spasticity.

Some disagreement exists, however, on the nature of the interdependence of the quadriceps and hamstring spasticity. Sutherland and Cooper argue, from their experience with four spastic diplegic children with crouch gait, that the prolongation of the quadriceps activity during stance is a secondary compensatory mechanism to check against increased knee flexion rather than a direct result of inherent spasticity.[67] Conversely, Perry et al. found that hyperactivity of the rectus femoris in some of their patients with crouch gait decreased in duration after surgical release, a finding more consistent with a mechanism of inherent spasticity.[51]

Tendon Transfers

EMG studies are similarly valuable in planning tendon transfers. Ideally, muscles used for transfer should show activation during the same phase of gait as the muscles that they are meant to assist.[14,50] Transfer of the posterior tibial tendon is a popular treatment for correcting varus posture of the hind foot when it can be demonstrated that the deforming forces during walking are caused by inappropriate phasing (i.e., activity present during swing phase) of this muscle's activity.[27,39] If on examination the posterior tibialis reveals a continuous spastic activation throughout the entire gait cycle, however, then tendon lengthening would be recommended.[50,59]

Figure 12-5 shows the preoperative EMG analysis of a cerebral palsy child for whom a posterior tibial tendon transfer is recommended. The activation of the posterior tibial muscle at the start of swing (toe-off) is maladapted, but it can be used to assist in elevating the forefoot during swing if that muscle's tendon is transferred to the dorsum of the forefoot.

This transfer has also been effective when gait studies demonstrated that the transferred muscle failed to contract actively during the swing phase.[26] In this

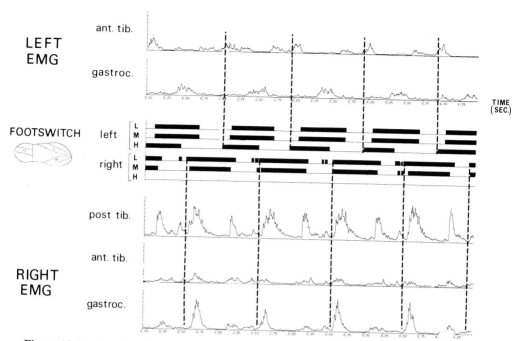

Figure 12-5. Display of processed EMG and footswitch data as a function of time in a child with spastic right hemiplegia. Footswitch plotted in center shows foot-to-floor contact patterns (stance events). The letters *L, M,* and *H* indicate lateral, medial, and heel tapes, respectively. Left foot shows near-normal foot-to-floor contact consisting of heel strike followed by contact of forefoot to achieve foot-flat. Next, the heel is lifted, leaving only forefoot contact, and finally toe-off occurs as swing-through is commenced. Right foot shows total absence of heel contact due to equinus foot posture. Intermittent contact just before the start of each stance phase indicates foot drag during swing. *Vertical dotted lines* in left EMG indicate stance markers from heel strike data. Note normal reciprocal activation of the tibialis anterior muscle during swing until just after heel strike followed by activation of gastrocnemius muscle during midstance. *Vertical dashed lines* in right EMG indicate stance markers taken from start of weightbearing contact of forefoot in the absence of any heel strike. Coactivation of gastrocnemius and tibialis anterior muscles is striking, as is the aberrant activation of the posterior tibial muscle at the start of swing.

case, the tension of the transferred muscle complex helped to inhibit plantar flexion during swing by a purely mechanical "check-rein" effect.

Another useful transfer for correcting nonfixed varus deformity is the split anterior tibial tendon transfer.[30] In this treatment, one section of the tendon is left intact at its natural medial insertion, and the other section is attached to the lateral dorsum of the forefoot (cuboid bone); thus a yoke effect is created that effectively balances the forefoot. Such surgery is properly indicated when the EMG gait study reveals that the tibialis anterior is continuously active throughout all phases of the gait cycle.

In their study of nine spastic cerebral palsy children with varus posture during gait, Perry and Hoffer studied the EMG activity of the anterior and posterior tibialis, gastrocnemius, soleus, and peroneus brevis and longus muscles.[50] The salient features of the EMG findings were that three children had phase-reversed or dysphasic activity of the posterior tibialis muscle, while in another two children this muscle was continuously active. The four remaining children all showed continuous spastic activity of the tibialis anterior muscle. These EMG studies thus distinguished three categories of muscle activity among the nine patients that the clinical examination alone could not distinguish.

A similar investigation of seven children with valgus foot deformity during gait produced two groupings: (1) the peroneus brevis (two children) or longus (one child) was active only during the stance phase, and this group was treated by a posteromedial

CLEVELAND V.A. MEDICAL CENTER--GAIT ANALYSIS REPORT

NAME: JLK

	06/16/81	14:19
SS #:	AGE: 6	SEX: M	HAND: L
HEIGHT: 1.150 M	WEIGHT: 23.60 KG	TREATMENT:	DIAGNOSIS:
BRACE: WITHOUT BRACE		COMPARISON RUN: 06/16/81	PERONEAL STIMULATOR

FREQUENCY DISTRIBUTION OF FOOT PLACEMENTS FOR LEFT FOOT

CURRENT

PLACEMENT	FREQUENCY	% OF ALL CYCLES
173456★	9	25.00
13456	7	19.44
1346	7	19.44
123456	1	2.78
17346★	9	25.00
132346	1	2.78
12346	1	2.78
13486	1	2.78

COMPARISON RUN

PLACEMENT	FREQUENCY	% OF ALL CYCLES
13456	10	28.57
1346★	12	34.29
173456	7	20.00
17346	4	11.43
134656	1	2.86
173456586	1	2.86

FREQUENCY DISTRIBUTION OF FOOT PLACEMENTS FOR RIGHT FOOT

CURRENT

PLACEMENT	FREQUENCY	% OF ALL CYCLES
83456	4	10.25
8234586	4	10.26
234586	2	5.13
23456★	9	23.08
8234586	1	2.56
13456	4	10.26
2346	5	12.82
8123456	1	2.56
82943456	1	2.56
83456	3	7.69
234586	1	2.56
234686	2	5.13
8345686	1	2.56
8234568686	1	2.56

COMPARISON RUN

PLACEMENT	FREQUENCY	% OF ALL CYCLES
13456★	16	44.44
23456	4	11.11
13456	13	36.11
2346	3	8.33

KEY

1=HEEL   5=MEDIAL
2=HEEL+LATERAL 6=SWING
3=FOOTFLAT   7=HEEL+MEDIAL
4=LATERAL+MEDIAL 8=LATERAL

○┼┼┼○ WITHOUT BRACE
■┅┅┅■ PERONEAL STIMULATOR
│ PREDICTED NORMAL MEAN AND STANDARD DEVIATION FOR CYCLE TIMES BETWEEN 1.0 AND 1.5 SEC

CADENCE (10⁻² STEPS/MIN)

VELOCITY (METERS/SEC)

STRIDE LENGTH (METERS)

LEFT	STANCE
	SWING
	DOUBLE SUPPORT 1

RIGHT	STANCE
	SWING
	DOUBLE SUPPORT 2

0.00 0.20 0.40 0.60 0.80 1.00 1.20 1.40 1.60 SEC.

transfer at the involved tendon, and (2) the peroneus brevis (three children) was continuously active or the peroneus brevis and the longus was continuously active (one child), and muscle release was performed.

More recently, Bennet et al. have suggested a different approach to the treatment of valgus foot deformity.[4] Their EMG studies of six cerebral palsy children with valgus foot posturing revealed that spasticity of the peronei was present in only one patient, and they argue that a more probable cause of pes valgus is a lack of function of the tibialis posterior, since nonfunctioning of this muscle was a consistent finding in all six patients. In order to restore muscle balance, the investigators transferred the peroneus brevis to the tendon of the tibialis posterior in two patients and report excellent early results.

FOOTSWITCH ANALYSIS

The concept of observing gait by noting when various parts of the foot touch the ground is actually quite old, and a technique that records the status of electrical contact between wires placed on the bottoms of a person's shoes and a conductive walkway was reported as early as 1932.[61] Although various combinations of electrode number and positioning along the bottom of the foot have been used by various investigators, one highly satisfactory arrangement, as diagrammed in the inset of Figure 12-6, is to affix 3 separate strips of 2.5-cm wide aluminum foil tape to the heel and to the medial and lateral borders of each of the person's shoes.

Using these three contacts, it is possible to define seven different foot-to-floor contact combinations during weightbearing: heel, heel plus lateral, heel plus medial, all three (foot flat), medial plus lateral (forefoot), medial, and lateral. These combinations are electrically coded so that each produces a distinct potential that can be transmitted to a computer system for automated processing and graphic analysis. The system provides an estimate of cadence (steps each minute), and, by noting the time taken by the patient to traverse the central 5-m span of the walkway, the patient's average forward velocity is calculated. The swing time, or time that the foot is in the air, and the stance time, or time that the foot is on the ground, is registered for each foot, and average values for the left and right foot are computed. Another parameter of gait that can be assessed is the duration of double support, which is the amount of time both feet are in contact with the ground. There are two components of double support in each step: the left heel in combination with the right toe, and the left toe in combination with the right heel. Average values for both components of double support are calculated, as are the individual average stride lengths for the left and right legs. Symmetry of movement can be readily assessed by comparing these results for both feet.

Gait data are collected over a 5-m length at the center of the walkway to eliminate effects of acceleration and deceleration, and the recording is initiated and terminated automatically, since the patient triggers photocells at either end of this predefined length. When the analysis is complete, the computer provides a printout of measurements and personal information along with a statistical analysis and graphic display of the results. A sample printout is shown in Figure 12-6. Different types of braces may also be compared, as may gait performance before and after var-

---

Figure 12-6. Standard clinical footswitch analysis report form of the Cleveland V.A. Medical Center. Header includes patient personal data and experiment identification information. Use of a trielectrode footswitch permits registration of seven possible foot-to-floor contacts (see text). The occurrence and temporal ordering of these contact patterns during stance are registered for each step, and a frequency distribution of the patient's foot placement pattern is furnished based on about 30 successive steps (approximately 6 traverses of the walkway). The most frequently occurring foot placement pattern is identified for each foot by an *asterisk,* and average values based on this most frequent pattern are computed and graphed for several parameters, including double support, stride length, stance duration, and swing duration. Symmetry between the left- and right-foot placement patterns is readily assessed with these measures. The computer-generated display permits a comparison of the patient's current performance (without brace) with previous data recorded while the patient walked with a gait-synchronized peroneal nerve stimulator. Patient is six years of age with spastic right hemiplegia resulting from a cerebrovascular accident during open heart surgery. Note the reduction in variability of the right-foot placement pattern when the stimulator was used and the conversion of the onset of stance to a normal heel strike on almost all the foot steps.

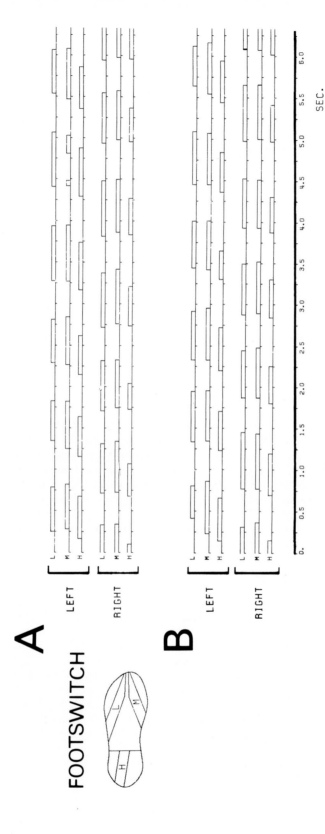

Figure 12-7. Raw Footswitch display of data used for Figure 12-6. In part A the patient walks with a foot-drop on the right side and this is clearly indicated by the fact that the lateral foot contact slightly precedes that of the heel. The left footswitch pattern is normal. In part 'B' the foot-drop has been corrected by having the patient walk with a gait synchronized peroneal nerve stimulator. The presence of a normal heel strike on each step is readily apparent.

126

ious treatments. For example, preoperative and post-operative surgical evaluation is possible and is usually done in conjunction with the dynamic EMG. Figure 12-7 shows some of the raw foot contact data that was used to prepare the printout shown in Figure 12-6. A considerable amount of qualitative information may be obtained from this type of presentation.

Another example to further illustrate the use of the footswitch information is shown in Figure 12-8. The foot–contact parameter that is displayed is the average interval between contact of the heel and the first contact of the forefoot for about 6 traverses of the walkway (approximately 30 steps). Analysis for this parameter is an extension of the foot–contact studies already described and was developed to provide a quantitative evaluation of the effectiveness of various treatments to correct equinus gait in cerebral palsy children with dynamic ankle-extensor spasticity.[55–57]

It is known that in a certain percentage of the patients whose equinus gait has been corrected with tendo-Achilles lengthening (TAL) surgery, the abnormality may reappear, necessitating repeat surgery.[74] By following all the patients treated with TAL with periodic gait evaluation, a better understanding of the factors responsible for these remissions and the general time course involved may be obtained. If the responsible variables can be identified, then perhaps physical therapy techniques or some other measures may be used to improve the long-term success of the operation.

Perry and associates have developed a portable footswitch system that uses a microprocessor and desk-type printing calculator for analysis and graphic readout of the footswitch information.[8,52] This system is commercially available at reasonable cost and allows a small hospital to obtain a considerable amount of quantitative and clinically useful gait information.

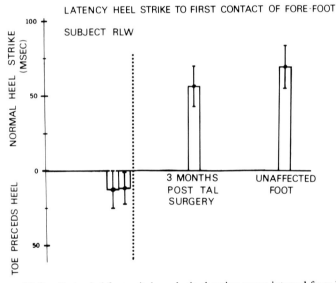

Figure 12-8. Extended footswitch analysis showing mean interval from heel-strike to first contact of the forefoot (plotted upward) or from initial forefoot contact to heel contact (plotted downward) as occurs in abnormal "toe-first" stance. In the absence of significant changes in the hip and knee function, the time interval from heel contact to the initial contact of the forefoot is a function of: the elevation of the forefoot as heel strike is approached; the ability of the ankle dorsiflexors to resist foot slap; and the degree of relaxation of the ankle extensors. About 30 footsteps are studied for each evaluation session. *Vertical tick marks* denote ± standard deviation. Patient data to left of *dotted line* was taken on two successive occasions about one week apart and preoperatively. As shown from these data, the patient walked mainly with a toe-first gait. After TAL operation, patient's equinus is corrected and a normal heel strike is seen at start of stance. (Unaffected leg is shown for addition comparison.)

ADDITIONAL GAIT STUDIES

Limb Motion

More elaborate studies can detail the child's kinematics or actual joint motions. Methods of evaluation include electrical measuring devices called goniometers that are strapped to each joint, television systems that scan for the position of small light bulbs fastened to the patient, movie film systems that photograph the position of reflective markers and then locate their positions on each frame, and the Selspot system which notes the three-dimensional position of light-emitting diodes fastened to the patient at strategic points.[29,35-37,62,72] This type of information is most useful when specific abnormal joint motions and postures are being treated. Examples include crouch stance, scissoring, and hip subluxation.

Through such limb motion studies of the gait of cerebral palsy children, Mann et al. have concluded that the technique of proximal release of the hamstring muscles to allow increased knee extension is a poor treatment for hamstring contractures because this procedure also causes an undesirable increase in anterior pelvic tilt and a decrease in hip extension.[41]

With similar cinemagraphic techniques, improvement in early swing phase knee flexion after rectus femoris release has been objectively shown for patients who walked with a stiff-knee gait due to rectus femoris spasticity.[71]

Force Analysis

The final major component of gait analysis is the determination of the various forces that are present in the bones, joints, and muscles. The forces on the foot are estimated by having the patient walk across a pressure-sensitive device in the walkway called a *Force Plate*. Generally, fore–aft as well as lateral shear forces and a vertical force component are resolved individually and may be transmitted to the computer concurrently with all the other gait data. The magnitudes and directions of the forces acting on the foot are then calculated. By combining these data with EMG information about when particular muscles are working, plus knowledge of the geometry of the patient's body including the joints and muscles, it is possible to calculate estimates of the joint, muscle, and ligament forces present during walking.

This information is useful in supplementing the subjective techniques generally used for deciding on a treatment plan. For example, a patient with complex gait deficiencies may exhibit numerous compensatory maneuvers to facilitate walking. Force analysis in combination with the other gait data should make these readily apparent and reduce the very real possibility of an unfortunate result occurring when a major compensatory mechanism is removed as an unexpected consequence of treatment designed to improve gait. The force analysis is also useful in predicting joint or ligament damage due to prolonged unreasonable stress levels. Such techniques, for example, have revealed the presence of excessive knee-flexion torque in spastic diplegics with progressive crouch gait.[67]

*   *   *

There are, at present, about 22 well-instrumented gait analysis centers across the country, and new installations will undoubtedly be added.[66]

REFERENCES

1. Basmajian JV: Electrodes and electrode connectors, in Desmedt JE (ed): New Developments in Electromyography and Clinical Neurophysiology, vol. 1. Basel, Karger, 1973, pp 502–510
2. Basmajian JU, Stecko GA: A new bipolar indwelling electrode for electromyography. J Appl Physiol 17:849, 1962
3. Bekey GA, Chang C, Perry J, et al: Pattern recognition of multiple EMG signals applied to the description of human gait. Proc IEEE 65:674, 1977
4. Bennet GC, Rang M, Jones D: Varus and Valgus Deformities of the Feet in Cerebral Palsy. Proceedings of the Canadian Society for Biomechanics and Human Locomotion. From Pathological Gait to the Elite Athlete. London, 1980, pp 27–29
5. Blanton PL, Lehur RP, Martin JH, et al: Further observations on the histologic response of skeletal muscle to EMG fine wire-electrodes. Significance of insulation. Electromyography 11:475, 1971
6. Bleck EE: The hip in cerebral palsy. Orthop Clin North Am 11:79, 1980
7. Bleck EE, Ford F, Stevick HC, et al: Electromyographic telemetry study of spastic gait patterns in cerebral palsied children. Dev Med Child Neurol 17:307, 1975
8. Bontrager EL, Barnes L: Footswitch stride analyzer, in annual report, Rancho Los Amigos Hospital, Downey, Cal., 1979, pp 45–50
9. Bouisset S, Goubel F: Interdependence of relations between integrated electromyography and diverse bio-

mechanical quantities in normal voluntary movements. Electromyography (suppl 1) 8:151, 1968

10. Buchtal F, Guld C, Rosenfalck P: Multielectrode study of the territory of a motor unit. Acta Physiol Scand 39:83, 1957

11. Burnett CN, Johnson EW: Development of gait in childhood. I. Method. Dev Med Child Neurol 13:196, 1971

12. Burnett CN, Johnson EW: Development of gait in childhood. II. Dev Med Child Neurol 13:207, 1971

13. Caldwell CW, Reswick JB: A percutaneous wire electrode for chronic research use. IEEE Trans. Biomed. Eng 22:429, 1975

14. Close JR, Todd FN: The phasic activity of the muscles of the lower extremity and the effect of tendon transfer. J Bone Joint Surg 41A:189, 1959

15. Csongradi J, Bleck E, Ford F: Gait electromyography in normal and spastic children, with special reference to quadriceps femoris and hamstring muscles. Dev Med Child Neurol 21:738, 1979

16. Delgado JMR: Electrodes for extracellular recording and stimulation, in Nastuk WL (ed): Physiological Techniques in Biological Research, vol 5. New York, Academic Press, 1964

17. DeLuca CJ: Physiology and mathematics of myoelectric signals. IEEE Trans Biomed Eng 26:1979

18. DeLuca CJ, LeFever RS, Stulen FB: Pasteless electrode for clinical use. Med Biol Eng Comput 17:387, 1979

19. Ferris CD: Introduction to Bioelectrodes. New York, Plenum, 1972

20. Fischer G, Sayre GP, Bickford RG: Histologic changes in the cat's brain after introduction of metallic and plastic coated wire used in electro-encephalography. Proc Mayo Clin 32:14, 1957

21. Freeborn CW, Ross G, Barnes L, et al: Spectral Analysis of EMG Signals, in annual report, Rancho Los Amigos Hospital, Downey, Cal., 1979, pp 35–37

22. Gans C, Gorniak GC: Electromyograms are repeatable precautions and limitations. Science 210:795, 1980

23. Geddes LA: Electrodes and the Measurement of Bioelectric Events. New York, Wiley, 1972

24. Gottlieb GL, Agarwal GC: Dynamic relationship between isometric muscle tension and the electromyogram in man. J Appl Physiol 30:345, 1971

25. Gottlieb GL, Agarwal GC: Filtering of electromyographic signals. Am J Phys Med 49:142, 1970

26. Gritzka TL, Staheli LT, Duncan WR: Posterior tibial transfer through the interosseus membrane to correct equinovarus deformity in cerebral palsy. Clin Orthop 89:201, 1972

27. Gunn DR, Molesworth BD: The use of tibialis posterior as a dorsiflexor. J Bone Joint Surg 39:674, 1957

28. Hagy JL, Mann RA, Keller CW: Normal Electromyographic Data. San Francisco, Shriners Hospital for Crippled Children, 1973

29. Herman R, Wirta Blampton S, et al: Human solutions for locomotion, in Herman RM, Grillner S, (eds):

30. Neural Control of Locomotion, vol. 18. Advances in Behavioral Biology. New York, Plenum, 1976

30. Hoffer MM, Reiswig JB, Garrett AM, et al: The split anterior tibial tendon transfer in the treatment of spastic varus hind foot of childhood. Orthop Clin North Am 5:31, 1974

31. Hogan N, Mann RW: Myoelectric signal processing: Optimal estimation applied to electromyography. 1. Derivation of the myoprocessor. IEEE Trans Biomed Eng 27:382, 1976

32. Holt KS: Facts and fallacies about neuromuscular function in cerebral palsy as revealed by electromyography. Dev Med Child Neurol 8:255, 1966

33. Jonsson B, Komi PU: Reproducibility problems when using wire electrodes in electromyographic kinesiology, in Desmedt JE (ed): New Developments in Electromyography and Clinical Neurophysiology, vol. 1. Basel, Karger, 1973, pp 540–546

34. Jonsson B, Reichmann S: Displacement and deformation of wire electrodes in electromyography. A roentgenologic study. Electromyography 9:201, 1969

35. Kettelkamp DB, Johnson RJ, Smidt GL, et al: An electrogoniometric study of knee motion in normal gait. J Bone Joint Surg 52A:775, 1970

36. Lamoreux LW: Kinematic measurements in the study of human walking. Bull Prosthet Res 3:10, 1971

37. Larson LE, Sandlund B, Oberg PA: Selspot recording of gait in normals and in patients with spasticity. Scand J Rehabil (Suppl 6), 1978

38. Lindstrom LH, Magnusson RI: Interpretation of myoelectric power spectra: A model and its applications. Proc IEEE 65:653, 1977

39. Lipscomb PR, Sanchez JJ: Anterior transplant of the posterior tibial tendon for persistent palsy of the common peroneal nerve. J Bone Joint Surg 43A:60, 1961

40. Mann RA, Hagy JL: The function of the toes in walking, jogging and running. Clin Orthop 142:24, 1979

41. Mann RA, Larsen LJ, Mahoney M, et al: Proximal hamstring release in children with cerebral palsy. Presented at a meeting of American Academy for Cerebral Palsy, New Orleans, 1975

42. Mathews PBC, Muir RB: Comparison of electromyogram spectra with force spectra during human elbow tremor. J Physiol 302:427, 1980

43. Milner-Brown HS, Penn RD: Pathophysiological mechanisms in cerebral palsy. J Neurosurg Psychiatry 42:606, 1979

44. Murray MP, Guten GN, Sepic SB, et al: Function of the triceps surae during gait. Compensatory mechanisms for unilateral loss. J Bone Joint Surg 60A:473, 1978

45. Murray MP, Sepic SB: A comparison of free and fast speed walking patterns for normal men. Am J Phys Med 45:8, 1966

46. Okamoto T, Kumanoto M: Electromyographic study of the learning process of walking in infants. Electromyography 12:149, 1972

47. Peckham HP, Thrope GB, Marsolais EB: Percutaneous intramuscular excitation of paralyzed skeletal muscle: Electrode reliability. Proceedings of the Fourth Annual Conference on Rehabilitation Engineering. Washington, D.C., 1981, pp. 229–231

48. Perry J: Cerebral palsy gait, in Samilson RL (ed): Orthopaedic Aspects of Cerebral Palsy. Philadelphia, Lippincott, 1975

49. Perry J, Giovan P, Harris LJ, et al: The determinants of muscle action in the hemiparetic lower extremity. Clin Orthop 131:71, 1978

50. Perry J, Hoffer MM: Preoperative and postoperative dynamic electromyography as an aid in planning tendon transfers in children with cerebral palsy. J Bone Joint Surg 59A:531, 1977

51. Perry J, Hoffer MM, Antonelli D, et al: Electromyography before and after surgery for hip deformity in children with cerebral palsy. A comparison of clinical and electromyographic findings. J Bone Joint Surg 58A:201, 1976

52. Perry J, Antonelli DJ, Bontrager EL: Pathokinesiology service report number 4: VA-Rancho gait analyzer final project report. Rancho Los Amigos Hospital, Downey, Cal., 1976

53. Perry J, Hoffer M, Giovan P, et al: Gait analysis of the triceps surae in cerebral palsy. A preoperative and postoperative clinical and electromyographic study. J Bone Joint Surg 56:511, 1974

54. Reiner S, Rogoff JB: Instrumentation, in Johnson EW (ed): Practical Electromyography. Baltimore, Williams & Wilkins, 1980

55. Riso RR: Fourth Annual Progress Report. Cleveland, Case Western Reserve University Rehabilitation Engineering Center, Ohio, pp. 40–61, 1981

56. Riso RR, Sutin KT: Graphical displays for footswitch analysis in gait studies. Proceedings of the Fourth Annual Conference on Rehabilitation Engineering. Washington, D.C., pp. 156–158, 1981

57. Riso RR, Crago PE, Sutin K, et al: An Investigation of the carry-over or therapeutic effects of FES in the correction of drop foot in the cerebral palsy child. Proceedings of International Conference on Rehabilitation Engineering, Toronto, 1980, pp. 220–222

58. Roosth HP: Flexion deformity of the hip and knee in spastic cerebral palsy: Treatment by early release of spastic hip-flexor muslces. Technique and Results in Thirty-Seven Cases. J Bone Joint Surg 53A:1489, 1971

59. Ruda R, Frost HM: Cerebral palsy. Spastic varus and forefoot adductus, treated by intramuscular posterior tibial tendon lengthening. Clin Orthop 79:61, 1971

60. Samilson RL, Perry J: The orthopaedic assessment in cerebral palsy, in Samilson RL (ed): Orthopaedic Aspects of Cerebral Palsy. Philadelphia, Lippincott, 1975

61. Schwartz RP, Heath AL: The pneumographic method of recording gait. J Bone Joint Surg 14:783, 1932

62. Simon SR, Nuzzo RM, Koskinen MF: A comprehensive clinical system for four dimensional motion analysis. Bull Hosp Joint Dis 38:41, 1977

63. Simon SR, Mann RA, Hagy JL, et al: Role of the posterior calf muscles in normal gait. J Bone Joint Surg 60A:465, 1978

64. Statham L, Murray MP: Early walking patterns of normal children. Clin Orthop 79:8, 1971

65. Strayer Jr LM: Gastrocnemius recession. Five-year report of cases. J Bone Joint Surg 40A:1019, 1958

66. Sutherland DH: Gait analysis in cerebral palsy. Dev Med Child Neurol 20:807, 1978

67. Sutherland DH, Cooper L: The pathomechanics of progressive crouch gait in spastic diplegia. Orthop Clin North Am 9:143, 1978

68. Sutherland DH, Cooper L: Crouch gait in spastic diplegia. Orthop Trans 1:76, 1977

69. Sutherland DH, Cooper L, Daniel D: The role of the ankle plantar flexors in normal walking. J Bone Joint Surg 62A:354, 1980

70. Sutherland DH, Olshen R, Cooper L, et al: The development of mature gait. J Bone Joint Surg 62A:336, 1980

71. Sutherland DH, Larsen LJ, Mann R: Rectus femoris release in selected patients with cerebral palsy: A preliminary report. Dev Med Child Neurol 17:26, 1975

72. Sutherland DH, Hagy JL: Measurement of gait movements from motion picture film. J Bone Joint Surg 54A:787, 1972

73. Sutherland DH, Schottstaedt ER, Larsen LJ, et al: Clinical and electromyographic study of seven spastic children with internal rotation gait. J Bone Joint Surg 51A:1070, 1969

74. Truscelli D, Lespargot A, Tardieu G: Variation in the long-term results of elongation of the tendo achillis in children with cerebral palsy. J Bone Joint Surg 61B:466, 1979

75. Zuniga EN, Leavitt LA: Quantified gait characteristics of women. Arch Phys Med Rehabil 54:570, 1973

76. Zuniga EN, Truong XT, Simons DG: Effects of skin electrode position on averaged electromyographic potentials. Arch Phys Med Rehabil 51:264, 1970

Irwin B. Jacobs

13

Epilepsy

For the patient it is a state of continuing dread (usually shared by his friends and family) interrupted by recurring attacks of involuntary behavior.[7]

The overall aim of treatment of children with cerebral palsy is to enable them to grow and function as normally as possible. The addition of epilepsy to an already burdensome physical disability makes this goal more difficult to reach. This chapter will discuss the problems and management of epilepsy in children with cerebral palsy.

Although seizures are a common symptom of a variety of diseases in childhood, there is an increased prevalence in patients with cerebral palsy. This may range from 55–72 percent in cases of spastic hemiplegia to about 23 percent in the choreoathetotic or ataxic forms.[3] The estimate of the incidence of epilepsy (recurrent seizures) in the general population varies between 0.5–1.5 percent.[2]

It must be emphasized that seizures are a symptom of disease and not a diagnosis. It follows that treatment must be directed to the underlying disease, if this can be defined. Treatment of a particular disease manifesting seizures as part of its symptomatology frequently controls the seizures. Under these circumstances, treatment is determined by the nature of the underlying disease process. Thus, removal of a meningioma, not the administration of anticonvulsant drugs, is the *specific* therapy for the seizures related to this neoplasm. If anticonvulsant drugs are employed, they are used as a *symptomatic* measure and are not directed against the underlying disorder.

In the case of cerebral palsy, which is based on a irreversible lesion of the central nervous system (CNS) acquired in utero or shortly after birth, it is apparent that only symptomatic treatment is possible

for both the underlying disorder and the seizures to which it gives rise. All variety of seizures may complicate cerebral palsy; tonic–clonic generalized seizures with loss of consciousness (grand mal), focal motor–sensory seizures, and partial complex seizures (temporal lobe epilepsy) are the most common.

When epilepsy occurs in a child with cerebral palsy, problems in addition to the seizures themselves arise. These may range from the side-effects of anticonvulsant drugs to prejudices in the school and community that make it difficult for the patient to adjust to the underlying disability. The unpredictable nature of the seizure episodes may lead to anxiety in both child and parent(s) and may cause additional emotional difficulties.

PATHOPHYSIOLOGY

The exact pathophysiologic mechanisms that underlie seizures are not fully understood; nevertheless, the intelligent management of children with epilepsy requires at least a fundamental understanding of the genesis of seizures. One can define an epileptogenic focus as a group of abnormal cerebral cortical cells that initiates "an occasional, excessive and disorderly discharge." This was the postulation of John Hughlings Jackson, the eminent British neurologist of the 19th century, and current electrophysiologic data do not contradict this notion. Isolation (by partial surgical undercutting) of a cortical area will produce relative electrocerebral silence in normal cortical neurons. A major characteristic of the epileptogenic focus is that it can generate a discharge autonomously. The paroxysmal activity of epileptic neurons will not stop when such a focus is isolated from underlying subcortical structures. The pathologic states that cause previously normal neurons to develop this "independence" are, for practical purposes, the same states that cause the motor deficit in cerebral palsy. It is easy to understand, therefore, why patients with cerebral palsy whose motor deficit is secondary to pathologic lesions in the basal ganglia or cerebellum have a lower incidence of epilepsy than those whose lesions involve the cerebral cortex. In the general population, a significant percentage of patients appear to have an inherited predisposition to seizures; in patients with cerebral palsy, the seizures are more closely associated with the type and distribution of the underlying pathologic lesions.

The manifestations of epilepsy are, in part, reflections of the normal function of the area of the brain involved in the epileptic process. In the current international classification of epilepsy, the majority of seizures are classified as either generalized (nonfocal) or partial (focal). Penfield and Erickson have theorized that in the case of idiopathic generalized seizures (grand mal and petit mal), the abnormal discharge originates in deep subcortical structures, presumably the thalamus, and subsequently spreads to all cortical regions simultaneously—hence the term *centrencephalic epilepsy*.[7] These types of seizures are usually associated with immediate loss of consciousness, and most of the idiopathic or genetic epilepsies probably fall into this category. Partial (focal) seizures clearly imply underlying structural abnormalities. Such lesions are more easily demonstrated in patients with cerebral palsy than in patients without associated motor deficit. A discharge originating focally may spread to involve adjacent structures, in which case additional symptomatology, reflecting the function of the involved brain, will be added to the initial seizure manifestations. Another important concept is that the focal discharge may spread to subcortical structures, from which it is then mediated to all cortical areas as a secondary generalized discharge. In such instances, the initial focal symptomatology (either behavioral, sensory, or motor) will be followed by a loss of consciousness as the seizure discharge becomes generalized. On the basis of any remembered experience (aura) or observed manifestations occurring just before the loss of consciousness, and a knowledge of functional brain anatomy, the site of the seizure focus can be inferred.

It has long been known that well-defined areas of the brain subserve specific motor and sensory functions. A seizure that begins in the right toe, for example, can with fair certainty be assured to originate in the medial portion of the precentral gyrus of the contralateral cerebral hemisphere. A patient whose seizure begins with unusual psychic behavior (dreamy state, feelings of familiarity or strangeness) most likely has a temporal lobe focus. Thus, depending on the clinical manifestations of a seizure, particularly the initial ones, the anatomic site of the origin of the seizure discharge can be predicted.

Seizure manifestations may therefore be generalized or partial. The choice of anticonvulsant medication is made on the basis of the clinical pattern as determined by an accurate description of the attack and the character of the electroencephalographic (EEG) tracing. Since the physician seldom has an opportunity to witness the actual seizures, it is incumbent upon him to obtain a detailed account of the attack from a parent, relative, teacher, or therapist who spends a lot of time with the child and has witnessed the actual episode(s). In doing so, special attention should be paid to precipitating factors. Some seizures are "reflex in type" and may be precipitated by an unusual pattern of light or noise. Others are simply due to failure to take prescribed medication. This is the most common cause of loss of seizure control, especially in the adolescent. Questions to ask include, Was there an aura? How did the patient know an attack was about to take place? Was there any unusual taste, small, or behavioral change before the seizure started? Small children cannot articulate their feelings but have been noted to suddenly stop what they are doing and make their way to a parent to be held just before the development of overt seizure activity. Was there loss of consciousness during an episode or could the patient respond to some extent? Did the patient develop tonic (stiffening of the body) or clonic (rhythmic jerking of an extremity or the entire body) movements? Did the movements begin in one part of the body and spread to another? Was there difficulty with respiration or cyanosis? Did the head and eyes deviate in any particular direction? Did the patient bite the tongue or become incontinent? Inquiry should be made on the duration of each of these manifestations and the presence of characteristic residual symptoms such as weakness, headache, confusion, or the need to sleep.

CLASSIFICATION

Seizures in cerebral palsy can be classified along the lines suggested by Gastaut.[5] A simplified version is shown in Table 13-1. It must be emphasized that seizures in patients with cerebral palsy may be of any

Table 13-1

Classification of Epilepsy

Generalized seizures without focal onset
    Grand mal
    Absence (petit mal)
    Minor motor

Partial (or focal) seizures with or without generalization
    Partial seizures with elemental (simple) symptomatology
    Partial seizures with complex symptomatology

Adapted from Gastaut H: Clinical and electroencephalographic classification of epileptic seizures. Epilepsia 11:102, 1970

type and just as severe and frequent as in patients without underlying motor abnormalities. In fact, the seizures associated with spastic hemiplegia are often exceptionally difficult to control, and, not infrequently in these patients, as with spastic quadriplegics, a compromise is made between the cumulative side-effects of medication on one hand and complete siezure control on the other.

Generalized Seizures Without Focal Onset

Grand Mal Seizures

Grand mal seizures are major motor convulsions characterized by a sudden loss of consciousness, followed by generalized tonic or clonic spasms or both. Tongue biting, urinary and fecal incontinence, difficulty in handling saliva, and cyanosis occur frequently. Postictally, patients frequently complain of headache and muscle soreness. They are often confused, exhausted, and want to sleep. The frequency and severity of individual episodes is quite variable. Abortive attacks may consist of a brief lapse in consciousness or precipitous falling. If an aura (a subjective remembered experience) precedes the grand mal episode, the appropriate classification would be partial seizures with generalization.

Absence Seizures

The absence, or petit mal, episode is a sudden brief lapse of consciousness lasting anywhere from 5–30 sec. After the attack the patient is immediately alert. A very slight motor activity may be observed, such as rhythmic blinking of the eyelids or nodding of the head. Attacks may range in frequency from a rare episode to hundreds each day. Absence attacks are rare in patients with cerebral palsy.

Minor Motor Seizures

Minor motor seizures include myoclonic jerks, akinetic or atonic seizures with a sudden fall to the ground, or apparent episodes of tonelessness. There may be sudden involuntary movements of the trunk, or trunk and limbs, and these may be quite forceful. In infancy these attacks may be referred to as infantile spasms, salaam seizures, or jackknife convulsions.

Partial or Focal Seizures

Elemental or Simple Symptomatology

The site or origin of partial seizures is in the cerebral cortex. Those patients with elemental symptomatology are characterized by convulsive twitching of an isolated group of muscles with subsequent spread. This type of seizure may remain limited, and the patient may remain conscious. Progression of convulsive movements from one part of the body to another, a so-called march, may be observed, and once the opposite side of the body is involved, loss of consciousness usually occurs. Localized sensory symptoms rather than motor twitching may be present.

Complex Symptomatology

In partial seizures with complex symptomatology there is clouding of consciousness associated with automatic patterned movements such as chewing, swallowing, smacking of the lips, or fumbling with clothes. Attacks may be very brief but commonly last two or three minutes (rarely more then five). Brief episodes may be confused with absence attacks. Previously, complex partial seizures were referred to as psychomotor seizures because of the alteration in behavior, perception, and effect or as temporal lobe seizures because these seizures usually originate in that part of the brain.

INCIDENCE

Seizures may complicate all types of cerebral palsy. It is worth noting that the incidence varies among the different subtypes, a point of importance in respect to prognosis. This feature was studied by Crothers and Paine in 1959 during a reevaluation of a large series of patients seen between 1930 and 1950 (Table 13-2).[3]

Table 13-2
Incidence of Epilepsy in Patients
with Cerebral Palsy

Type of Cerebral Palsy	Incidence (%)
Hemiplegic	
Congenital	55
Acquired	72
Quadriplegic or triplegic	33
Extrapyramidal	23

Adapted from Crothers B, Paine RS: The Natural History of Cerebral Palsy. Cambridge, Harvard University Press, 1959

Whereas cerebral palsy of the spastic hemiplegic type carried the highest risk of associated epilepsy, a distinction exists between those with congenital (prenatal or natal) and acquired (postnatal) hemiplegia. Slightly over one half (55 percent) of the congenital, while nearly three quarters (72 percent) of the acquired group had a history of seizures. Further analysis of these data reveals that in the epileptic patients with acquired hemiplegia, more than three quarters still had episodes at the time of follow-up examination. In contrast, nearly half the patients with congenital hemiplegia and a history of epilepsy were seizure free at reexamination. The prognosis in quadriplegic and triplegic or extrapyramidal cerebral palsy is also good. Not only is the chance of seizures in these patients small (33 percent and 23 percent, respectively), but those patients who do develop seizures have an excellent chance for spontaneous resolution and no further need for anticonvulsant therapy (Table 13-3).

Table 13-3
Spontaneous Resolution of Seizures
in Cerebral Palsy

Type of Cerebral Palsy	Resolved (%)*
Hemiplegic	
Congenital	47
Acquired	24
Quadriplegic or triplegic	61
Extrapyramidal	91

Adapted from Crothers B, Paine RS: The Natural History of Cerebral Palsy. Cambridge, Harvard University Press, 1959
*Percentage of patients with history of seizures who were free of episodes at follow-up examination.

Also, the age of onset of the seizure disorder differs in patients with spastic hemiplegia, depending on whether the motor deficit is congenital or acquired. In the congenital form, seizures rarely occur in the newborn period; the vast majority begin with 4 yr, but occasional patients may not have their first seizures until 15 yr of age or even beyond. In the acquired type, seizures most often begin at the time of onset of the hemiplegia and may be associated with fever and coma. Frequently, the initial burst of seizures is prolonged for several hours or days (status epilepticus). Recurrent seizures begin within two years in the majority of patients, although the child must be considered at risk for an indefinite period. Children who acquire a hemiplegia after the age of 6 yr, are unlikely to develop an associated seizure disorder unless their initial presentation included convulsive activity.

ELECTROENCEPHALOGRAPHY

The EEG in patients with cerebral palsy correlates well with the underlying cerebral pathology. In the hemiplegic cases reported by Perlstein, two thirds of the abnormal discharges were focal, or limited to the affected side of the brain, while one third were bilateral.[8] In no patients was the predominent abnormality on the side opposite the cerebral lesion. The EEG also proved to be a reliable indicator of the presence of a seizure disorder. Of the 212 cases of cerebral palsy studied by Perlstein, 75 percent of those patients with seizures had an abnormal EEG, while in those without seizures, only 11 percent had abnormal recordings. Similarly, Aird and Cohen reported the presence of an EEG abnormality with convulsions in 88 percent of their group of 128 patients with the spastic form of cerebral palsy and in 61 percent of patients with the athetoid form.[1]

The characteristic EEG abnormalities in both spastic hemiplegics and quadriplegics consist of spike discharges, slow waves, fast activity, or voltage asymmetry, but the incidence of epilepsy cannot be correlated with the type of abnormality. The sole exception to this generalization is with wave complexes of the petit mal variant type; seizures occurred in approximately 80 percent of the patients with this type of EEG abnormality. The EEG abnormalities in the extrapyramidal forms of cerebral palsy are similar to those noted in the spastic types, although voltage asymmetry is much less common in the former.

The EEG is also important for its predictive value. In the absence of a history of seizures, the finding of an abnormal EEG suggests that clinical seizures may occur. Although this raises the question of prophylactic anticonvulsant therapy, my own practice is to treat only those patients with overt symptomatology.

EVALUATION

In the evaluation of cerebral palsy patients with epilepsy, as in all epileptics, a critical history and complete general physical and neurologic examination are of great importance. Since patients with cerebral palsy have a motor deficit to begin with, the neurologic examination will not be normal, and an attempt must be made to compare it to a previous neurologic assessment. Also, computed tomography (CT) scans of the skull should be obtained in order to help define the cerebral structural abnormality. As indicated above, the EEG is valuable in confirming the clinical impression of epilepsy and in localizing the site of the underlying lesion. It is also helpful in clarifying the type of seizure and in choosing the appropriate anticonvulsant medication. Serum electrolyte and liver and kidney function studies should be obtained along with a complete blood count (CBC) and urinalysis. These findings are rarely abnormal but serve as a baseline for the subsequent monitoring of adverse drug reactions.

TREATMENT

The management of epilepsy in patients with cerebral palsy is essentially the same as in patients without motor abnormalities, and standard texts should be consulted for details or choice of drugs and their doses, toxicity, and side-effects.[6,9] A brief summary of the medications used for various types of seizures is presented in Table 13-4. Further information about the commonly used drugs is presented in Table 13-5. Although a detailed discussion of these aspects of therapy is beyond the scope of this text, certain general principles in management, applicable to all forms of epilepsy in childhood, should be emphasized.

The goal of therapy through drug administration is the prevention of seizures, with freedom from all complications (including dose-related toxicity, side-effects, and idiosyncratic reactions). Such an ideal anticonvulsant drug is not yet available, and the best that one can achieve is a balance between effectiveness and adverse reactions. The physician must keep in mind that patients vary in their response to drugs and should constantly be alert for signs of toxicity.

Table 13-4
Specific Seizure Therapy

Generalized seizure focal onset
  Grand mal (major motor seizure)
    Principal drugs
      Phenobarbital
      Carbamazepin (Tegretol)
      Diphenylhydantoin (Dilantin)
      Primidone (Mysoline)
    Commonly included in therapy
      Clonazepam (Clonopin)
      Acetazolamide (Diamox)
  Absence seizure
    Principal drugs
      Ethosuximide (Zarontin)
      Clonazepam (Clonopin)
      Valproic acid (Depakene)
    Commonly included in therapy
      Phenobarbital
  Minor motor
    Principal drugs
      Valproic acid (Depakene)
      Clonazepam (Clonopin)
      Diazepam (Valium)
      Steroids
    Commonly included in therapy
      Phenobarbital
Partial seizures
  Partial seizures with elemental symptomatology
    Principal drugs
      Phenobarbital
      Diphenylhydantoin
      Carbamazepine
      Primidone
    Commonly included in therapy
      Clonazepam
      Acetazolamide
  Partial seizures with complex symptomatology
    Principal drugs
      Carbamazepine
      Diphenylhydantoin
      Primidone

Individualized regimens must be the rule rather the exception. A single appropriate medication, usually determined by seizure type, is selected and initiated at a dose that clinical experience suggests will result in a therapeutic blood level. The dose is gradually increased, if necessary, either until the seizures are controlled or troublesome side-effects appear. The time intervals between dose changes are a function

Table 13-5

Comparison of Drugs Used in Seizure Therapy

Drug	Therapeutic Range (μcg/ml)	Time to Reach Steady State (days)
Diphenyl-hydantoin	10–20	5–10
Phenobarbital	15–40	14–21
Primidone	5–12	4–7
Ethosuximide	40–100	5–8
Carbamazepine	40–120	2–4
Valporic acid	40–100	2–4
Clonazepam	0.013–0.072	4–10

of the frequency of seizure activity and the time it takes the drug to reach a steady-state blood level. If seizures continue, despite increased medication, to the point of adverse reactions, the dose is reduced to the level previously tolerated and another medication (preferably only one) is added and administered under the same principles of increasing dose.

An attempt should be made to use the fewest drugs at the lowest doses consistent with good seizure control. Blood levels should be monitored frequently to ensure that therapeutic levels have been reached and maintained. This is especially important for patients who are taking more than one drug and in whom compliance is suspect.

Anticonvulsants should be maintained for a minimum of four seizure-free years. Although many patients may eventually become free of seizures and not require further therapy (see Table 3), no clear guidelines exist which allow one to predict which children with cerebral palsy can safely discontinue their medication. The absence of associated mental retardation, late onset of seizures, and a normal EEG recording before medication is discontinued are good prognostic signs, and in such patients therapy can be terminated without significant risk of recurrence of seizures.[4] Anticonvulsant drugs should be discontinued slowly (one at a time) over several months.

An occasional patient may be resistant to all forms of medical therapy, including the use of steroids, adrenocorticotrophic hormone (ACTH) or a ketogenic or medium chain triglyceride diet. Such patients, if the underlying epileptic lesion is well localized, may be candidates for surgical extirpation of the focus. Extirpation should be undertaken only if severe and frequent seizures persist despite a sustained period of intense medical therapy and only in centers that are specially equipped for this type of neurosurgery.

HELPING CHILDREN AND PARENTS UNDERSTAND EPILEPSY

Although the use of anticonvulsant drugs is the cornerstone of treatment epilepsy, the physician must also be sensitive to social and psychologic factors. Enough time must be spent with parent(s) and child during their initial visits to help them deal with their feelings and provide them with an intelligent grasp of the disorder. Their recognition of the fact that seizures are usually short and do not further damage the brain helps to calm their anxiety. Parents need a great deal of reassurance and must be helped to feel confident in their ability to appropriately manage the acute symptoms of an individual episode. They must be instructed not to move the child during a seizure unless the location might cause injury. Tight clothing, especially around the neck, should be loosened, and the child gently turned to the side so that mucus, saliva, or emesis will flow freely out of the mouth rather than be aspirated. Tongue blades or similar objects should not be used, because the risk of breaking a tooth that might subsequently be aspirated outweighs any possible benefit from this type of intervention.

Many children are interested in and curious about their seizures as well as frightened by them. Obviously, the best way to answer their questions and relieve their anxiety is to talk clearly and in a straightforward manner about the epileptic episodes. In explaining epilepsy to children, one should try to avoid the standard cliches, which use the concept of electrical discharges suddenly occuring in the brain. Such analogies unfortunately enable children to conjure up a variety of erroneous or magical images of "sparks and lightning storms" taking place inside the skull.

My major aim is to help the child develop a concept of *brain* as being that organ that enables him or her to think, understand, and control the body. Throughout the discussion I try to convince the child of the intactness of his or her brain and to distinguish it from certain anatomic areas (of brain) that have specific functional significance. These areas can be referred to as *nerves* (a term that has meaning for a child); they can be explained as initiating movement but under the control of the brain. Epilepsy occurs when the nerves begin to act independently. Thus, rather than emphasize any impairment of brain, I simply speak about the occasional independence of some focal areas. This helps the child to conceptualize that an epileptic seizure can be caused by a very tiny focus. (In the actual discussion with the child, I usually begin by asking questions about how I am able to move my finger. It is from this starting point that the above concepts, which are easy for even a young child to understand, are developed.) One can even expand this approach, which is initially limited to motor symptomatology. It is possible to say that there are nerves that control consciousness, and if these nerves act independently, a person with epilepsy might lose consciousness. The concept of cerebral palsy can also be explained in this same way. If a child has difficulty moving his right arm and leg, it is not because his brain is abnormal, but, rather, because those nerves that control his right arm and leg are damaged. Even though the (normal) brain is telling the nerves to move the right side, they are not able to do so. In this way, the concept of *brain* is left intact, although the child recognizes small areas called *nerves* are not functioning appropriately.

Frequently the stress and anxiety associated with recurrent seizures are more of a problem than the epilepsy itself. It is only when parents are comfortable with their own feelings about their child's seizures that they will be able to understand and deal with similar feelings in their child. The assistance of a social worker, nurse, or psychologist especially knowledgeable about epilepsy and its treatment can be invaluable in helping the child and the family. It is only with total and comprehensive consideration and management of all problems associated with epilepsy and cerebral palsy that the child can be helped to achieve the fullest potential and thus learn to lead a useful, independent, and productive life.

REFERENCES

1. Aird RB, Cohen P: Electroencephalography in cerebral palsy. J Pediatr 37:448, 1950
2. Epilepsy Foundation of America: Basic Statistics on the Epilepsies. Philadelphia, F. A. Davis, 1975
3. Crothers B, Paine RS: The Natural History of Cerebral Palsy. Cambridge, Harvard University Press, 1959
4. Emerson R, D'Souza BJ, Vining EP, et al: Stopping medication in children with epilepsy. Predictors of Outcome. N Engl J Med 304:1125, 1981
5. Gastaut H: Clinical and electroncephalographic classification of epileptic seizures. Epilepsia 11:102, 1970
6. Livingston S: The Comprehensive Management of Epilepsy in Infants, Children and Adolescents. Springfield, Ill., Charles C Thomas, 1972
7. Penfield W, Erickson TC: Epilepsy and Seizure Localization. London, Bailliere, Tindall and Cox, 1941
8. Perlstein MA, Gibbs EL, Gibbs FA: The EEG in infantile cerebral palsy. Proc Am Res Nerv Ment Dis 26:377, 1947
9. Schmidt RP, Wilder BJ: Epilepsy. Comtemprary Neurology Series, Philadelphia, F. A. Davis, 1975

Paul R. Mitchell

14

Ophthalmologic Problems

Children with cerebral palsy require a thorough, careful eye examination, repeated when necessary, in order to diagnose problems that may benefit from early identification and treatment. Because of diffuse central nervous system (CNS) damage, associated dysfunctions, including visual ones, are common.[20] According to Perlstein, any child with abnormalities of the eye at birth should be considered to have brain damage until proven otherwise, and a complete neurologic examination is recommended.[19]

In addition to the history, a thorough eye examination would include inspection for orbit asymmetry and evaluation of eyelids, conjunctiva, cornea, anterior chamber, and pupillary response to light and accommodation. Visual acuity, eye position and movement, detection of strabismus, presence of fusion potential, stereoacuity, color vision, visual fields, refraction, fundus examination, and intraocular pressure measurements would complete an ideal ophthalmologic examination. The child's intelligence, ability, and cooperation determine the quality and quantity of information that can be successfully obtained.

OCULAR DEFECTS

Although there is extensive literature on cerebral palsy, little was published in the ophthalmic literature until Guibor presented data in 1953.[10] Since then, many authors have described the ocular abnormalities in cerebral palsy in 50–92 percent of patients studied.[5,8,10,14,15,17,18,22–24,27] The most common ocular abnormality is strabismus, reported in 15–62 percent of patients. Strabismus types include esotropia (inward deviation of the eyes) and exotropia (outward

deviation of the eyes). Esotropia is seen more frequently than exotropia in most reported studies.[3,5,10,12,16,17,22,27] Many other defects have been reported. Nystagmus has been reported in up to 16 percent, amblyopia in up to 37 percent, and optic atrophy in up to 17 percent of patients in different series.[12,17] Significant refractive errors have been reported in 25–76 percent of patients studied.[3,5,17,18,22–24,27]

Other less common ocular defects are congenital cataracts, ptosis, and corneal defects.[5,15,22,27] Retinal abnormalities have included retinitis pigmentosa, chorioretinitis, retrolental fibroplasia, and macular coloboma.[10,15,17,27] Spastic eyelids, coloboma of the iris, paresis of upward gaze, external ophthalmoplegia, papilledema, and abnormal head posture have also been reported.[5,7,8,23]

Many of these eye anomalies result in loss of binocular coordination (the simultaneous use of both eyes) and depth perception. Hand and eye coordination, walking, and reading may be less well developed because of abnormal ocular conditions.[2]

Strabismus is the most commonly seen of all ocular defects associated with cerebral palsy, but it may not always be the major ocular handicap. In order of educational or physical impedance, rather than order of frequency, the following ocular abnormalities offer the greatest hindrance to successful education and rehabilitation of the cerebral palsied child.[7] The following defects must be recognized and interpreted:

1. Blindness, bilateral subnormal vision, and high refractive errors that limit the ability to see, which is the most severe ophthalmologic handicap

139

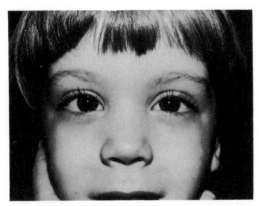

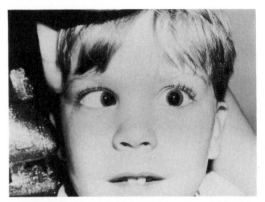

Figure 14-1. Straight eyes by corneal light reflex test. Light reflection is centered on each cornea. This is a 2-yr postoperative photograph of the child in Figure 14-2.

Figure 14-2. Esotropia of right eye by corneal light reflex test. Light reflection is centered on left eye but on temporal side of right cornea, demonstrating esotropia. This is a preoperative photograph of the child in Figure 14-1.

2. Ocular motility disturbances, strabismus, nystagmus, and abnormal head postures, making normal use of the eyes difficult or partially or severely limited
3. Amblyopia due to differences in refractive error or to strabismus and the suppression of one eye
4. Defects in visual fields, interfering with central vision and the ability to read
5. Combinations of the above defects
6. Associated developmental congenital or neurologic defects

BASIC SCREENING TESTS

Any person involved in the treatment of children with cerebral palsy should be aware of some basic screening tests to aid in the detection of ocular motor defects or vision abnormalities. If defects are suspected or diagnosed, the patient can be referred to an ophthalmologist who is interested in children's eye diseases and their associated motor anomalies.[2,10] Ocular motor defect screening consists of corneal light reflection and ocular rotation testing.

Ocular Motor Defect Screening

Corneal Light Reflexes

Testing for corneal light reflexes may be helpful in determining the presence of strabismus (deviation of the eyes). From several feet away a pen light or flashlight is shined at the child's eyes, and he or she

is encouraged to gaze at a distant target. The position of the light's reflection from each corneal surface is noted.

If the reflection is centered on each cornea, the eyes are considered to be straight (Fig. 14-1). When a light reflex is centered on one cornea and the reflex is on the temporal aspect of the other cornea, the child has esotropia, an inward crossing of the eyes (Fig. 14-2). If the reflex is placed on the nasal aspect of the other cornea, the child has exotropia (Fig. 14-3), an outward deviation or divergence of the eyes. Each millimeter of displacement of light reflex from the corneal center of the turned, or nonfixating, eye is equal to 15 diopters (7.5 degrees) of deviation. The importance of this will be discussed later in the chapter.

Some forms of strabismus are intermittent, and this test will not always reveal its presence if performed when the eyes are straight. Some children demonstrate only a phoria, or tendency, for the eyes to be misaligned, contrasted with a tropia, when the eyes demonstrate frank misalignment. Similarly, a phoria may not be detected by light reflex testing only.

The examiner must carefully observe the light reflex and avoid being deceived by a wide nasal bridge. *Pseudoesotropia* is the condition simulating esotropia. On adduction, or moving an eye toward the nose, the nasal sclera and part of the cornea may be covered by the epicanthal folds and nasal bridge. The eye may appear crossed, but if the light reflex is centered on each eye, there is no deviation but only the illusion of crossing.

Ocular Rotation Tests

Ocular rotation tests are performed to determine any disorder of eye movement by comparing vergence (the two eyes moving in opposite directions) and version (the two eyes moving in the same direction) movements. Disorders of vergence (including strabismus) and version (including nystagmus), difficulty in rotation, and paralysis of vertical movements are reported in 25–75 percent of patients in several studies.[5,10,22]

A pen light, a small toy, or a puppet is waved before the child's eyes in up, down, left, right and diagonal directions. Disturbances in ocular movements may involve one or both eyes.

If both eyes cannot move together in all directions, or if lateral position of gaze cannot be maintained for more than three seconds, a conjugate defect is present.[11] Conjugate ocular deviations are eye movement disturbances associated with irritative or destructive lesions of the CNS, usually in the cerebral cortex in children. The two eyes may be deviated upward (supraversion), toward the right (dextroversion), toward the left (levoversion) or downward (infraversion).[10] In a series of 142 patients with cerebral palsy, Guibor reported that 33 percent had horizontal conjugate defects, although other authors have reported lower percentages.[3,5,10,22]

Vision Screening

Vision screening may be performed with an illiterate E or alphabet chart at 20 ft. Vision is recorded separately in each eye if possible. Vision less than 20/30 with a cooperative child is considered abnormal, and referral to an ophthalmologist is recommended. Those children in whom vision cannot be easily screened should have a complete ophthalmologic examination.

OPHTHALMOLOGIC EXAMINATION

The complete ophthalmologic examination has been previously described. The most important parts will be discussed in greater detail, including visual acuity, stereoacuity, motility, refraction, fundus examination, and visual fields.

Visual Acuity

The ophthalmologist uses the previously described techniques of vision screening but in greater

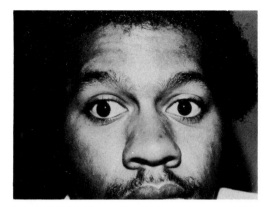

Figure 14-3. Exotropia of right eye by corneal light reflex test. Light reflection is centered on left eye but on nasal side of right cornea, demonstrating exotropia.

depth and detail. The presence of mental retardation will alter the child's capability to be tested. In a review of 234 patients, Hiles found that 33 percent had no mental retardation.[12,13] Mild retardation was found in 20 percent, moderate retardation in 22 percent, and severe retardation in 25 percent of the patients studied. Similar relationships were found among those patients seen with cerebral palsy at the Newington Children's Hospital, Newington, Conn.

The ophthalmologist must try to develop rapport with the child before undertaking the eye examination.[27] The young child should sit in the lap of the parent or a familiar person. Small toys are helpful in allaying fear.

Because the visual acuity measurement is the most important subjective part of the examination, it may be delayed until the child is at ease. After testing extraocular motility while the child has been looking at a movie or puppet, or after careful inspection of the child while he or she is playing with small toys, the ophthalmologist may then attempt a visual acuity determination.

The child is shown a visual acuity target appropriate for the age group. Below two years of age, a hand-held finger puppet, which may be illuminated internally with a pen light, may be used. The ophthalmologist observes the fixation pattern, or the child's ability to follow the target in all gaze directions. An attempt is made to cover each eye separately to determine any preference for seeing with one eye. In addition, a distant fixation target is used, such as an animated puppet or cartoon on a continuous loop reel

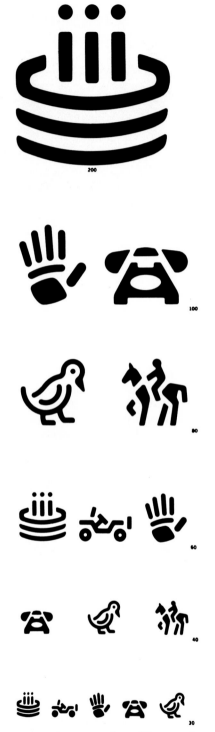

Figure 14-4. Picture eye chart. (Courtesy American Optical Corporation, Buffalo, N.Y. 14215)

that is activated by a remote control foot switch. The Sheridan Test for Young Children and Retardates (STYCAR) described in Chapter 10, can also be useful in children with significant cognitive and motor impairment.

If the child does not object to either eye being covered, vision may be considered to be approximately equal. A child with amblyopia or an organic visual defect in one eye will allow that eye to be covered; however, any attempt to cover the better-seeing eye will cause anxiety, crying, or frustration. The child will try to avoid the cover or attempt to remove it from the better-seeing eye. This simple test rapidly reveals significant differences in visual acuity between the two eyes long before the patient is capable of reading an eye chart. Treatment may then be instituted at an early age.

As the child grows, more sophisticated and reliable tests are used. With normal intelligence, children between two and three years of age are often capable of recognizing pictures on an eye chart (Fig. 14-4). Between three and five years of age, depending on the child's proficiency, an illiterate E (Fig. 14-5) or alphabet chart (Fig. 14-6) is used. Most children beyond the age of five with normal intelligence have little difficulty with these charts.

Precise visual acuity measurements are less reliable with increasing degrees of mental retardation. When a response to an eye chart is not possible, estimates of visual acuity must be made. By observing the retarded child's response to a movie or an animated puppet when each eye is covered separately, amblyopia may be detected, as previously described.

The child with impaired speech may be able to recognize the letters or pictures on an eye chart. A communication board, either made at school (Fig. 14-7) or commercially available (Fig. 14-8), with letters, words and numbers is placed before the child (Fig. 14-9). The child may point to a picture or letter on the response board corresponding to the picture or letter shown on an eye chart; this provides an accurate evaluation of visual acuity.

Visual acuity is measured with the following standard nomenclature, adapted from the American Medical Association (Table 14-1).[4] Vision measured or estimated to be worse than 20/70 will significantly limit the child's educational performance. Schooling will require large-print books, low-vision aids, and possibly Braille textbooks. Closed circuit television with magnification of books and reading materials may be necessary for the severely visually handicapped child.

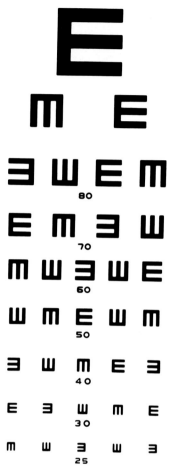

Figure 14-5. Illiterate E eye chart (Courtesy American Optical Corporation, Buffalo, N.Y. 14215)

Binocular Vision

Binocular vision, the simultaneous use of the eyes together, is measured with the Worth 4 Dot test and the Titmus Stereo Acuity Test[+] or the Random Dot Stereo Acuity Test.[†] The Worth 4 Dot test uses a flashlight with four small illuminated circles or dots. One circle is red, two are green, and one is white. A pair of special testing glasses is placed over the patient's eyes, with a green filter over the right eye and a red filter over the left eye. Because of the colored filters, the white circle appears green when

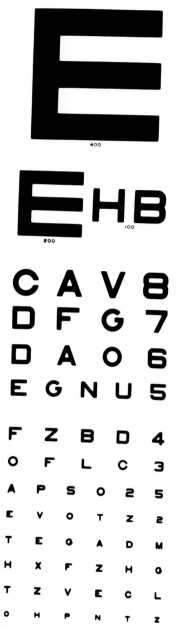

Figure 14-6. Alphabet eye chart. (Courtesy American Optical Corporation, Buffalo, N.Y. 14215)

seen by the right eye and red when seen by the left eye.

If both eyes are used together, the child reports seeing four circles or dots. If the child reports seeing either two or three dots, then one of the eyes is not being used because the brain is suppressing the im-

---

[+]Titmus Optical Co., Inc., Petersburg, Va.
[†]Stereo Optical Co., Inc., Chicago, Ill.

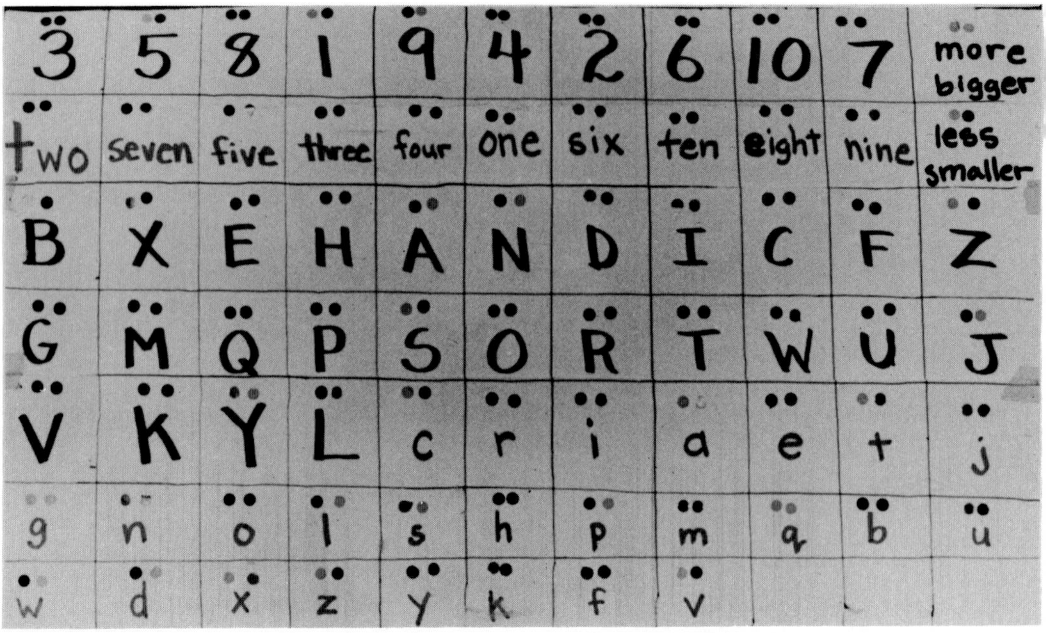

Figure 14-7. Communication board, noncommercial.

age. A report of five dots reveals that there is no suppression and that both eyes are being used at the same time because of double vision.

A test of stereo acuity, or fine binocular vision, is the Titmus test or Random Dot Test. It uses Polaroid eyeglasses and a specially calibrated series of disks. The patient is asked to report which disk appears elevated from the page, with increasing degree of difficulty. Stereoacuity to the level of 20 sec of arc is measurable. This test is extremely difficult to perform with less than normal intelligence. A separate section with cartoons and a picture of a fly is useful for the younger child who is able to cooperate.

Ocular Motility

Ocular rotation testing has been previously described. Evaluation for strabismus includes cover testing for both distant and near targets. The child is asked to read the symbols on an eye chart while the right eye is covered and uncovered. The examiner observes the right eye for any change in alignment when uncovered. Movement toward the nose indicates that the eye has been deviating outward under cover and is now returning to its straight-ahead position. This is exophoria, as found on the cover–uncover test. Movement in the opposite direction indicates

esophoria. The test is repeated on the left eye and with a small accomodative target for near testing.

The cross cover test measures tropia, or frank misalignment. As the right eye is covered, the left eye is observed for movement. A shift to the left indicates esotropia, while a shift to the right indicates exotropia. The cover is then placed over the left eye, and the right eye is observed for movement. By continuing to do the cross cover test and by placing prisms of various power over one eye, the exact measurement of the deviation is made (see Fig. 14-11). When the eye stops moving, the prism power equal to the diopters or degrees of deviation has been found. An accommodative target is also used for a near measurement. No eye movement indicates no strabismus.

Eye muscle rotations are also performed to detect inferior or superior oblique overacting, which is often associated with esotropia or exotropia.

Refraction

Refraction is a method of measuring any optical abnormality of the eyes to determine whether eyeglasses are necessary. Dilation of the pupil and paralyzing of accommodation (focusing ability) is best achieved with 1 percent cyclopentolate, 1 percent tropicamide, 2.5 percent phenylephrine, or a com-

I CAN HEAR PERFECTLY	PLEASE REPEAT AS I TALK (THIS IS HOW I TALK BY SPELLING OUT THE WORDS)	WOULD YOU PLEASE CALL
A AN HE	AM ARE ASK BE BEEN BRING CAN	ABOUT ALL
HER I IT ME	COME COULD DID DO DOES DON'T	AND ALWAYS
MY HIM SHE	DRINK GET GIVE GO HAD HAS HAVE	ALMOST AS
THAT THE THESE	IS KEEP KNOW LET LIKE MAKE MAY	AT BECAUSE
THEY THIS WHOSE	PUT SAY SAID SEE SEEN SEND SHOULD	BUT FOR FROM
WHAT WHEN WHERE	TAKE TELL THINK THOUGHT WANT	HOW IF IN
WHICH WHO WHY	WAS WERE WILL WISH WON'T WOULD -ED	OF ON OR
YOU WE YOUR	-ER -EST -ING -LY -N'T -'S -TION	TO UP WITH

A	B	C	D	E	F	G	AFTER AGAIN
	H	I	J	K	L	M	ANY EVEN
N	O	P	Qu	R	S	T	EVERY HERE
	U	V	W	X	Y	Z	JUST MORE
1	2	3	4	5	6	7	ONLY SO
	8	9	10	11	12	30	SOME SOON
							THERE VERY

| SUN. MON. TUES.
WED. THUR.
FRI. SAT. BATHROOM | PLEASE   THANK YOU   GOING OUT
MR.   MRS.   MISS   START OVER
MOTHER   DAD   DOCTOR   END OF WORD | $¢½(SHHH!!)?

———
IS MY NAME |

Figure 14-8. Communication board, commercially available. (Courtesy Trace Center, 314 Waisman Center, 1500 Highland Avenue, University of Wisconsin, Madison, Wisc. 53706)

bination. In young or retarded children, no subjective response is expected. In older children or those with minimal retardation, subjective response may help refine the refractive error during testing.

Eyeglasses are prescribed if the refractive error is of significant magnitude and if it is felt that the child will benefit from correction.

Significant refractive errors requiring correction have been found in 25–76 percent of patients.[3,17,18,22–24,27] Because refractive errors are known to cause fatigue and limited visual acuity, it is advisable to search for this ocular problem when evaluating handicapped children.[18] Hyperopia (farsightedness), myopia (nearsightedness), and astigmatism (abnormal corneal curvature) have been reported in different ratios in various studies.[3,17,18,22,23,27] Fantl and Perlstein found that most of the children they studied, with or without cerebral palsy, demonstrated hyperopia until age nine.[8,9] Non-cerebral-palsied children tend to become myopic later, while those with cerebral palsy remain hyperopic until the middle or late teens. This difference seems to be an inherent characteristic of cerebral palsy.[8,9]

Fundus Examination

Examination of the retina and optic nerve is best done through a dilated pupil, usually after refraction. The direct ophthalmoscope, used by most physicians, provides a magnified view of the optic nerve and posterior retina, but the total area seen at any given time is only several millimeters in diameter. The value of this instrument is limited with an uncooperative or retarded child who will not allow the examiner to get close to the eyes.

The ophthalmologist uses an indirect ophthalmoscope, placed on his head, with a hand-held biconvex lens of 20 to 30 diopters placed before the

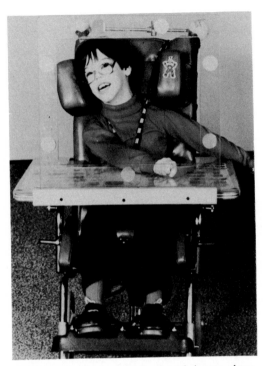

Figure 14-9. Communication board, in use, showing child with cerebral palsy pointing to a letter corresponding to letter shown on eye chart.

is observed. The peripheral retina may be examined anterior to the equator of the eye without difficulty. When retardation or fear of examination occurs, assistance in holding the patient's head may be necessary for a more meaningful view of the fundus. Examination under anesthesia is occasionally needed for the uncooperative child.

The most important intraocular finding with cerebral palsy is the presence of optic atrophy.[17] Retinal abnormalities are less common.[10,15,17,27] The etiology of optic atrophy is usually secondary to cerebral agenesis or hydrocephalus when associated with cerebral palsy.[5]

Visual Fields

The visual field describes the central and peripheral field of view, usually tested at a distance of 1 m from the patient. A tangent screen or a perimeter allows precise localization of visual field defects. This equipment has limited application in the normal pediatric population because of the child's tendency to follow the testing targets rather than gaze at a fixation target directly before the eyes. For similar reasons, this equipment has less application for testing cerebral palsied and retarded children.

Of all methods of visual fields testing, the confrontation method is probably the most widely used. It is a rapid, qualitative screening test of the visual fields. The patient looks directly at the examiner's eyes. Each eye is examined separately. The ophthalmologist displays several fingers on each hand and asks the patient to count the number of fingers seen. All four quadrants are tested: superior, inferior, nasal,

patient's eyes. The ophthalmologist uses both of his eyes simultaneously with the indirect ophthalmoscope; this provides a more satisfactory view of retinal and optic nerve detail. Less magnification is provided, but a much wider field of view of the retina

Table 14-1
Visual Acuity Definitions

Visual Acuity	Definition		% Loss of Central vision	
NLP	No light perception		100	
LP	Light perception		100	
LP with P	Light perception with projection		100	
HM	Hand motion		98–99	
CF	Counts fingers at (no. of) feet	Blind	95–97	Estimated
3/400	Must be 3 ft from 20/400 symbol to see clearly			
20/400	Legal blindness		90	
20/200	Legal blindness		80	
20/70	Visually handicapped		40	
20/40	Driver's license		15	
20/20	"Normal"		0	

and temporal. Gross field defects, such as hemi-anopsias, may be detected in this manner. This method of testing is also unreliable with nonverbal or retarded children, however.

Visual field defects may not be detected early, and a subsequent examination, months to years later, may first demonstrate a significant visual field defect. Tizard et al. studied 106 patients with hemiplegia selected from a larger group of children with cerebral palsy.[25] Almost 25 percent were found to have hom-onomous hemianopsia, and most of these children had sensory defects. If perimetry or confrontation fields could not be used, the child was placed before the mother, who attempted to attract the child's attention. The examiner, located behind the child, passed attractive objects around the child's head. Almost uncontrollable shifting of the eyes toward the side affected with hemianopsia was frequently seen. Even in infants, if a bright or attractive target is brought into the peripheral field, the child will often make a conjugate gaze movement toward the object. A hom-onomous hemianopsia may be suspected if this gaze movement is lacking on one side.[7]

MANAGEMENT

Strabismus, amblyopia, nystagmus, and optic atrophy, the most common ocular defects, require specific treatment.

Strabismus

Strabismus treatment is first discussed in patients without cerebral palsy. Esotropia describes a crossing inward of the eyes. Congenital esotropia occurs at birth or within the first few months of life. Amblyopia or poor vision from disuse of one eye is uncommon because of the alternate fixation usually found; however, if amblyopia is present, patching over the eye with better vision before surgery is indicated. Refractive error is not usually significant, and eyeglasses usually provide little benefit. Treatment is surgical, preferably within the first year of life. With congenital esotropia, the opportunity for binocular vision development gradually diminishes with age if surgery is delayed beyond the first year of life.

Accommodation is the normal focusing of the eyes, including miosis or pupil constriction, increase in the anterior–posterior diameter of the lens, and convergence or crossing of the eyes.

Accommodative esotropia describes an excessive amount of inward turning of the eyes when the effort is made to focus on a target. Accommodative esotropia occurs usually at approximately two and a half years of age, although onset may occur from six months to seven or eight years of age.

Treatment of accommodative esotropia is usually eyeglasses, if the patient is hyperopic (far-sighted), or anticholinesterase medication (isofluro-phate or echothiophate iodide), which constrict the pupil. These medications are useful for the young child or the child who is unable or refuses to wear eyeglasses. Either treatment relaxes the focusing effort the child makes, producing less convergence effort and reducing the amount of esotropia. Bifocal eyeglasses may be necessary if the amount of esotropia at near testing significantly exceeds the esotropia at distance testing. Any residual esotropia not corrected by eyeglasses or anticholinesterase medication is called nonaccommodative esotropia. If this esotropia at distance testing is 15 diopters or more despite the above corrections, then surgery is helpful for this nonaccommodative esotropic component.

Exotropia is rarely present at birth. In young children, intermittent exotropia is more common and presents with a divergence only part of the time, often becoming constant later. Stereopsis is usually normal when the eyes are straight but absent when the eyes are divergent. Treatment is surgical if the exotropia still occurs in the presence of a corrected refractive error and measures 15 diopters or more.

Conservative management of cerebral palsy and strabismus has been advocated by different authors. In 1953, Guibor recommended conservative treatment with atropine eye drops, prisms, and eyeglasses.[10] He believed that early surgery for esotropia was usually unsuccessful before eight years of age and required repeated operations. Surgery at eight years or older was reported as usually successful. Some patients displayed improved walking, talking, and writing after an improvement in ocular stability. In 1960, Abercrombie suggested early surgery to achieve the best possible binocular vision, which would be of special advantage to handicapped children.[1]

In 1966, however, Altman et al. recommended delaying treatment for refraction and motility problems beyond that for a normal child because of poor cooperation and problems with understanding.[3] Since some children tended to improve with age, strabismus surgery was often delayed.

Pigassou-Albouy and Fleming reported that therapy, prognosis, and gravity of amblyopia and strabismus differed considerably between normal children and those with cerebral palsy.[21] In normal children, amblyopia and strabismus showed response if treat-

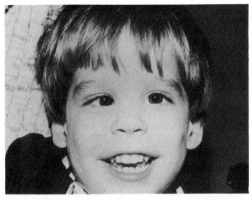

Figure 14-10. Preoperative photograph of patient aged three years eight months with esotropia and cerebral palsy.

ment was started before age six or seven. In children with cerebral palsy, the same treatment may give less satisfactory results because the amblyopia is partly due to neurologic brain lesions. Depending on the lesion, prognosis for improved vision is variable. The neurologic lesions are generally not curable and show resistance to therapy. Pigassou-Albouy and Fleming formerly treated strabismus in cerebral palsied children but have discontinued this and treat only the amblyopia when the child is at least four years old.[21]

Because of the lack of clearly defined guidelines in the management and treatment of strabismus in cerebral palsy, Hiles et al. undertook the treatment of a series of 234 children with cerebral palsy, using standard principles of strabismus therapy as applied to neurologically normal children.[12,13] Results of therapy in this series indicated that satisfactory alignment could be achieved in the majority of patients,

even in the presence of severe motor involvement or retardation.

Ninety percent of those children treated for accommodative esotropia with eyeglasses or anticholinesterase therapy achieved satisfactory alignment. Seventy-seven percent of those children with non-accommodative esotropia, or crossing of the eyes that could not be completely improved with glasses or anticholinesterase therapy, had successful eye muscle surgery. Eighty-six percent of patients who underwent surgery for exotropia achieved satisfactory results. Only 2 percent of patients showed spontaneous reduction of their strabismus to cosmetically acceptable ranges.

In patients with esotropia, the average age of initial surgery was 3.9 years, while in exotropic patients the average age of initial surgery was 5.7 years. Neurologically abnormal children require a more conservative approach before surgical intervention in order to allow for development of a stable preoperative ocular alignment. Although functional binocular alignment was not likely because of the age at which surgery was performed, cosmetically acceptable results were obtained in a high percentage of patients.[12,13] Other authors agree with Hiles.[16,24] At the Newington's Children's Hospital, children with cerebral palsy are similarly managed. A three-year-old boy with cerebral palsy and esotropia is seen in Figure 14-10. Note the light reflex displacement on the corneas. Figure 14-11 shows that the esotropia is neutralized by the prism. The amount of eye muscle surgery depends on the degree of deviation. Figure 14-12 shows the straight eyes 22 mo after surgery.

It is well known that patients with cerebral palsy have a high incidence of strabismus. On the other hand, the entity of congenital esotropia traditionally

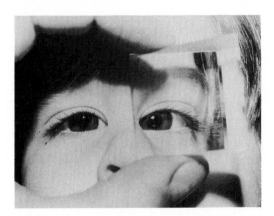

Figure 14-11. Esotropia, measured with prism and light reflex, in patient in Fig. 14-10.

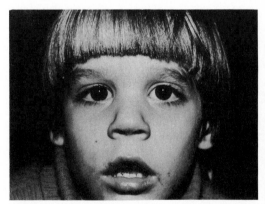

Figure 14-12. Straight eyes, 22 mo postoperatively, in patient in Fig. 14-10.

has been handled by the ophthalmologist as an isolated oculomotor problem requiring surgical treatment. A recent study by Wheeler et al. at the Newington Children's Hospital, using the Bayley Scales of Infant Development before and after surgery for congenital esotropia, has identified patients with mild and previously unsuspected cerebral palsy.[26] This earlier detection of cerebral palsy than otherwise would have occurred has allowed intervention therapy to be started earlier.

Amblyopia

Amblyopia can be detected as early as six months of age and should be treated as soon as diagnosed. A patch is placed over the eye with better vision, known as the fixating eye, in order to stimulate vision in the nonfixating, or amblyopic, eye. Commercially available eye occlusion patches, e.g., Opticlude[+] and Coverlet,[†] are most satisfactory. Patching is usually done during most of the child's waking hours until significant improvement in vision occurs. Part-time patching is then done to maintain satisfactory vision. Patching is more successful in the young child and is less successful as the child approaches age nine, when visual maturation occurs; patching is then usually discontinued. The most common reasons for amblyopia are lack of use of one eye from strabismus or from unequal refractive errors. Eyeglasses are often required in addition to patching.

Nystagmus

The presence of nystagmus may affect a child's head posture. With pendular or jerk nystagmus, there may be a null, or resting, point that allows clearest vision. If this null point is not in the primary or straight-ahead position, the child may turn the head to the side, up, or down to find the position of least nystagmus. Marked head posture may require eye muscle surgery for elimination of the head and face turn by moving the eye muscles to shift the null point to the primary position.

Nystagmus with associated retinal abnormalities may require magnifying eyeglasses, low vision aids, and special enlarged-print reading material.

[+]Opticlude Home Health Care Products, Medical Products Division of 3M, 3M Center St. Paul, Minn.

[†]Beiersdorf, Inc., P.O. Box 5529, South Norwalk, Conn.

Optic Atrophy

Optic atrophy is not reversible and has no treatment. The level of visual impairment may require no treatment in mild cases of optic nerve atrophy. More severe optic atrophy may require the use of low-vision aids, closed circuit television, and even Braille texts when blindness occurs.

REFERENCES

1. Abercrombie MLJ: Perception and eye movements; some speculations on disorders in cerebral palsy. Cerebral Palsy Bull 2:142, 1960
2. Aiello JS: Ocular problems in cerebral palsy. Arizona Med 15:415, 1958
3. Altman HE, Hiatt RL, Deweese MW: Ocular findings in cerebral palsy. South Med J 59:1015, 1966
4. American Medical Association: Estimation of loss of visual efficiency. Chicago, Council on Industrial Health, 1955
5. Breakey AS: Ocular findings in cerebral palsy. Arch Ophthalmol 53:852, 1955
6. Breakey AS, Wilson J, Wilson BC: The relationship between visual disorders and visual-perceptual deficits in cerebral palsy. Dev Med Child Neurol 10:251, 1968.
7. Diamond S: Ocular evaluation of the cerebral palsied child. Am J Ophthalmol 48:721, 1959
8. Fantl EW, Perlstein MA: Ocular refractive characteristics in cerebral palsy. Am J Dis Child 102:36, 1961
9. Fantl EW, Perlstein MA: Refractive errors in cerebral palsy. Their relationship to the causes of brain damage. Am J Ophthalmol 63:857, 1967
10. Guibor GP: Some eye defects seen in cerebral palsy, with some statistics. Am J Phys Med 32:342, 1953
11. Guibor GP: Cerebral palsy: A practical routine for discerning oculomotor defects in cerebral palsied children. J Pediatr 47:333, 1955
12. Hiles DA, Wallar PH, McFarland F: Current concepts in the management of strabismus in children with cerebral palsy. Ann Ophthalmol 7:789, 1975
13. Hiles DA: Results of strabismus therapy in cerebral palsied children. Am Orthopt J 25:46, 1975
14. Kalbe U, Berndt K, de Decker, et al: Klin Monatsbl Augenheilkd 175:367, 1979
15. Landau L, Berson D: Cerebral palsy and mental retardation: Ocular findings. J Pediatr Ophthalmol 8:245, 1971
16. Levy NS, Cassin B, Newman M: Strabismus in children with cerebral palsy. J Pediatr Ophthalmol 13:72, 1976
17. Lossef S: Ocular findings in cerebral palsy. Am J Ophthalmol 54:1114, 1962
18. Pearlstone AD, Benjamin R: Ocular defects in cerebral palsy. Eye Ear Nose Throat Monthly 48:437, 1969
19. Perlstein MA: Medical aspects of cerebral palsy. Nerv Child 8:128, 1949

20. Perlstein MA, Barnett HE: Nature and recognition of cerebral palsy in infancy. JAMA 148:1389, 1952

21. Pigassou-Albouy R, Fleming A: Amblyopia and strabismus in patients with cerebral palsy. Ann Ophthalmol 7:382, 386, 1975

22. Schachat E, Wallace HM, Palmer M, et al: Ophthalmologic findings in children with cerebral palsy. Pediatrics 19:623, 1957

23. Schrire L: An ophthalmological survey of a series of cerebral palsy cases. South A Med J 30:405, 1956

24. Seaber JH, Chandler AC: A five-year study of patients with cerebral palsy and strabismus, in Moore S, et al.

(eds): Orthoptics: Past, Present, Future New York, Grune & Stratton, 1976, pp 271–277

25. Tizard JPM, Paine RS, Crothers B: Disturbances of sensation in children with hemiplegia. JAMA 155:628, 1954

26. Wheeler M, Stonesifer K, Kenny M: Developmental evaluation of congenital esotropia. Ophthalmology 86:2161, 1979

27. Wiesinger H: Ocular findings in mentally retarded children. J Pediatr Ophthalmol 1:37, 1964

Stephanie S. Neuman

15

Intellectual Disabilities

The finding of intellectual disability within the general population has been variously estimated at 3–5 percent, depending on the definition of retardation applied. Estimates derived from a normal distribution of levels of intellectual functioning (Fig. 15-1) suggest that 3 percent of the population would have intellectual levels falling more than 2 standard deviations from the mean, i.e., intellectual quotients (IQ) of 69 and below. Table 15-1 indicates the relative proportion of the retarded to be found in each of the varying categories, based on standard deviation units of 15.

There is an increased prevalence of mental retardation in children with cerebral palsy as compared to the general population. Mental retardation has been found to be associated with cerebral palsy at rates of 40–55 percent.[5,9,11] O'Reilly suggested a continuum of deficits, including both mental and physical handicaps, among cerebral palsied children in the United States.[14] This research suggested that only 38 percent of these children functioned intellectually within the average-to-superior range, with or without serious physical deficits.

An accurate and valid psychologic assessment of the handicapped child is of primary importance in a comprehensive evaluation. The psychologist encounters several difficulties in providing this valid assessment, yet relatively little attention has been given to these difficulties or to defining appropriate procedures for assessing multihandicapped children and adults.

PROBLEMS IN ASSESSMENT

The following case study provides an example of problems in assessment.

James resided in a state institution for 12 of his last 15 yr. He was admitted to the hospital for an orthopaedic procedure. This young man carried the diagnoses of profound mental retardation, left spastic hemiparesis, and moderate hearing loss. He was nonambulatory, and many of his activities seemed limited to grabbing at people and angrily throwing materials. Yet without the benefit of any formal educational program or organized stimulation, he had developed an amazing facility with puzzles. How could this best be understood? Was it possibly an overlooked functional skill or, rather, a rote skill without use?

Assessment with James was very productive. Nonverbal measures were used throughout and his manipulation of the new and foreign hospital environment was observed. On all measures he achieved successes consistent with a six- to eight-year level of functioning. When watching television, his system of gestures and excitement objectively indicated that he was interpreting the content and context of the visual stimuli to outside references. He related, attended, maintained a focused attention, worked hard, smiled at his own mastery, and became exceedingly angry when the staff had to leave him. Some Bliss symbols for communication of his basic needs were provided and taught during this admission. He responded well to this intervention. Certainly, this individual was delayed in his development, cognitively within the moderate range of retardation, and hindered by expressive aphasia. These diagnoses were previously overshadowed by the enormity of his other handicaps.

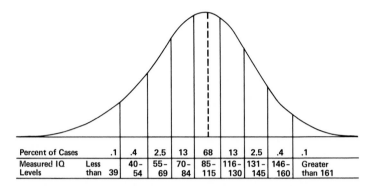

| Percent of Cases | | .1 | .4 | 2.5 | 13 | 68 | 13 | 2.5 | .4 | .1 |
| Measured IQ Levels | Less than 39 | | 40-54 | 55-69 | 70-84 | 85-115 | 116-130 | 131-145 | 146-160 | Greater than 161 |

Figure 15-1. Normal distribution of intellectual levels. (From Diagnostic and Statistical Manual of Mental Disorders, (Third Ed), American Psychiatric Association, 1980.)

Cases like the one cited are unfortunately not unique within the multihandicapped population.[4,6,20] The term *differential diagnosis* is often bantered glibly; however, it is never more acutely needed than with children who are motor, as well as possible intellectually, limited.

STANDARD MULTIFACTORED PSYCHOLOGIC ASSESSMENT

Public Law 94-142 has mandated that school-aged children are entitled to appropriate education to meet their individual needs. School systems attempt to meet this mandate but are often ill equipped. Larger urban areas often have special multidisciplinary resources to aid in psychologic evaluation. The "typical" psychologic battery of tests frequently administered to handicapped children usually includes the following:

1. An overall cognitive measure such as the Wechsler Intelligence Scale for Children–Revised (WISC–R) or the Stanford Binet–Revised[16,17]
2. A measure of independence in self-care such as the Vineland Social Maturity Scale or the Adaptive Behavior Scale[2,7]

Table 15-1

Levels of Mental Retardation in Relation to Measured Intelligence

Range in IQ Scores on Tests with Standard Deviation of 15	Terms Used in DSM III*	Relative Percentage	Educational Classification
70–84	Borderline intelligence	14	Slow learner (sometimes included in educable range)
55–69	Mild retardation	2.5	Educable retarded
40–54	Moderate retardation	.4	Trainable retarded
25–39	Severe retardation	.1	Trainable retarded
Below 25	Profound retardation	.1	Total-care group

*DSM III, American Psychiatric Association: Diagnostic and Statistical Manual of Mental Disorders (ed. 3) Washington, D.C. The Association, 1980.

3. Academic mastery as assessed by the Wide Range Achievement Test and the Peabody Individual Achievement Test[8,12]
4. Personality variables as explored through the Draw-A-Person Test and sentence completion[13,15]

This "typical" battery may be inappropriate, erroneous, and even invalid in certain children with chronically handicapping disorders, however, if all other pertinent variables are not considered simultaneously. Assessment of James (see the case study) with such a standard battery would have given further credibility for placing his function within the profound range of retardation. The cognitive measures require verbal reception and verbal expression of problem-solving tasks. The nonverbal, perceptual–motor, or performance items are timed. With no speech and very little manipulative ability due to his spasticity, he would have met with little but anger and frustration. His independence in daily activities was also "profoundly" limited, requiring assistance in all areas of self-care. Academic testing would have been futile. These paper and pencil tasks were completely foreign for this patient. Obviously, typical psychologic tests and standard assessment procedures fall short for many handicapped children. A multifactorial assessment is significantly more important in these children.

MULTIFACTORIAL ASSESSMENT

A multifactorial assessment defines strengths as well as deficits. The concept of the multifactorial assessment itself must be achieved and maintained. Additionally, one must understand the total child—both limitations due to disabilities and strengths. The objective is to reinforce these strengths to support and compensate for the areas of deficit.

Several principles in testing multihandicapped children are (1) the avoidance of preconceptions, (2) the establishment of communication, (3) a clear understanding of the use of standard measures, (4) teaching and learning, and (5) the recognition of defense mechanisms. The goal is to provide a valid assessment of capabilities and potential for learning and to suggest modalities for further growth.

Avoidance of Preconception

The clinician must not bring preconceptions to the evaluation. An open mind, attuned to nuances of behavior, functional play, and social development,

will provide important areas for exploration. Any preconception of "What most children with cerebral palsy are like" or "Blind people can't . . ." will only diminish one's own ability to process information objectively.

Establishment of Communication

An avenue of communication must be established. Multimodal exploration is a prerequisite here. Establishing a method of relating and communicating with a nonverbal, hearing-impaired, spastic child with strabismus can challenge one's creativity. All avenues should be examined (auditory, visual, motor, tactile, kinesthetic) to locate a reliable, consistent, mutually understood stimulus–response pattern.

These sensory channels must also be differentiated, since there can be discrete deficits in output or input processing. This problem is often most clearly seen in children with perceptual–motor problems. One child may process visual stimuli adequately (input) yet have difficulty coordinating the fine motor movements to copy geometric designs (output). A second child may not visually process external stimuli (input) adequately and therefore, despite age-adequate fine motor skill (output), be unable to put a peg in a hole with ease. Both children perform poorly on these perceptual–motor tasks for quite different reasons. The two case studies below illustrate this point.

Linda, aged 16, was accompanied by her mother, who replied to all conversation directed toward her daughter. Linda had little effective motion in any extremity and required the full support of a specially adapted care chair. She did not have intelligible speech and had frequent athetoid movements. Her receptive verbal skills, however, were at least in the 10–12 yr level, as assessed by her appropriate smiles to remarks and casual conversation. When both Linda and her mother seemed comfortable, the mother was asked to sit in the waiting room so that Linda and the examiner could get better acquainted. The first task was to find a way to communicate, and Linda was enthusiastic to try. Although she did not have enough motor coordination to grasp a pencil or fat crayon or to place a block on an X, she spotted a typewriter in the office and looked at it encouragingly. This required a high level of independent dexterity, but by holding her elbow on the chair pad and supporting her wrist, with painstaking care she typed out "hello," and her assessment began.

The evaluation of a second child with cerebral palsy, developmental delays, and significant emotional disturbance led to a quite different resolution. Frank, aged four and one half years, could reliably respond by hitting a xylophone and was actually assessed by his mastery of simple and complex tone, rhythm patterns, and tunes. He enjoyed this "game" so much that he put the examiner to the test in "Name That Tune." He would applaud when the correct tune was named and the music repeated for him.

Standard Measures

Standard measures cannot be abused. All psychologic tests have been validated and standardized with specified administration techniques. Divergence from these methods invalidates the results. Some latitude is essential, however, in using these tools with handicapped children. The clinician must be well grounded in the research base and design of the test in order to obtain reliable, relevant, and valid estimates of a child's functioning.

Obviously, verbal measures for a nonverbal child are inappropriate, as are visual tasks for a blind child; however, some items of all sensory modalities are necessary to explore the degree of deficit the child experiences in these channels as well as to find avenues the child may use to compensate. For example, a child with a visual processing deficit might be encouraged to try the task with his or her own verbal supports or "talking through the problem," e.g., "the crayon line goes up here, then over, then down."

A complete listing of tests commonly used for assessing children with specific deficits is beyond the scope of this chapter, but a few of the most widely used nonverbal scales, tests, and assessment measures are discussed below.

Leiter International Performance Scale

The Leiter International Performance Scale (LIPS) test requires neither examiner verbal direction nor child verbal response.[1] The LIPS assesses conceptual development on increasingly difficult match-and-sort-to-sample tasks. Blocks are presented and demonstrated to the child; they must be placed in a tray to solve the problem presented on a stimulus strip. Children find it interesting, fun, and nonthreatening. The scale is useful for children of mental age 24 mo to 7–8 yr. For children without the requisite motor ability to place the blocks in the tray, the blocks can be set on or next to the stimulus strip.

Columbia Mental Maturity Scale (CMMS)

The Columbia Mental Maturity Scale (CMMS) has recently been restandardized and presents to the child 93 large, different pattern sequences requiring increasing difficulty of conceptual problem-solving

skills.[3] The test is useful with children of mental age three to nine years.

Hiskey Nebraska Test of Learning Aptitude

The Hiskey Nebraska test has norms for both hearing and deaf children aged 3–16 yr.[10] It is a performance-oriented scale with several subtests that evaluate visual–motor coordination, sequential memory, visual discrimination and association, and matching and conceptual relationships.

Normed Toys

An important adjunct in assessing multihandicapped children is the child's level and quality of play. Evaluating the level of functional play skills is often quite helpful. A child psychologist's toys should be carefully selected to allow for a wide range of developmental skills. They should, of course, be of interest to children. Levels of toy play have been validated to differentiate between diagnostic groups and have been found to have practical use.[18,19]

A child who can roll a large ball but cannot throw it has functioning motorskills with this toy below the 12-mo level. Completing a simple seven-piece wooden Charlie Brown puzzle is consistent with a five-year level of functioning (four years if the child needs help with the tricky purple strip for the pants). Copying rhythms and tone patterns is not a standard assessment tool but can be broken down into the auditory short-term memory skill level required. All toys can be broken into the developmental levels necessary for successful mastery and the discrete abilities that are tapped.

Teaching and Learning

Assessment should also include both teaching and learning. Psychologists are trained in understanding the cognitive processes involved in the mastery of a particular task. Failures are said to represent a lack of development in that area. Understimulation or deprivation as an interference to development is either overlooked completely or sought out so diligently that it leads to spurious expectation for the child. A more moderate approach, it would seem, is to take the opportunity to teach a child a task once he or she has demonstrated difficulty with it. Additionally, this can provide diagnostic information in several respects. Obviously, the child is not credited with successful completion if taught.

Questions the examiner should explore in regard to teaching a task to a child include the following:

1. How difficult was it to teach the child? Was a quick demonstration presented or was it necessary to break the task down into lower developmental levels? If so, what mental age levels?
2. Once the skill was learned, was the child able to generalize it to another similar task, reflecting integrated learning rather than rote?
3. Did the child retain the concept and skill level necessary to independently master the task at the next visit?

If the child is able to master the task with a simple demonstration, retain the skill over time, and generalize the concept to other like materials, a case would then be more logically made for deprivation. Reconsider James (see the case study on page 151). He demonstrated mastery with interlocking puzzles sent with him from his residential setting. The WISC–R puzzles were presented and appeared quite foreign to him. All were beige tone, lacking color variation, and had straight edges without the rounded interlocking joints. After giving the standard directions, the first puzzle—a three-piece apple—was completed and removed by the examiner. The first actual test puzzle, a picture of a girl, was presented but James was bewildered. A return to the apple, which was completed together, and the girl, also jointly arranged, led to James's demonstrating a growing sense of confidence. The last three test puzzles were presented and completed slowly but accurately. The following day, thus testing out the above hypothesis, James completed the puzzles with alacrity and was able to tackle other new and complex puzzles quite adequately.

Defense Mechanisms

The multihandicapped child often meets the psychologist with his or her own set of misperceptions. There is frequently a sense of forboding and failure and an overriding negative sense of self-worth. This may overtly be registered through a feigned act of boredom or disinterest or, conversely, by angry, out-of-control behavior. Children develop a wide range of compensatory mechanisms to deal with their handicaps: Some are adaptive and serve as appropriate coping devices; others are maladaptive and attempt to "hide the problem." The examiner's task is not only to understand and empathize but also to facilitate the child's participation in the evaluation. For this, patience and flexibility in procedures, timing, and the allowance for several visits are necessary (see the following case study).

The case of Robert, aged 15, posed such a problem. He had lived at home and attended school sporadically until the third grade, at which time he moved to a residential facility. He was nonambulatory and had good range of motion in his upper extremities. His speech was dysarthric and, at first, almost unintelligible. During the opening discussion or monologue with the psychologist, Robert's speech productivity and intelligibility improved. Clearly, his dysarthria was more pronounced when he was anxious, but he also seemed to be using it as an avoidance mechanism. As the meeting progressed, his very low self-image became more evident. He was well entrenched in failure, feigned ignorance for each question asked or task presented, and required substantial and frequent support to tackle anything. The assessment necessarily was quite lengthy and required several sessions.

After completing the assessment, a significant amount of time was spent in conversation about his life, the institution, and other personal interactions. He was able to become animated, even ebullient at times, and knew multitudes of details about the routine, staff functions, and hospital gossip. He had been attending inservice presentations for the staff and could discuss medical problems with a wealth of well-founded knowledge.

On the WISC–R, Robert was found to be functioning within the mild range of retardation. This was a low estimate because of the degree of his avoidance. At one session he mentioned an interest in sports; when the local paper was brought to him, he was asked to read it to himself. When he finished he replied to questions accurately and went on to summarize fan reaction to the defeat, replete with details. He had kept his abilities well concealed for many years.

REFERENCES

1. Arthur G: Arthur Adaptation of the Letter International Performance Scale: Instruction Manual. Chicago, Stoelting, 1952
2. Balthazar EE: Balthazar Scales of Adaptive Behavior. Palo Alto, Consulting Psychologists Press, 1976
3. Burgenmeister BB, Blum LJ, Lorge I: Columbia Mental Maturity Scale: Guide for Administering and Interpreting. New York, Harcourt Brace Jovanovich, 1972
4. Campbell J, Magda R: Kleinfelter's Syndrome in a three-year old severely disturbed child. J Autism Child Schizo 2:34, 1972
5. Conley RW: The Economics of Mental Retardation. Baltimore, The Johns Hopkins University Press, 1973
6. Cox S: The learning disabled adult. Acad Ther 13:79, 1977
7. Doll EA: The Measurement of Social Competence. Princeton, Educational Test Bureau, 1953

8. Dunn LM, Markwardt FC: Peabody Individual Achievement Test: Manual. Circle Pines, Minn., American Guidance Service, 1970

9. Greenbaum M, Buehler JA: Further Findings on the Intelligence of Children with Cerebral Palsy, Am J Ment Defic 65:261, 1960

10. Hiskey MS: Hiskey-Nebraska Test of Learning Aptitude: Manual, Lincoln, Neb., Union College Press, 1966

11. Hohman LB, Freedheim DK: Further Studies on Intelligence Levels in Cerebral Palsied Children, Am J Phys Med 37:90, 1958

12. Jastak JK, Jastak S: The Wide Range Achievement Test, Manual of Instructions (1978 Revised Edition). Wilmington, Jastak Associates, 1978

13. Koppitz EM: Psychological Evaluation of Children's Human Figure Drawings. New York, Grune & Stratton, 1968

14. O'Reilly DE: The future of the cerebral palsied child. Dev Med Child Neurol 13:635, 1971

15. Rotter JB, Wellerman B: The incomplete sentence test as a method of studying personality. J Consult Psychol 11:43, 1947

16. Terman LM, Merrill MA: Manual for the Stanford-Binet Intelligence Scale (Third Revision, Form L-M). Boston, Houghton Mifflin, 1973

17. Wechsler D: Manual for the Wechsler Intelligence Scale for Children—Revised. New York, The Psychological Corp., 1974

18. Weiner BJ, Ottinger DR, Tilton JR: Comparison of the toy–play behavior of autistic, retarded, and normal children: A re-analysis. Psychol Rep 25:223, 1969

19. Weiner EA, Weiner BJ: Differentiation of retarded and normal children through toy-play analysis. Multivariate Behav Res 9:245, 1974

20. Wing L: Differentiation of retardation and autism from specific communication disorders. Child Care Health Dev 5:57, 1979

Janet Yost
Pamella McMillan

16

Communication Disorders

This chapter offers an overview of speech, language, and hearing problems associated with cerebral palsy. The cerebral palsied child and the family require a multifaceted, cooperative effort from many professionals. Pediatric health care providers must be aware of the type and degree of the communication impairments that may be present in their patients and understand the habilitation contributions that the speech–language pathologist and audiologist can make.

SPEECH AND LANGUAGE DISORDERS

Early Speech and Language Development

Human speech does not occur in a simple or isolated way. It is a marvelously delicate and complex balance of neuromuscular movements made audible, which depend upon reliable sensory input, a central nervous system (CNS) adequate for attention, memory, and conceptualization, an intact motor system, and an environment that provides something to talk about as well as listeners and speakers with whom to interact.

The child's experiences in the first year of life have a great deal of bearing on what the developing speech system will be like. Although all children learn language in the same kind of developmental sequence, certain aspects are culture specific. The child's immediate language environment will provide speech models from whom to learn the specific speech sounds (phonemes) of the culture. Through time and

experience the child will mature and learn, given an accepting and stimulating environment. These experiences come to the child through sensations of vision, hearing, touch, smell, and body kinesthesia. At the same time the child is experiencing and learning through motor exploration.

Discrimination and perception (the ability to derive meaning from sensations) appear surprisingly early and form the vehicle for language learning. Eventually the young child begins to perceive and discriminate auditory stimuli, such as the spoken word *dog* when paired with the visual stimulus of an actual dog. He soon makes the giant leap in understanding that the spoken word *dog* represents the four-legged animal in the next room. The word (symbol) *dog* is now in the child's listening (receptive) vocabulary, well before he is able to say the word. He will soon begin to generalize his new word *dog* to all dogs of different sizes and shapes and may overgeneralize it to all animals or all furry things. In order to say the word, he must not only have the concept and name of *dog* but also the necessary neuromuscular power to produce the correct speech sounds that constitute the acoustic event *dog*.

Speech and Language Variations in Cerebral Palsy

Infants born with cerebral palsy, whether due to anoxia or a multitude of less common causes, are considered to have static, nonprogressive damage to affected areas of the brain. One of the most common and pervasive sequela of such lesions is disordered and delayed speech and language development. The

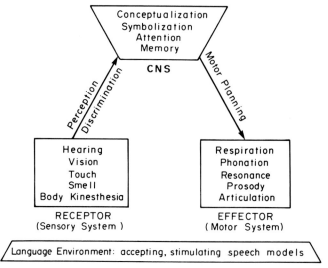

Figure 16-1. Levels of speech and language development vulnerable to disruption and impaired function.

range of these disorders covers the full spectrum from near normal to complete anarthria (lack of speech). Many specific areas of functioning necessary for normal speech and language development may be impaired at any or all levels in the child with cerebral palsy. Figure 16-1 shows how many levels are vulnerable to disruption and impaired fuction.

Limited Sensory System (Receptor)

The cerebral palsied infant very often lacks the auditory, visual, tactile, and kinesthetic stimulation that underlies early language development. Hearing loss is common and will be further discussed in the section on hearing disorders. Tactile sensitivity and perception are usually disturbed in cerebral palsied children.[5] In addition, sensory input from distorted muscles and abnormal posture probably have a detrimental effect on both cognitive and motor learning. Disturbance of body awareness may be severe enough to result in body agnosia.[15] The oral sensory functions so essential both to babbling and to feeding may be lacking. In some cases, lack of oral sensations may actually produce a rare instance of oral stereognosis. Visual problems are also common among cerebral palsied children (see Chap. 14). All these sensory limitations, especially those of hearing, will adversely affect the child's acquisition of language.

Limited Conceptualization

The higher-level functions of attention, memory, conceptualization, and symbolization may also be deficient in the cerebral palsied child. The inci-

dence of mental retardation is high and seems to be related to topography of the CNS damage. Spastic quadriplegics are most likely to have cognitive, as well as language, deficits. Athetoid patients are least likely to be impaired intellectually but almost always have defective speech articulation. It is important to differentiate between *language* deficits (comprehension and use of words and sentences) and *speech* impairments (speech sound production).

Limited Motor System (Effector)

It is in the motor area that cerebral palsy provides the most frequent and disabling sequelae. Motor speech is no exception. The motor limitations of the cerebral palsied child have a specific impact on speech articulation development, usually an area of particular deficit for most. Even when language comprehension is relatively intact, expressive skills may be severely disordered, largely because of neuromuscular impairment, which affects the functioning of the articulators as well as other organs of speech. Difficulties with biting, sucking, swallowing, and chewing have been found to coexist with poor articulation.[14] Verbal apraxia (poor coordination of the articulators) may occur even in the absence of paresis of the musculature. The most common problem, dysarthria, deserves a more complete discussion.

Dysarthria. Dorland's Illustrated Medical Dictionary defines dysarthria as "imperfect articulation of speech due to disturbance of muscular control which results from damage to CNS or PNS."[7] This traditional medical definition has considered dysarthria to be a disturbance of speech *articulation* alone. By contrast, from the work of Darley et al. at the Mayo Clinic, a broadened definition has evolved. They define dysarthria as follows: "A collective name for a group of related speech disorders that are due to disturbance in muscular control of the speech mechanism resulting from impairment of any of the basic motor processes involved in the execution of speech."[6]

Dysarthria is complex, just as speech is complex. It involves not only articulation, but the entire effector system for speech: respiration, phonation, resonance, articulation, and prosody (Fig. 16-2). These five elements of motor speech are inextricably woven together and must function as a unified whole for speech to be produced normally. They may also be thought of as taking place through a unified system of tubes and valves. For purposes of discussion we will briefly examine each component individually, bearing in mind that this is a purely artificial separation.

Respiration.   Respiration provides the energy source for speech. In normal breathing, rhythmic inspiration and expiration occur at the rate of 16–20 cycles/min (cpm). In cerebral palsy there are many possible breakdowns in this process. Inspiration may be too shallow, decreasing the quantity of air for speech. The child may be able to inhale deeply but unable to control exhalation. The rhythm of breathing is often affected.[2] Increased rate of respiration is common in cerebral palsy. Rates above 30 cpm will result in poor speech production and may well interfere with babbling in infancy. Asynchrony of the diaphragmatic–abdominal musculature is often seen in children with cerebral palsy.[15] In addition, they usually have decreased vital capacity or reduced reserves of lung volume.[5] Expiratory reserve is reportedly the most reduced function in cerebral palsied children and precisely the one most needed for speech, since speech occurs on exhaled air.

Phonation.   Phonation, or voicing, takes place in the glottis at the level of the larynx. As exhaled air leaves the lungs, the first valve in the speech effector system is the glottal valve of the larynx, with its vocal folds that adduct during speech. In normal speech the adducted vocal folds are set into vibration by the regular cycle of exhaled air from the lungs. Voice disruptions common to cerebral palsy result from irregularities of rate or amount of air flow and irregular tension of the vocal folds, caused by paresis or spasms of the muscles of the larynx. Changes in the tension of the folds result in inappropriate pitch and loudness deviations. A common problem is lack of coordination of exhaled air and phonation. Air may escape before the folds are adducted and set into vibration, causing breathy or aspirate voice quality and short, choppy phrasing of speech.

Resonance.   Resonance is the acoustic process by which components of the vocal tone are damped or amplified as they pass the pharyngeal, oral, and nasal cavities. Many resonance problems are the result of aberrant patterns of neuromuscular function of the valving of these cavities, particularly the velopharyngeal valve, which separates the pharynx from the nasal cavity. In normal speech the velum, or soft palate, moves to close this valve, preventing air from escaping through the nose (except for the nasal sounds *m* and *n*). Persons who lack the musculature to close this valve will have inefficient control of the air flow for speech and will be perceived as hypernasal.

Articulation.   The processes of articulation and resonance cannot be separated, since they occur simultaneously during speech. The valving process oc-

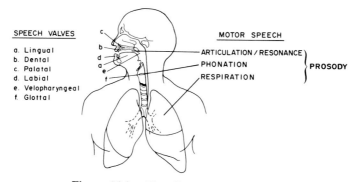

Figure 16-2.   The effector system for speech.

curs not only at the level of the soft palate but also at many points of contact by the tongue, hard palate, teeth, lips, and mandible (Figure 16-2). These articulators modify the airstream by the valving process into specific speech sounds, known as *phonemes*. The rapid coordinated movement patterns of the articulators are obviously extremely susceptible to neuromuscular breakdowns, as occur in cerebral palsy. Distorted consonants are the most common result of poor control of the musculature of the articulators. Vowel production may also be affected. In addition to the tongue, lips, and palate, the mandible becomes an important factor in the speech of cerebral palsied youngsters. Many have difficulty in keeping the mandible raised. Others cannot control the range of mandibular movement. A displaced mandible can affect the tongue's position, thus interfering with its movements and valving function. Lip control is extremely deficient in many cerebral palsied children, affecting not only sucking and feeding but also articulation.

Prosody.   Prosody, the fifth component of speech production is interwoven with the other four. Prosody refers to the rate and rhythm of speech. Intonation, stress, and melodic variations in individual speech patterns are all elements of prosody. Weak and particularly irregular muscle movements will severely affect prosody, whether on the level of respiration, phonation, or articulation.

Spastic versus athetoid dysarthrias.   The work of Darley et al. with adult neurology patients clarified and classified several clinically identifiable dysarthrias.[6] The clusters of speech symptoms that characterize neurologic disorders unfortunately do not apply to neurologically involved children. The developmental nature of cerebral palsy means, in effect, that speech patterns change over time through growth and maturation, language development, and a myriad of other factors. Darley et al., however, do give a means of approaching and analyzing dysarthric speech. Although the dysarthrias of spastic versus athetoid or other categories of cerebral palsy are not discrete or clear cut, some clinical distinctions can be observed.[2-4] (Note that most of our data comes from clinical observations rather than experimental or longitudinal studies.) A study of over 1000 patients in New Jersey in 1951 revealed that 68 percent of the cerebral palsied children had speech impairments. Dysarthria was present in 88.7 percent of the athetoid group and in 51.9 percent of the spastic group.[11] A slightly lower incidence (44 percent) has been cited

for spastic diplegics.[12] Wolfe found that 100 percent of his group of athetoid children had neuromuscular involvement of the articulators, larynx, and lungs, causing 40 percent of the children to have "severe unintelligibility."[17] By contrast, of the spastic children in the same study, only 28 percent were found to have significant unintelligibility.

A number of observers, including Kent and Netsell, have reported the following characteristics of athetoid speech: poor respiratory control, slow rate of speech, weak voice, low pitch, monotone, irregular valving of the velopharyngeal port, poor tongue and lip control, and excessive jaw movements.[13] Compared to spastics, athetoids as a group have measurably more deficits in all these parameters.[2,3] We can thus infer that respiration, phonation, resonance, articulation, and prosody are all more affected in the athetoid group. Despite these observations, workers still lack an adequate corpus of well-documented data on the actual speech characteristics of large numbers of cerebral palsied children over time. Much more work is needed in this area, as is investigation into the *language* potential and performance of these same children. When factors such as hearing loss, mental retardation, or restricted language environment are present, one must suspect deficient or delayed comprehension and expression of language (vocabulary and grammar) as well. One must be particularly alert to the child whose comprehension of language is good but whose expressive language is severely impaired by dysarthria.

INTERVENTION AND REMEDIATION

Because of the complex, developmental nature of cerebral palsy, early intervention on the part of several professionals is essential. Early involvement of an occupational and a physical therapist is necessary to ensure maximum gross and fine motor development. The speech–language pathologist as a rule becomes actively involved with the cerebral palsied child during infancy, even before first words emerge. The occupational therapist and speech–language pathologist may profitably work together on goals of stimulating the musculature of feeding and babbling.[2,5,10] Parent education on normal speech and language development, auditory development, and expected norms of development for cerebral palsied infants must be presented. Simultaneous or concurrent social work counseling of parents is most helpful during this stage, since parents may be unrealistic about their child's language (and other) development or may be unable to cope with the realities they face.

Such an ideal interdisciplinary approach to the child and family has become more of a reality in recent years, with the evolution of centers offering early intervention in the form of parent–infant programs and special preschools. Federal and state legislation now mandates early identification and intervention for handicapped youngsters. In such programs, it has now become the rule rather than the exception for the physical and occupational therapists, psychologist, speech–language pathologist, audiologist, and social worker to work closely on behalf of the child and family.

The role of the speech–language pathologist has shifted away from the traditional one of *speech therapist* (or *speech correctionist*) to that of language-development specialist. His or her role has been broadened to include assessment and facilitation of such nonspeech behaviors as babbling, attention and eye contact, optimal positioning for respiration and phonation, and turn taking. Many of these prespeech goals are worked on in close association with physical and occupational therapists. During this early stage, any one of the team members may take the lead in implementing the joint goals and interpreting them to the parents. This enables the parents to have one primary person with whom to build a bond of trust and ensures their active cooperation and follow-through.

With school-aged cerebral palsied children, the speech–language pathologist's role includes that of ongoing evaluation and therapy for the child's speech impairments as well as language deficits. He or she must carefully analyze the elements that may be contributing to the dysarthric speech (e.g., respiration, phonation, articulation, resonance, and prosody) as well as the child's comprehension and use of vocabulary, grammar, and sentence structure.

Both the pediatrician and speech–language pathologist should be especially alert to the element of hypernasality in the cerebral palsied child's speech. This may be caused by inadequate musculature of the velopharyngeal port, resulting in "cleft palate–like" speech.[8] The contribution of a prosthodontist may be significant in these cases. Hardy et al., at the University of Iowa, found very favorable results with palatal lifts versus pharyngeal flap surgery.[9] They summarize their findings by stating that "clearly, prosthetic management of palatal paresis in children with cerebral palsy is the procedure of choice. Not only is there no surgical risk to the child, but there appears to be a greater probability of success with the prosthetic program than with the surgical procedure."[9] Just as every cerebral palsied child should be considered at risk for hearing loss, so also should every cerebral palsied child with hypernasal speech be considered a candidate for prosthetic management.

It must be stated that even with optimal early intervention in prespeech, language, and speech areas, many cerebral palsied children remain essentially nonverbal or severely unintelligible. At some point a decision must be made on alternate or supplemental modes of communication. Supplementary communication systems may include sign language, Bliss symbols, communication boards, a variety of electronic devices based either on the alphabet or on a picture–symbol system, and newly emerging synthetic speech devices.[1,16] In recent years the trend has been toward early introduction of nonverbal communication modes for cerebral palsied children to serve initially as a supplementary system (and language–intellectual stimulus), which later may become the child's primary means of communication if speech does not develop adequately. Nonverbal communication may be encouraged when speaking skills are lagging behind comprehension. Pointing, gesturing, sign language, and symbol systems (such as Bliss) are all felt to be important forms of communication, even for a child who will eventually develop adequate verbal language. Early interaction with others and motivation to communicate (by any means available) is felt to be a primary goal for the development of receptive and expressive language. Early introduction of the concept of the importance of "communication" skills versus "speech" skills often results in ease of acceptance on the parents' part if alternate modes of communication must become primary for their child rather then supplementary. This is especially true for the cerebral palsied child whose communicative functioning is complicated by mental retardation, severe motor involvement, or hearing loss.

HEARING DISORDERS

The prevalence of hearing loss in the cerebral palsied population is very high compared to that in the general population. Most of the causes of cerebral palsy can also produce hearing loss. A discussion of the implications and classification of hearing loss will precede specific information on hearing loss in cerebral palsy.

Importance of Early Identification

Hearing loss interferes with communication and is therefore a significant handicap at any age. Hearing loss present from birth or early infancy is especially handicapping because it prevents normal exposure to, and learning of, verbal language. A child who cannot hear speech normally will not learn to understand or produce it normally. If the hearing loss is severe enough, it will prevent the achievement of verbal language competence, and an alternative language system, usually sign language, will be necessary for meaningful communication.

Early identification is a critical factor in the hearing-impaired child's habilitation. The child's ability to learn language, whether verbal, sign, or some other symbol system, is greatest in infancy and early childhood. The earlier a hearing loss is diagnosed and habilitation started, the greater the potential for language development. Maximizing auditory input through an appropriate hearing-aid fitting during the critical language learning period maximizes the probability that the child will learn to understand and produce speech.

A child who cannot learn verbal language and who is not exposed to an alternative communication system will be an extremely handicapped individual. Without a language system, learning in general will be impaired and psychosocial and emotional development will likely suffer as well.[29,35,38]

Hearing can be tested in children of any age and habilitation since a hearing problem can begin immediately. Because of the importance of early identification and habilitation on long-term functioning of the congenitally or neonatally hearing-impaired

child, much attention has been focused on developing newborn hearing screening programs. A committee was established in 1969 to develop guidelines for hearing screening in newborns. Members included representatives from the American Speech and Hearing Association, the Academy of Ophthalmology and Otolaryngology, and the Academy of Pediatrics. This Joint Committee on Hearing Screening in Infants recommended that newborns who are at risk for hearing loss, based on medical and family history, be seen for audiologic evaluation by two months of age.[18] The factors that place an infant at high risk for hearing loss, according to the Joint Committee, are listed in Table 16-1. Some hospitals now have newborn hearing screening programs. More often, however, the primary health care provider must refer the child to an audiologist for audiologic evaluation. The primary health care provider should ensure that children at risk for hearing loss are evaluated, and he or she should be alert to the possibility of hearing loss in every child.

Approximately 40 percent of children with congenital or early-onset hearing loss will *not* be included on the high-risk register.[23,36] Some of these hearing-impaired children have less common associated abnormalities, such as pigmentary or renal disorders, which might alert the primary health care provider to the possibility of hearing loss.[27,28] Most of them, however, show no clue to the presence of hearing loss in the most careful history and physical examination.[20,33] These children are felt to have genetically determined hearing losses, in most cases with undetected prenatal and postnatal illnesses accounting for some of the losses. Careful attention to parent report, and skilled health care provider observation, is needed to detect these hearing losses early. Children who are suspected of not responding to sound normally should be referred for audiologic evaluation as soon as possible.

The pediatric health care provider should be aware of what information can be obtained through audiologic evaluation. Several audiologic assessment methods are available. Children can usually be evaluated audiologically with behavioral test techniques. Observation of reflexive behavior in children under six months, and classic and operant conditioning techniques with older children, can usually be used to obtain reliable information about hearing acuity. Impedance audiometry is an electroacoustic measure that provides information about middle ear status and hearing. Tympanometry and acoustic reflex testing, the components of impedance audiometry, are noninvasive tests that allow measurement of the sound-

Table 16-1
Infants at High Risk for Hearing Loss

History of hereditary childhood hearing impairment

Rubella or other nonbacterial intrauterine fetal infection (e.g., cytomegalovirus [CMV] and herpes infections)

Defects of ear, nose, or throat; malformed, low-set, or absent pinnae; cleft lip or palate (including submucous cleft); any residual abnormality of the otorhinolaryngeal system

Birth weight less than 1500 g

Bilirubin level greater than 20 mg/100 ml serum

conducting properties of the outer and middle ear through a probe placed in the ear canal. Electrophysiologic measures are sometimes used in testing hearing acuity. Averaged electroencephalographic (EEG) potentials can be measured through scalp electrodes in response to auditory stimuli. Further discussion of pediatric test techniques and the information that can be obtained through audiologic evaluation may be found in several references.[26,32]

Classification

Hearing loss is classified according to degree and type. Degrees of hearing loss are grouped into four categories: mild, moderate, severe, and profound. The term *deafness* is sometimes used to refer to severe or profound hearing loss. It is also used imprecisely in medical literature to refer to any degree of hearing loss. There are three types of hearing loss: conductive, sensorineural, and mixed.

The severity or degree of a hearing loss is defined by how intense auditory test stimuli must be before they are perceived. The effect on verbal language development becomes more marked with greater degrees of hearing loss. Sign language is often the primary mode of communication for severely and profoundly hearing-impaired people; however, a great deal of variability in verbal language competence is seen among individuals with the same degree of hearing loss.

Conductive

Conductive hearing loss occurs when an abnormality in the outer or middle ear interferes with or blocks the conduction of sound energy from the environment to the cochlea. Conductive hearing losses are usually treatable. They cannot be worse than moderate, since, at this intensity, sound will pass through the bones of the skull to the cochlea. With conductive hearing losses speech can be understood easily if it is loud enough. A person with a conductive hearing loss that is not medically or surgically treatable will hear and understand speech well with a hearing aid.

Sensorineural

Sensorineural hearing loss occurs when there is an abnormality of the cochlea or eighth cranial nerve. Sensorineural hearing loss is generally much more handicapping than conductive hearing loss. This type of hearing loss cannot be medically or surgically remedied and is associated with difficulty understanding speech as well as hearing acuity problems. Coch-

lear or eighth cranial nerve damage results in a distorted, incomplete signals' reaching the auditory cortex. Even when speech is made loud enough to be *heard* well, it cannot necessarily be *understood* well. For this reason, a hearing aid may provide less than optimal benefit for the sensorineurally hearing–impaired person, although in most cases a hearing aid is helpful. Generally, the more severe the hearing acuity loss, the greater the accompanying understanding problem, although a great deal of variability is seen.

Mixed

A person can have both a sensorineural and a conductive hearing loss. For example, ossicular abnormalities and cochlear damage might be observed in a rubella child, resulting in a conductive and a sensorineural component to the hearing loss.

Hearing Loss in Cerebral Palsy

The hearing loss associated with cerebral palsy is almost always sensorineural. Table 16-2 lists the known noninherited causes of early childhood sensorineural hearing loss; most of them are recognized as etiologic factors for cerebral palsy as well.[19] The degree of sensorineural hearing loss seen with cerebral palsy varies a great deal. In general, children with athetoid cerebral palsy due to Rh incompatibility demonstrate the most severe hearing losses, while lesser degrees of hearing loss are seen in spastic cerebral palsied children.[24,30] Many different configurations of hearing loss are seen, but typically, hearing acuity is less impaired for low-frequency sounds than for high-frequency sounds (frequency corresponds to pitch). The hearing loss may be mild for low-frequency test stimuli and severe-to-profound for high-frequency test stimuli. In some cases a severe-to-profound hearing loss may be present at all frequencies.[21,37]

Cerebral palsied children are at least as likely to have conductive hearing loss as the general pediatric population. Middle ear effusion is the most common cause of conductive hearing loss, and although these losses are usually mild, they can be educationally significant. A mixed hearing loss may occur when a conductive problem is present in a sensorineurally hearing–impaired child. A moderate sensorineural hearing loss may become a severe mixed hearing loss in the presence of middle ear effusion. Periodic temporary decreases in hearing acuity may easily go unnoticed in an already hearing-impaired child, especially when there are other handicaps and

Table 16-2

Known Exogenous Causes of Prelingual
Sensorineural Hearing Loss

Preconception and prenatal

  Rubella
  CMV
  Ototoxic and other drugs; maternal alcoholism
  Hypoxia
  Syphilis
  Toxemia, diabetes, other severe systemic
    maternal illnesses
  Parental irradiation
  Toxoplasmosis

Perinatal

  Hypoxia
  Traumatic delivery
  Maternal infection
  Ototoxic drugs
  Premature delivery

Neonatal and postnatal

  Hypoxia
  Infection
  Meningitis
  Encephalitis
  Ototoxic drugs
  Erythroblastosis fetalis
  Infantile measles or mumps

Reprinted from Bergstrom L, Hemenway WG, Downs MP:
A high-risk registry to find congenital deafness. Otolaryngol
Clin North Am 4:369, 1971. With permission.

communication is impaired. Special effort should be
made to minimize conductive hearing loss overlay in
such sensorineurally hearing–impaired childen, since
every bit of residual hearing is needed for optimal
learning. Periodic build up of cerumen may be a
problem for hearing aid users, since earmold use tends
to impact cerumen and cause a conductive component.

Widely varying prevalence figures for hearing
loss in cerebral palsied children have been reported.[24,30,31] A number of factors may have contributed to the divergence of findings:

1. *Biased samples.* Most studies have sampled from
   restricted populations, such as children in special
   schools, athetoid children, or children who were
   readily testable.

2. *Differing or unreliable measures of hearing loss.*
   Parent reports or case reviews have been used as
   the measure of hearing loss in some studies, and,
   where hearing testing was performed, stimuli have
   varied considerably.

3. *Varying definitions of hearing loss.* Investigators
   have used different cutoff points for sensitivity in
   determining abnormal hearing.

A study by Morris in 1973 provides the best
estimate of the prevalence of hearing loss in the cerebral palsied population.[30] He evaluated 97 percent
of known cerebral palsied preschool and school children 0–15 yr of age in northwest England. Twelve
percent of this population had a sensorineural hearing
loss considered to be serious in that it affected the
normal development of verbal language. Another 2
percent had educationally significant conductive hearing losses.

Table 16-3 shows the prevalence of educationally significant sensorineural hearing loss in cerebral
palsied children by age. These data suggest that the
prevalence has decreased over the last 5–15 yr. Morris points out that the lower prevalence reported in
the group aged 0–4 yr may actually be due to undiagnosed hearing loss.

Exactly comparable prevalence figures for "educationally significant" sensorineural hearing loss in
the general pediatric population are not available. The
National Census of the Deaf Population in the United
States, however, provides some comparative data
(Table 16-4).[34] Among children aged 0–16 yr in the
general population, the prevalence of bilateral significant hearing loss was 0.66 percent. This category
of hearing loss included very mild hearing loss and
conductive as well as sensorineural types. The prevalence of severe-to-profound sensorineural hearing
loss in this population was 0.14 percent. This figure
is consistent with other investigators' findings for
much smaller populations.[22,23,36] The available data
suggest that the prevalence of significant hearing loss
in the cerebral palsied population is at least 20 times
that in the general pediatric population.

Table 16-5 shows the prevalence of sensorineural hearing loss in athetoid and nonathetoid cerebral palsied children of different ages. These figures
include hearing loss of lesser degree not believed to
be interfering with normal verbal language development. A much higher prevalence of hearing loss
in the athetoid group is apparent and is consistent
with other studies. Also shown is the sharp decrease
in prevalence of hearing loss in the athetoid group in
more recent years, while prevalence in the nonath-

Table 16-3

Prevalence of Educationally Significant Sensorineural Hearing Loss in Cerebral Palsied Children According to Age

	Age (yr)			
	0–4	5–9	10–15	0–15
No. of cerebral palsied children	71	126	79	276
No. with educationally significant sensorineural hearing loss	6	14	13	33
Prevalence (%)	8.4	11.1	16.4	12.0

Reprinted from Morris T: Hearing impaired cerebral palsied children and their education. Public Health 88:27, 1973. With permission.

Table 16-4

Comparative Prevalence of Hearing Loss Figures in Percentage*

In general population of children aged 0–16 yr (Schein and Delk[34])		
Bilateral significant hearing loss	0.66	(0.660–0.664)
Severe-to-profound sensorineural hearing loss	0.14	(0.141–0.143)
In cerebral palsied population of children aged 0–15 yr (Morris[30])		
Educationally significant sensorineural hearing loss	12.0	(8.1–15.8)

*Ninety-five percent confidence intervals shown in parentheses.

Table 16-5

Prevalence of Sensorineural Hearing Loss in Athetoid and Nonathetoid Forms of Cerebral Palsy According to Age

		Age (yr)			
		0–4	5–9	10–15	0–15
Nonathetoid	*No. of cases*	65	113	66	224
	No. with sensorineural hearing loss	5	13	8	26
	Prevalence (%)	8	11	12	11
Athetoid	*No. of cases*	6	13	13	32
	No. with sensorineural hearing loss	1	6	7	14
	Prevalence (%)	17	46	53	43

From Morris T: Hearing impaired cerebral palsied children and their education. Public Health 88:27, 1973. With permission.

etoid group has remained essentially unchanged. The decline in the prevalence of hearing loss with athetoid cerebral palsy is thought to be due to the control of Rh incompatibility.

Education and Audiologic Habilitation

Vernon investigated the educational and achievement handicaps evidenced by the hearing-impaired cerebral palsied population.[37] Deafness (used here to mean severe-to-profound sensorineural hearing loss) alone is a severe educational handicap, and although the distribution of intelligence in the deaf population is the same as that in the general population, academic progress of the deaf child is about one third to one half that of normal hearing children. Vernon found that deaf cerebral palsied children as a group were grossly retarded educationally even when compared to non-cerebral-palsied deaf children. A comparison between hearing cerebral palsied children and deaf cerebral palsied children was not reported. Vernon noted, however, that among deaf cerebral palsied children, deafness poses a more significant barrier to communication and learning than motor involvement does. Cunningham and Holt also stated that the cerebral palsied hearing-impaired child's educational needs that result from hearing loss may be more critical for educational achievement than those related to motor problems.[21] Accurate assessment of intelligence is certainly important for educational placement and may be difficult with the hearing-impaired cerebral palsied child. The importance of assessing the severely hearing–impaired child's intelligence appropriately with nonverbal intelligence tests has been discussed by Hine, Vernon, and Vernon and Mindel.[25,37,38]

Several investigators have discussed the problem in educational placement for cerebral palsied hearing-impaired children.[21,30,37] Schools for the hearing impaired often have not been designed or staffed for the physically handicapped, and schools equipped to educate the physically handicapped rarely have the sound amplification systems, sound treatment, or staff needed for the education of the hearing impaired. Educational programs that provide resources in both areas to the cerebral palsied hearing-impaired child are available in some areas, however. The team following the cerebral palsied hearing-impaired child may need help in deciding which handicap determines school placement and ensure that other needed therapy is obtained outside of school.

Sign language is a visual–manual language that can be used by most cerebral palsied hearing-impaired children. Significant visual or motor problems, however, may prevent the learning and use of standard sign language. Modification may be needed to maximize a child's ability to communicate. A tactile–manual sign language is used by deaf–blind people, and a number of other communication systems, some involving electronic equipment, can facilitate language learning and communication by the physically handicapped. Team members working with a cerebral palsied hearing-impaired child might work together to choose, or even design, an appropriate system.

Thorough audiologic evaluation and appropriate hearing-aid fitting may be an extended process with the cerebral palsied child. Motor involvement may obscure subtle behavioral responses to sound in the infant and prevent the use of standard test techniques with older children. Impedance audiometry measures may be difficult to obtain in even relatively cooperative children because of movement. The presence of vision problems or developmental delay may also complicate the audiologic diagnosis and habilitation process. The parents' acceptance of the hearing loss and hearing aid are basic to the child's own adjustment to the hearing handicap and habilitation. Parent education, counseling, and support from the audiologist—and often the social worker or psychologist—are important parts of the habilitation process. Annual audiologic reevaluation is generally obtained for hearing-impaired children, and some may need to be seen more often. The life span of hearing aids for active children may be even less than the usual three to five years. Careful troubleshooting and maintenance of the aid is critical.

Audiologic evaluation and habilitation can be accomplished in the cerebral palsied hearing-impaired child *who is referred for evaluation*. The delay seen in diagnosis of hearing loss is not due to test difficulties but to failure of the health care provider to refer. Cunningham and Holt documented this failure to refer, even in the face of parental concern about hearing, in their review of cases, and it is the experience of many audiologists working with children.[21] Certainly, a delay in diagnosis of hearing loss should not occur for children known to have cerebral palsy. Hearing loss should be ruled out or documented very early in their health care program, since they are known to be at high risk for hearing loss. Early coordinated evaluation and management of the hearing-impaired cerebral palsied child maximizes habilitative potential.

REFERENCES

Speech and Language Disorders

1. Beukelman D, Yorkston K: A communication system for the severely dysarthric speaker with an intact language system. J Speech Hear Disord 42:265, 1977
2. Blumberg ML: Respiration and speech in the cerebral palsied child. Am J Dis Child 89:48, 1955
3. Byrne MC: Speech and language development of athetoid and spastic children. J Speech Hear Disord 24:231, 240, 1959
4. Clement M, Twitchell TE: Dysarthria in cerebral palsy. J Speech Hear Disord 24:118, 1959
5. Cruickshank WM (ed): Cerebral Palsy, a Developmental Disability. Syracuse, Syracuse University Press, 1976
6. Darley F, Aronson A, Brown J: Motor Speech Disorders. Philadelphia, Saunders, 1975
7. Dorland's Illustrated Medical Dictionary (ed 26): Philadelphia, Saunders, 1981
8. Hardy JC: Intraoral breath pressure in cerebral palsy. J Speech Hear Disord 26:309, 1961
9. Hardy JC, Netsell R, Schweiger JW, et al: Management of velopharyngeal dysfunction in cerebral palsy. J Speech Hear Disord 34:123, 1969
10. Hoberman SL, Hoberman M: Speech rehabilitation in cerebral palsy. J Speech Hear Disord 25:111, 1960
11. Hopkins T, Bice HV, Colton K: Evaluation and Education of the Cerebral Palsied Child. Washington, D. C., International Council for Exceptional Children, 1954
12. Ingram TTS: Pediatric Aspects of Cerebral Palsy. Edinburgh, Edinburgh Press, 1964
13. Kent R, Netsell R: Articulatory abnormalities in athetoid cerebral palsy. J Speech Hear Disord 43:353, 1978
14. Love RJ, Hagerman EL, Taimi EG: Speech performance, dysphasia and oral reflexes in cerebral palsy. J Speech Hear Disord 45:59, 1980
15. McDonald E, Chance B: Cerebral Palsy. Englewood Cliffs, N. J., Prentice-Hall, 1964
16. McDonald E, Schultz A: Communication boards for cerebral palsied children. J Speech Hear Disord 38:78, 1973
17. Wolfe WA: A comprehensive evaluation of 50 cases of cerebral palsy. J Speech Hear Disord 15:234, 1950

Hearing Disorders

18. American Speech and Hearing Association, American Academy of Ophthalmology and Otolaryngology, and American Academy of Pediatrics: Supplementary statement of joint committee on infant hearing screening. Am Speech Hear Assoc 16:160, 1974
19. Bergstrom L, Hemenway WG, Downs MP: A high risk registry to find congenital deafness. Otolaryngol Clin North Am 4:369, 1971
20. Brown KS: The genetics of childhood deafness, in McConnell F, Ward P, (Eds): Deafness in Childhood. Nashville, Vanderbilt University Press, 1967
21. Cunningham C, Holt KS: Problems in diagnosis and management of children with cerebral palsy and deafness. Dev Med Child Neurol 19:479, 1977
22. Downs MP: Report of the University of Colorado screening project, in Mencher GT (ed): Early Identification of Hearing Loss. Basel, Karger, 1976
23. Feinmesser M, Tell L: Evaluation of methods of detecting hearing impairment in infancy and early childhood, in Mencher GT (ed): Early Identification of Hearing Loss. Basel, Karger, 1976
24. Gerber SB: Cerebral palsy and hearing loss. Cerebral Palsy J 27:6, 1966
25. Hine WD: Psychological assessment of a group of cerebral palsied children with hearing impairments. Public Health 88:35, 38, 1973
26. Jerger J (ed): Handbook of Clinical Impedance Audiometry. Dobbs Ferry, N.Y., American Electromedics, 1975
27. Konigsmark BW: Hereditary deafness in man. N Engl J Med 281:714, 774, 827, 1969
28. Konigsmark BW, Gorlin RJ: Genetic and Metabolic Deafness. Philadelphia, Saunders, 1976
29. Mindel BD, Vernon M: They Grow in Silence: The Deaf Child and His Family. Silver Spring, Md., National Association of the Deaf, 1971
30. Morris T: Hearing Impaired cerebral palsied children and their education. Public Health 88:27, 1973
31. Nober EH: Hearing problems associated with cerebral palsy, in Cruickshank WM (ed): Cerebral Palsy: Its Individual and Community Problems Syracuse, Syracuse University Press, 1966
32. Northern JL, Downs MP: Hearing in Children, Baltimore, Williams & Wilkins, 1978
33. Proctor CA, Proctor B: Understanding hereditary nerve deafness. Arch Otolaryngol 85:23, 1967
34. Schein JD, Delk MT: The Deaf Population of the United States. Silver Spring, Md., National Association of the Deaf, 1974
35. Schlesinger HS, Meadow KP: Sound and Sign: Childhood Deafness and Mental Health. Berkley, University of California Press, 1972
36. Tell L, Levi C, Feinmesser W: Screening of infants for deafness in baby clinics, in Bess FH (ed): Childhood Deafness: Causation, Assessment and Management. New York, Grune & Stratton, 1977
37. Vernon M: Clinical phenomenon of cerebral palsy and deafness. Exceptional Children 36:743, 1970
38. Vernon M, Mindel EE: Psychological and psychiatric aspects of profound hearing loss, in Rose DE (ed): Audiological Assessment, Englewood Cliffs, N.J., Prentice-Hall, 1971

Part IV

Therapeutic and Surgical Management

Frederick B. Palmer   Renee C. Wachtel
Bruce K. Shapiro   Arnold J. Caputo

17

Primitive Reflex Profile

A complete developmental diagnosis is a necessary prelude to treatment in cerebral palsy or any other developmental disability. The assessment must include all four major streams of development: language, nonlanguage problem solving, social, and motor. Emphasis should be placed on defining the nature and degree of delay and describing any associated deficits. As one component of a complete developmental diagnosis, this chapter will discuss an expanded assessment of neuromotor development in infancy and childhood. The concepts and practical items discussed are of value in the routine monitoring of normal development in a general pediatric practice, in the assessment of the infant at risk for developmental problems, and in the motor evaluation of the child with apparent motor delay. The approach leans heavily on the assessment of primitive reflexes, postural responses, and motor milestones as supplements to the more traditional neurologic examination.

ASSESSMENT OF EARLY NEUROMOTOR DEVELOPMENT

Motor Milestone Scales

The traditional approach to evaluation of early motor development is through assessment of the child's developmental competence in relation to a standard motor milestone scale, such as that in Table 17-1. The definition of *delay* then becomes clear, at least for individual motor milestones. (Whenever milestones are used to monitor developmental progress, close attention must be paid to their accurate definition. For example, *sitting* may be interpreted as

sitting with support, sitting alone, or independently assuming the sitting position, skills spanning three full months).

Neurologic Examination

The next diagnostic step is a classic neurologic examination, which, with its emphasis on deep tendon reflexes, Babinski sign, muscle tone, and strength, is often unrewarding because (1) it does not stress the developmental changes in these phenomena that occur with central nervous system (CNS) maturation, particularly in the first year, and (2) it does not correlate with motor function. The pediatrician is faced with defining an abnormality that changes with age. For example, the normal newborn has increased flexor tone in the extremities that gradually diminishes during the first six months of life; however, truncal and nuchal tone are often quite low early on and increase gradually with the development of head and truncal stability. Babinski sign is not abnormal in the early months and is thus of little value (unless asymmetric). The developing reach of a normal six-month-old can at times look disturbingly athetoid. When one relies *only* on the classic neurologic examination, particularly in the child with mild involvement there is little wonder it is said that cerebral palsy cannot be diagnosed before 12, 18, or even 24 mo of age.[19]

Maturational Precursors

A more appropriate clinical approach to motor delay demands a detailed understanding of the nature of early motor development. Milestones are observ-

Table 17-1
Gross Motor Milestones Up to 18 Mo*

Position	Age (mo)
Prone	
Chin up	1
Chest up	2
On elbows	3
On wrists	4
Rolls	3–5
Sits with support	6
Sits without support	8
Comes to sitting	9
Pulls to stand, cruises	10
Walks two hands held	11
Walks one hand held	12
Walks alone	13
Runs	18

*See Illingworth[10] and Knobloch and Pasamanick[11] for more detailed listing.

able and measurable endpoints of CNS maturation, but many developmental factors leading up to the ultimate attainment of motor milestones can also be measured reliably. Among these maturational precursors are the primitive reflexes and postural responses. Attention to these factors, in addition to the classic examination, can result in earlier and more accurate motor diagnosis.

Primitive Reflexes

The primitive reflexes are brain stem–mediated, whole-body motor reflexes that develop during gestation and are present at birth. As a general rule, they clinically disappear during the first six to nine months of life. They are not easily elicitable in the older child or adult except after brain injury. It can be assumed that with developmental maturation of higher neural structures, the primitive reflexes become inhibited or suppressed, to reappear only when the higher inhibition is removed.

Postural Responses

Postural responses are maturational motor skills, that develop during the first year of life and form the basis for the attainment of functional motor skills, i.e., the motor milestones. Commonly used examples are the development of head, trunk, and body righting, upper extremity protective extension, and equilibrium reactions.

Developing Motor Skills

Figure 17-1 graphically summarizes the relationship between the primitive reflexes, postural responses, and developing motor skills. With maturation, the dominant effects of the primitive reflexes diminish and the developing postural responses are manifested. The postural responses, in turn, form the immediate precursors for development of identifiable motor skills—the motor milestones. Thus, a delay in disappearance of primitive reflexes will be reflected in a delay in appearance of postural reflexes and related motor milestones. In many instances the relationship between individual primitive reflexes, postural responses, and motor acts is clinically apparent; however, it is clear that combinations or profiles of primitive reflexes and postural responses are more important determinants of motor development than individual reflexes or responses alone.

CLINICAL APPLICATION

The clinical application of an evaluation of primitive reflex activity falls into four major areas:

1. Early motor (and nonmotor) diagnosis
2. Development of a motor prognosis
3. Design of therapy programs
4. Markers of gestational maturity

Recognition of the relationship of the primitive reflexes and postural reactions to CNS maturation is paramount to the understanding of their clinical use. They are markers of neurologic integrity or abnormality. Deviation from normal maturation patterns of primitive reflexes, postural responses, or both can be a valuable clinical tool for the early detection of CNS dysfunction.

Early Motor (and Nonmotor) Diagnosis

Abnormalities in the appearance and suppression of the primitive reflexes in the first year of life reflect CNS dysfunction. Thus, attention to the primitive reflexes in the early months allows an abnormality to be recognized before delay in postural maturation or motor milestone attainment is clinically apparent. Two major abnormalities are noted, often together: (1) an abnormally strong reflex in the first six months of life

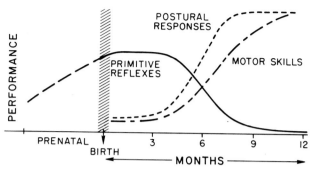

Figure 17-1. An idealized composite of the interrelationships of primitive reflexes, postural responses, and motor milestones. (Modified from Capute A, Accardo P, Vining E, et al: Primitive Reflex Profile. Baltimore, University Park Press, 1978.)

and (2) persistence of a reflex beyond the time of its normal clinical disappearance or inhibition. Such an approach to early motor diagnosis was emphasized by Paine but has not been universally applied because of the difficulties in gathering objective information about reflex intensity and persistence.[15] Because of these difficulties, Capute and associates have developed a scale to quantify reflex activity during the first two years of life.[4] This scale has been adapted to 9 different reflexes and is being applied prospectively to a sample of 450 children during sequential routine well-child visits in the first 2 yr. of life. The scale, conceptually very simple, consists of a 5-point grading scale (0,1,2,3,4) of reflex intensity. Table 17-2 presents the general format for the scoring. The adaptation of this scale to the individual reflexes is presented elsewhere.[5] Several reflexes will now be discussed, with emphasis on their developmental nature and clinical usefulness.

Asymmetric Tonic Neck Reflex

The asymmetric tonic neck reflex (ATNR) is one of the original primitive reflexes described by Magnus and de Kleijn in the first part of this century and is now familiar to most clinicians as the "fencer's position."[13] The reflex is easily elicited with the child in the supine position. With rotation of the head 45°–90° to either side, there is active flexion of the extremities on the occiput side and extension on the chin side (Fig. 17-2). Afferent pathways for this brain stem reflex are the first three cervical roots, which carry proprioceptive information from the joints and muscles of the upper cervical vertebrae.

The relationship between the primitive reflexes, postural responses, and motor acts as described in Figure 1 is easily seen in the case of the ATNR. The presence of this reflex interferes with the development of volitional rolling, sitting, and upper extremity midline activity. In the presence of a strong ATNR, the child who initiates rolling from the supine position by rotating the head to one side is prevented from completing the maneuver by the reflexively extended arm. Since reflex activity decreases with maturation, the motor act becomes possible and is recognized as an achieved milestone. Independent sitting requires the development of certain postural reactions, including the propping or protective reactions of the upper extremities, which aid in readjusting disturbed balance. If the upper extremities are reflexively maintained in flexion or extension, depending on the position of the head, the rapid extension needed for these propping responses will be impossible and effective sitting not attainable. Similarly, it can be seen

Table 17-2

Quantitative Reflex Scale

0	Absent
1+	Appropriate tone changes elicited but position changes not seen
2+	Appropriate position change seen (physiologic)
3+	Pronounced or prolonged, more exaggerated than normally seen, not readily habituated
4+	Obligatory, infant unable to break out of reflex for a minimum of 30 sec (pathologic)

Modified from Capute A, Accardo P, Vining E, et al: Primitive Reflex Profile. Baltimore, University Park Press, 1978.

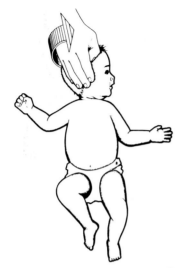

Figure 17-2. ATNR. (Reprinted from Capute A, Accardo P, Vining E, et al: Primitive Reflex Profile. Baltimore, University Park Press, 1978. With permission.)

Table 17-3
Scoring System for Asymmetric Tonic Neck Reflex

0	No reflex activity
1+	With passive head rotation, no visible response, but increased extensor *tone* noted in extremities on chin side or increased flexor *tone* on occiput side
2+	Visible partial flexion or extension
3+	Visible full flexion or extension (unsustained)
4+	Obligatory (more than 30 sec) flexion or extension

From Capute A, Accardo P, Vining E, et al: Primitive Reflex Profile. Baltimore, University Park Press, 1978.

how a strong ATNR can interfere with upper extremity midline activity unless the head is aligned perfectly in the midline. Thus, reaching and hand-to-mouth activity characteristic of the infant aged four to six months depend on the diminution of the reflex.

The above paragraph is a simplification of the effects of reflexes on individual motor acts. It is clear that a number of different reflexes and postural responses affect the development of individual motor acts. For example in addition to the ATNR, the tonic labyrinthine and Moro reflexes, as well as the development of derotational righting, a postural response, are important in the attainment of rolling from the supine to the prone position. Preliminary work suggests that different combinations of reflexes may influence the development of different motor skills.[7] Further definition of the natural history of individual reflexes and their interactions will be important in the development of realistic therapy goals for the child with a motor handicap.

The natural history of the ATNR can be summarized from preliminary data from a group of 180 normal infants followed sequentially through the first 2 yr of life.[4] The 5-point grading scale has been adapted to the ATNR, as shown in Table 17-3

A number of clinical points deserve mention. First, the reflex has its maximum activity during the first six months of life, with gradual diminution thereafter; visible activity (2+,3+) is uncommon at 9 mo

and rare after 12 mo. Tone changes (1+) may persist for a number of months and are not indicative of significant *motor handicap*. It remains to be seen, however, whether persistence of tone change of this or other reflexes indicates *subtle CNS abnormality*.

Second, the obligatory reflex (4+), from which the child cannot escape for over 30 sec, was never seen in this group of normal children, although it is common in children with brain damage. Any infant with an obligatory sustained ATNR should therefore be regarded as at extreme risk for CNS abnormality. This is a finding common to most of the primitive reflexes and a key to the early recognition of cerebral palsy.

Third, there is a slight increase in level of reflex activity in the first three months of age. This is probably related to the strong flexor positioning of the normal newborn, which inhibits the manifestation of the ATNR. A child may thus have a rather mild manifestation of the reflex (1–2+) as a newborn but at 2–3 mo develop a 3+ response. This pattern is normal.

Fourth, reflex manifestation appears to be stronger when the child voluntarily rotates the head as opposed to the head's being passively rotated by the examiner. A so-called 2+ response may thus be seen at 12 mo with active head rotation when passive rotation yields no visual response.

Fifth, the ATNR may influence findings on the classic neurologic examination. When there is significant ATNR activity, the child's head should be held in the midline when evaluating deep tendon reflexes and Babinski's sign to avoid confusing asymmetries.

Tonic Labyrinthine in Supine and Prone Positions

The tonic labyrinthine reflexes in the supine (TLS) and prone (TLP) positions were also described by Magnus and de Kleijn and shown to originate from labyrinthine afferent nerves.[13] They are not as well known as the ATNR but equally as important clinically. When eliciting the TLS, the child is placed in a supine position and the neck is hyperextended. There is reflexive tonic extension of the trunk and lower extremities with tonic shoulder retraction and adduction, generally with elbow flexion (Fig. 17-3). The reflex is broken by flexion of the neck upon the chest and an observable decrease in extension and shoulder retraction. When the child is placed in the prone position for elicitation of the TLP, with neck flexion there is active flexion of the trunk and lower extremities, with active protraction of the shoulders (Fig. 17-4). When the head is then passively extended in the prone position, the active flexion diminishes and there may be active extension. The TLS and ATNR show similar developmental patterns. The time of greatest activity is during the first 4–6 mo, with rapid decrease thereafter such that occasional position change is seen at 9 mo, with normal children rarely showing more than subtle tone changes after 12 mo. Again, as in the ATNR, sustained obligatory responses are virtually never seen in normal children at any age.

The TLP shows a somewhat different natural history and is rather difficult to evaluate. Active flexion when the head was flexed in the prone position in our sample persisted well into the second year of life. Furthermore, the overlap with the symmetric tonic neck reflex and Landau righting reaction, which are both active in the prone position, make evaluation of the TLP difficult.

The TL reflexes interfere with the development of upper-extremity weight bearing in the prone position. The child with strong TL reflexes is not able to bear weight on extended arms in the prone position when the head and neck are extended because of reflexive shoulder retraction when the neck is extended. Similarly, if the TLS is active in the supine position, there will be tonic shoulder retraction and the inability to roll over the retracted shoulders. The tonic trunk extension also interferes with the development of segmental truncal derotation, a postural response. The TLS thus must diminish before volitional rolling from the supine position is possible. A strong TLS interferes with stable sitting because of the truncal extension that occurs when the head is lifted, resulting in the infant's falling backward.

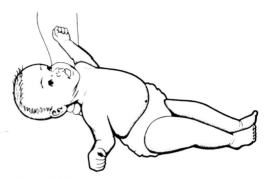

Figure 17-3. Tonic labyrinthine in supine position. (Reprinted from Capute A, Accardo P, Vining E, et al: Primitive Reflex Profile. Baltimore, University Park Press, 1978. With permission.)

It may be evident that there is a similarity between bilateral decorticate posturing and the TLS position of trunk and lower extremity extension, elbow flexion, and shoulder retraction. This has given rise to the idea of "physiologic decorticate posturing" in the first few months of life and further emphasizes the drawbacks of the classic neurologic examination when not seen in developmental context.[6] True decerebrate posturing with truncal and lower extremity extension, shoulder retraction, and upper extremity *extension* may also be related to the TLS but is not seen in normal children.

Moro Reflex

The Moro reflex, familiar to most pediatricians as a valuable part of the newborn's examination, is elicited in a variety of manners. A reliable method is to simply place the child in the supine position on a padded surface and allow the head to fall back

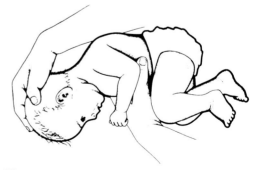

Figure 17-4. Tonic labyrinthine in prone position. (Reprinted from Capute A, Accardo P, Vining E, et al: Primitive Reflex Profile. Baltimore, University Park Press, 1978. With permission.)

approximately 3 cm onto the surface. Alternate methods include striking the surface (Moro's original method) or holding the child supine in one's arms and allowing the head to rapidly extend a few centimeters. With this sudden extension of the neck, there is immediate symmetric abduction of the arms and opening of the hands and a subsequent flexion and adduction of the arms into a position of embrace. There may also be lower extremity extension and, in extreme instances, opisthotonic positioning of the entire trunk and extremities. Our preliminary data conform closely with smaller, previously reported series and show rapid diminution of the Moro reflex during the first six months.[18] Few children have a Moro response at the six-month examination or later. Again, the obligatory (opisthotonic) response is not seen in normal children.

Clearly, a strong Moro reflex will interfere with the development of almost all early motor acts if rapid change in head position or sudden noise cause such a whole-body reflexive motor response. In normal children the Moro response has largely diminished before volitional rolling is attained.

The Moro reflex can easily be confused with the startle response, which is a normal reflexive withdrawal of *flexion* to any sudden stimulus. This is present from infancy throughout life and should not be regarded as a persistent Moro reflex.[17] Absence or asymmetry of the Moro response in the first two months of life is an exquisite sign of abnormality. Absence may be due to profound hypotonia, severe CNS insult, or severe systematic illness. Asymmetry may indicate underlying hemiplegia, brachial plexus injury, or clavicular fracture.

Symmetric Tonic Neck Reflex

The symmetric tonic neck reflex (STNR), also described by Magnus and de Kleijn, is similar to the ATNR because head position influences extremity flexion or extension, but it differs in that there is no side-to-side asymmetry.[13] When the neck is extended, the upper extremities extend and the lower extremities flex. Correspondingly, when the head is flexed, the upper extremities flex and the lower extremities extend. This reflex, clearly present in infants with brain damage is not readily elicited in normal infants. Our preliminary findings suggest that subtle position or tone changes are present in only about 10 percent of the normal population, with a maximum prevalence around 4–6 mo. Strong manifestation or persistence of the STNR is an important indicator of CNS abnormality.

In children with cerebral palsy the STNR interferes with activities in the prone position, where head flexion induces upper extremity flexion, thereby interfering with upper-extremity weight-bearing activities. Similarly, reciprocal-extremity activities such as creeping or crawling are not possible when the extremities are strongly influenced symmetrically by head position.

Placing Reflexes

The lower-extremity placing reflex is present at birth and is elicited by holding the infant in vertical suspension and touching the dorsum of the foot to the edge of a surface, e.g., a table top. Presence of the reflex is indicated by flexion and then extension of that extremity as if placing the foot on the surface. Like the Moro reflex, absence or clear asymmetry of placing should be recognized as abnormal. A similar placing reflex appears in the upper extremities by three months and should also be evaluated for presence and symmetry. These reflexes gradually merge into visually mediated volitional behavior, and their disappearance cannot easily be assessed. When evaluating placing, the secondary extensor phase of the reflex must be present and is the key component of the placing response. It allows one to differentiate simple withdrawal of the extremity.

The evaluation of primitive reflexes as a component of early motor diagnosis should thus be directed toward findings in several areas:

1. The persistence of significant reflex activity beyond the time in which it is normally seen should be noted.
2. The presence of obligatory (sustained) reflex activity at any age is not seen in normal infants. This is best noted through evaluation of the ATNR and TLS and recognition of opisthotonic posturing in an exaggerated Moro response.
3. Absence of reflex activity at a time when it is normally present is an important indicator and often reflects generalized hypotonia that may be due to severe CNS dysfunction.
4. Marked reflex asymmetry is not seen in normal infants. This is easily assessed through attention to the Moro, placing, and grasp reflexes but can be also seen in other areas. Evaluation of the TLS may show asymmetric shoulder retraction in children with developing hemiplegias.
5. Discrepancies between upper- and lower-extremity activity in a child may aid in the topographic subclassification of cerebral palsy. For example, children with spastic diplegia, where the lower extremities are more involved than the upper ex-

tremities, may show more lower-extremity tonic involvement with the ATNR and TLS and delay in the appearance of lower-extremity placing until after the appearance of upper-extremity placing.

As the natural history of the primitive reflexes is better understood, the earlier diagnosis of cerebral palsy should become a reality. The grading of reflexes may be equally effective in identifying children with milder degrees of persistent or asymmetric reflex activity, however. These children may have little or no early motor delay, just atypical reflex activity. Nevertheless, these variations from normal may be indicators of subtle CNS dysfunction and early neurologic markers of minimal cerebral dysfunction, central communicative disorders, and learning disabilities. Milder abnormalities in reflex activity thus may be analogous to the "soft" neuromotor signs of the school-aged child in that they are markers of CNS dysfunction in nonmotor areas.[8]

Development of a Motor Prognosis

Since primitive reflexes are an integral part of a complete infant neuromotor examination and an aid in identifying CNS dysfunction, they also may be of use in distinguishing degrees of abnormality. Examination of primitive reflexes at an early date can help distinguish the child with mild to moderate cerebral palsy from the child with severe cerebral palsy. An accurate assessment of motor prognosis is important in parent counseling and establishing realistic long-term therapeutic goals. It is also a key factor in the evaluation of long-term effects of intervention strategies. In recent years the traditional therapeutic modalities (physical therapy, occupational therapy, orthopaedic surgery) have become more and more entrenched, making their efficacy increasingly difficult to evaluate. The practical difficulties in performing a randomized, controlled study of different treatment strategies (and indeed of no formal treatment) are becoming almost insurmountable. Treatment evaluation in the future may depend on the comparison of experimental outcome versus a well defined, previously established prognosis.

The primitive reflexes offer considerable help in this area. Studies by Paine of children with cerebral palsy have demonstrated close correlation between level of reflex activity (ATNR) and motor development.[15] Bleck extended these findings to develop a prognosis score based on the presence of certain obligatory primitive reflexes and the absence of certain postural reflexes in cerebral palsy.[2] With this prognosis score, subsequent ability to ambulate was accurately predicted in 94.5 percent of the children.

In a similar study of 233 children, all initially evaluated before 1 yr of age, Molnar and Gordon were able to confirm the ability of early primitive reflex activity to predict later motor function.[14] They found the best predictor of ultimate ambulation was a child's ability to sit independently by 24 mo of age. All children with spastic quadriplegia, diplegia, choreoathetosis, or mixed cerebral palsy who sat independently by 24 mo ultimately walked. Those who did not sit by 24 mo did not necessarily fail to walk, however. In these children, the presence or absence of obligatory reflexes (including ATNR, STNR, and TLS) clearly predicted the child's ultimate ability to walk. Any persistent obligatory reflexes precluded walking.

In our experience, these findings are borne out, although a rare exception deserves mention. There are a few children, almost always with good cognitive abilities, who are able to use their primitive reflexes to aid in performing certain motor skills, albeit in an extremely deviant fashion. For example, we have seen children with choreoathetosis and an extremely strong ATNR who can control the flexion and extension of their legs (and canes in the upper extremities) by rotating their head first to one side and then to the other, thereby producing a peculiar but functional gait. These are rare exceptions, however, and serve largely to emphasize the prognostic value of primitive reflexes in the majority of cases.

If the presence or absence of obligatory primitive reflexes can predict the ultimate presence or absence of ambulation, intermediate levels of reflex activity might predict intermediate levels of motor competence. The grading system described above might aid in refining prognosis in the child with motor-impairment. To test this hypothesis, Capute and associates evaluated 53 children with cerebral palsy and compared reflex activity with current motor functioning.[5] They evaluated four reflexes (ATNR, STNR, TLS, positive support) and added the scores. They compared this total score with the child's ambulatory status: ambulators without assistance, ambulators requiring assistance (braces, canes, walkers), and nonambulators. The nonambulators had consistently higher scores and were completely discriminated from ambulators. The intermediate group had an intermediate reflex score but showed some overlap with the other two groups. Although this information is preliminary, it implies that a more quantitative prognosis is possible and suggests future research directions.

Sustained primitive reflex activity over time is associated with the ultimate development of orthopedic deformity. For example, a child with an obligatory ATNR that is asymmetric to one side will often lie in that position continuously. Secondary deformities such as scoliosis (concave to the occiput side), subluxation-dislocation of the occiput hip, and flexion contractures on the occiput side are frequently seen. Children with a strong TLS in the upper extremities may develop contractures in shoulder retraction and elbow flexion. An obligatory positive support, the child who is *persistently* on tiptoe when held standing, is very likely to lead to tendo Achilles contractures that require surgery. This should be distinguished from the child who goes up on tiptoe only transiently, who may not require surgery, and who perhaps will benefit from orthotic management alone.

Design of Therapy Programs

Many of the traditional physical therapy disciplines emphasize the inhibition of reflex activity by careful positioning of the child.[3,9] As the effects of the primitive reflexes are being inhibited in a therapy or positioning program, the therapist should be alert to the early appearance of the various postural responses. As these responses appear, the therapist should facilitate them in order to encourage the development of related motor acts. The techniques used for inhibiting these primitive reflexes and facilitating the postural responses, although based on general guidelines of the various schools of treatment, are largely determined by the therapist's clinical experience and knowledge of the individual patient. No carefully designed scientific studies have looked at these various therapeutic treatments.

The importance of primitive reflexes in therapy programs can be appreciated when considering positioning techniques. A child with a strong TLS will be positioned in a chair that induces partial flexion of the neck, hips, and lower extremities to prevent triggering and subsequent activity of the TLS. Similarly, a child with a strong ATNR will be positioned with the head in the midline, where interfering flexion or extension of extremities will not be manifest. Attention to primitive reflexes alone is insufficient. Most therapists also focus on facilitation of developing postural responses. These responses of righting, equilibrium, and protection serve as the immediate precursors to functional motor acts (see Fig. 17-1). Two postural reactions may be used as illustrations.

Landau Reaction

The Landau reaction is a chain of midline righting responses.[12] When the child is held in prone suspension, voluntary head and neck extension is followed by truncal extension. Hip and knee extension may also occur but are not a part of the originally described reaction. The infant's ability to right himself or herself against gravity begins around two months of age and is complete by six months. It is felt that the truncal stability represented by a mature Landau reaction is one of the postural prerequisites to volitional rolling and independent sitting. An obligatory TLP, with its reflexive flexion in the prone position, interferes with the expression of the Landau reaction.

Upper Extremity Propping Reactions

The propping or "protective extension" reactions are best evaluated with the examiner supporting the child in the sitting position. By six months, when the trunk is displaced anteriorly, the child will extend the arms to the surface anteriorly and support his or her weight. This reaction is a prerequisite to the six-month ability to sit in the tripod position. By eight months, when displaced laterally, the child will extend the arms laterally and bear weight. This reaction is necessary for more independent sitting and movement in and out of the sitting position. Posterior propping emerges at 10–12 mo or later and may be related to walking and pivoting while sitting. Activity of any primitive reflex that influences upper-extremity mobility, especially the ATNR and TLS, will preclude the development of the propping reactions.

Further definition of the relationship between primitive reflexes, postural responses, and motor action should be of considerable aid in developing an objective rationale for treatment of the child with cerebral palsy. For example, postural prerequisites should be defined for important individual motor acts. Thus, when the child has reached a certain postural stage of readiness, it would be realistic to expect that intensive therapy would result in attainment of a specific motor skill. If these postural prerequisites were not present, the therapist would recognize, at least for the time, that attempts to develop that skill would be unrealistic and instead emphasize earlier skills.

Gestational Markers

The gestational onset of observable primitive reflexes is an area of potential clinical application. Limited specific information is available on the natural history of the primitive reflexes in the preterm neonate, but several small studies suggest that some reflexes—the Moro response and the plantar and palmar grasps—are present at 29 wk of gestation and perhaps earlier. Other reflexes—ATNR, TLS, and TLP—appear to emerge during the last two or three months of fetal life.[1,20] Ultimately, assessment of reflex activity in the premature newborn may contribute to the definition and description of *risk* as well as aid in the estimation of gestational age.

REFERENCES

1. Amiel-Tison C: Neurologic evaluation of the maturity of newborn infants. Arch Dis Child 43:89, 1968
2. Bleck E: Locomotor prognosis in cerebral palsy. Dev Med Child Neurol 17:18, 1975
3. Bobath K: A Neurophysiological Basis for the Treatment of Cerebral Palsy. London, Spastics International Medical Publications. 1980
4. Capute A, Accardo P, Vining E, et al: Primitive Reflex Profile. Baltimore, University Park Press, 1978
5. Capute A, Accardo P, Vining E, et al: Primitive reflex profile: A pilot study. Phys Ther 58:1061, 1978
6. Capute A: Identifying cerebral palsy in infancy through study of primitive reflex profiles. Pediatr Ann 8:589, 1979
7. Capute A, Shapiro B, Wachtel R, et al: Motor functions: Associated primitive reflex profiles. Dev Med Child Neurol 24:662, 1982
8. Capute A, Shapiro B, Palmer F: Spectrum of developmental disabilities: Continuum of motor dysfunction. Orthoped Clin North Am 2:3, 1981
9. Fay T: The neurological aspects of therapy in cerebral palsy. Arch Phys Med Rehabil 29:327, 1948
10. Illingworth R: The Development of the Infant and Young Child: Normal and Abnormal. Edinburgh, Churchill Livingstone, 1980
11. Knobloch H, Pasamanick B (eds): Gesell and Amatruda's Developmental diagnosis: The Evaluation and Management of Normal and Abnormal Neuropsychologic Development in Infancy and Early Childhood (ed 3). Hagerstown, Harper & Row, 1974
12. Landau A: Über einen tonischen Lagereflex beim alteren Säugling. Klin Wochenschr 2:1253, 1923
13. Magnus R, de Kleijn A: Die Abhängigkeit des Tonus der Extremitätanmuskeln von der Kopfstellung. Arch Ges Physiol 145:455, 1912
14. Molnar GE, Gordon SU: Cerebral palsy: Predictive value of selected signs for early prognostication of motor function. Arch Phys Med Rehabil 57:153, 1976
15. Paine R: Evolution of infantile postural reflexes in presence of chronic brain syndromes. Dev Med Child Neurol 6:345, 1964
16. Paine R, Brazelton T, Donovan D, et al: Evolution of postural reflexes in normal infants and in the presence of chronic brain syndromes. Neurology 14:1036, 1964
17. Parmelee A: The critical evaluation of the Moro reflex. Pediatrics 33:773, 1964
18. Peiper A: Cerebral Function in Infancy and Childhood. New York, Consultants Bureau, 1963
19. Skatvedt M: Cerebral palsy. Acta Pediatrica Uppsala (supp 11) 46:1958
20. Wachtel R, Starrett A: Primitive reflexes in premature infants. (in preparation)

Mary C. Lawlor
Anita Zielinski

18

Occupational Therapy

The role and principles of occupational therapy in the comprehensive management of patients with cerebral palsy encompass a broad range of services in a variety of settings. The types of service include evaluation, treatment, participation as a health care team member, consultation and education of the patient, the family, and other service providers.

The scope of occupational therapy deals primarily with the complex interrelationship between meaningful activity and human performance. It strives to enhance performance through the provision of selected treatment activities designed to facilitate neuromuscular growth and the development of functional skills necessary for the achievement of maximal independence. The concepts of purposeful activity, developmental sequence, and quality of performance collectively comprise its framework. Therapists use their abilities in these three areas to perceive simultaneously the different aspects of performance and to develop a comprehensive clinical profile that pertains to the patients' overall performance in relationship to the environment.

EVALUATION

Before conducting an evaluation, the therapist must obtain important clinical information through a careful medical and developmental history from the parents, physician, and/or guardian. This information should include primary diagnosis and related medical concerns, precautions, allergies, current medications, psychologic and behavioral history, developmental milestones, method of communication, hearing and visual status, type of diet, reason for evaluation, previous treatment, and current living environment.

Separating the evaluation process into two specific phases—screening and comprehensive—has proven effective.

The *screening evaluation* is performed to obtain a generalized assessment of how an individual functions. It consists of securing the relevant background information and a brief review of overall performance. Areas requiring further assessment are identified and are then addressed in the comprehensive evaluation.

The *comprehensive evaluation* assesses specific areas of performance and allows the therapist to determine what types of services the patient will require. Once the evaluative baseline data have been gathered, they are processed into a composite clinical profile of abilities and limitations. This information is used in the formulation of treatment goals.[30]

Comprehensive evaluation can include many areas of performance. The major areas are sensorimotor, perceptual motor, upper extremity, activities of daily living, adaptive equipment, play and leisure, and educational and work readiness skills. It should be remembered that these areas overlap and are separated for purposes of evaluation and discussion. The specific aspects of each of these areas will be considered later in this chapter.

Factors Affecting the Evaluation Process

Administration of standardized tests, including developmental evaluations of cognition, perceptual motor abilities, and fine motor performance, is frequently limited in children with cerebral palsy and other developmental disabilities. Standardized testing should be used selectively. The severity of the movement disorder and initial anxiety of the patient may affect the validity of testing.

Observations of the child or adult who is performing a variety of activities and movements based on a developmental framework can provide the most valuable information on capabilities. Conducting certain portions of the evaluation in varying environments and at different times of the day is recommended. This gives insight on how environmental factors and demands of daily routine affect performance. Pertinent information on performance can also be obtained through an interview with the patient and family.

Reassessment

Although the actual central nervous system (CNS) damage in children with cerebral palsy is nonprogressive, the resulting physical handicaps and developmental delays change as the child grows, requiring reassessment at regular intervals. These intervals may depend on several factors, including the child's specific diagnosis, rate of growth, specific requirements, nature of treatment, and organization of the treatment center. The use of movies or videotapes can be a valuable tool to allow comparative clinical observations over time.

Through the course of various evaluations, problems may be observed that require other specialized intervention. These problems can include, but are not limited to, increased contractures, structural deformities, lack of performance or regression, possible seizure activity, and many others.

TREATMENT

Information related to specific areas of delay or limitation must be integrated and correlated to determine specific interventions. The type of treatment intervention may be direct or indirect depending on each individual's specific requirements. *Direct treatment* with regard to performance will be discussed later in this chapter. *Indirect services* can include consultation to parents and other care providers, educational staff, and vocational staff. Goals that are established should be realistic, i.e., based not only on the patient's clinical profile but on the living and working environment and available resources. A combination of direct and indirect service delivery is often used, e.g., the parents of a child receiving therapy work with the therapist to carry out certain portions of the program at home. Parents, family, and other care providers often play a key role in generalizing treatment goals into the normal daily routine. The therapist is able to educate family members on handling and positioning techniques to facilitate the provision of basic care. This is an extremely important factor, since long-range therapy goals are established to increase function in daily, educational, or vocational tasks. Through working closely with parents and other care workers, the therapist can help to establish realistic expectations of the outcome of a specific treatment program.

CLINICAL APPLICATIONS

There are a number of theories and proposed treatment approaches for cerebral palsy. It is the therapist's responsibility to understand and delineate the rationale for treatment activities within each performance area.[3]

Sensorimotor Performance

The term *sensorimotor* may be broadly defined as an individual's use of sensory information, including visual, auditory, tactile, olfactory, proprioceptive, and kinesthetic, to produce an adapted motor response. Adapted responses are purposeful, goal-directed actions that comprise the functional component to movement.[4,5]

The interrelationship of sensation and movement necessitates consideration of sensorimotor functioning when one evaluates motor performance of any type. Evaluation and treatment of motor performance in cerebral palsy goes beyond the attainment of developmental milestones to assessing the quality of movement and determining whether the motor response is adaptive. Within this framework, therapists are concerned specifically with reflex maturation and the influence of abnormal muscle tone on the patient's ability to use sensory information effectively.

Reflex Maturation

The neonatal and early childhood reflexes can be thought of as adapted responses. These primitive reflexes form the basis for purposeful motor activity.[8-10,14] Initially, they allow the infant to swallow, grasp, and they adjust the head to breath; later they allow the infant to roll over, sit, assume a quadriped position—posturally adjusted to maintain balance—and, finally, stand and walk. These reflexes begin as involuntary patterns of flexion and extension, influencing many muscle groups. They develop sequentially and become increasingly refined, leading to voluntary control. Through sensorimotor development, they become modified by CNS maturation and by the infant's movement experience. The sensory feedback that the infant receives from movement, particularly kinesthetic and proprioceptive, plays a key role in building increasingly higher sensorimotor skills.[19] Primitive reflexes retained beyond age ranges established as norms can indicate sensorimotor delay. (see chapter 17)

Postural reflexes and responses do not disappear as the child grows, but are modified and retained into adulthood and become important components of co-ordinated movement. These are first seen and de-scribed as righting reactions, which enable the infant to assume a normal position of the head in space and normal trunk alignment. They are integrated and become part of more complex equilibrium reactions. Equilibrium reactions provide a valuable mechanism for postural adjustments and accompany all volitional movements. They orient and prepare people for pur-poseful movements as well as allow them to maintain balance throughout the executed movement. The presence and quality of these reflexes are assessed.

Abnormal Muscle Tone

Damage to the CNS in the developmental period can result in the retention of primitive and abnormal reflexes, poor or absent postural reflexes, and ab-normal muscle tone. Although modern neurophysi-ology is not yet able to explain completely the reasons for abnormal muscle tone, neurodevelopmentalists postulate that reflex activity, particularly the postural reflexes, plays an important part in regulating muscle tone.[19] Normal muscle tone is essential for the body to make spontaneous movements and adjustments to adapt to environmental demands. In cerebral palsy, where the primitive reflexes are not integrated and abnormal tonic reflexes persist, abnormal tone, such as spasticity and athetosis, is displayed.

In assessing muscle tone, the muscle groups most affected, the degree of severity, and the factors that influence tone must be described. Observations of movement should occur in a variety of situations and positions, since abnormal tone and movement may appear under more stressful situations. Other aspects of assessment should include functional strength, en-durance, the presence of associated reactions, and tremors.

Treatment

Treatment of motor performance problems should include challenging and varied activities that provide a mixture of sensory and movement experiences (Fig. 18-1.). The focus of treatment is to increase senso-rimotor function through the integration of reflexes to gain an adapted response comprised of normal movement patterns.[19]

Parents are shown how certain positions and handling techniques based on sensorimotor principles can assist them in bathing, dressing, and feeding the child. Activities should be designed and adapted so that the desired movements are spontaneous and au-tomatic rather than the result of concentrated effort. This ensures that the learned actions become incor-porated into the child's overall movement patterns and generalized to other skills rather than being rote, isolated, or splintered skills. We have found this ap-proach also effective in the adolescent and adult pop-ulation. The therapist must set realistic and functional goals to which to apply the adaptive responses, e.g., increasing eye–hand coordination so that the patient can eat without assistance. Treatment results may require longer periods with the older patient. Patient cooperation and motivation are most necessary for this approach to be effective. Careful decisions must be made with the patient who attempts to use ab-normal movements in accomplishing certain tasks.

In treating the adolescent and adult with cerebral palsy, other factors arise that are often not found in young children. Severe soft-tissue contractures and osseous deformities of the spine and extremities may exist.[29] This can be especially true in those persons who have not received adequate previous treatment or have been institutionalized for long periods. Mus-cle weakness and atrophy may be present from years of disuse. These problems must be taken into account in designing treatment programs.

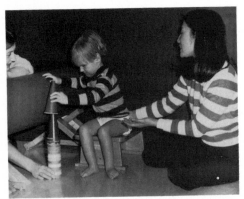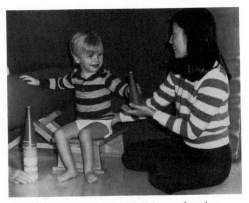

Figure 18-1. Boy aged two years with spastic diplegia and poor sensorimotor abilities performing activities (A) Stacking cones are used to improve vision coordination, depth perception, sensation, and reaching abilities. (B) Transfer of cones allows integration of sensory input as well as improved coordinate trunk movement, posture, eye–hand function, and fine motor skills.

Perceptual Motor Performance

The interrelationship between perceptual motor performance and sensorimotor performance is an important one. Although some experimental data suggest that elements of perception exist at birth, further sensorimotor development is essential for these elements to mature and become functional.[22] As the

Table 18-1
Components of Perceptual Abilities

Visual

    Depth perception
    Figure–ground discrimination
    Spacial relations
    Position in space

Visual motor

Auditory

    Localization
    Figure–ground discrimination
    Memory
    Sequential memory

Motor planning

    Body scheme
    Proprioception
    Kinesthesia
    Directionality
    Laterality

---

child moves about and explores the environment, he or she develops and refines perception. Adequate sensorimotor development provides the necessary head control, trunk stability, and rotation to free the extremities to enable exploration. The child's cognitive level and motivation are also important. Most children are intrinsically motivated to explore and become independent to varying degrees. The degree and quality of their movement and exploration affect perceptual abilities.

Assessment

Perceptual abilities have a direct effect on activities of daily living and on educational, vocational, and leisure activities. They can be divided into four basic categories: visual, visual motor, auditory, and motor planning. The basic components of each category are shown in Table 18-1.

Visual perception. Elements of visual perception include depth perception, figure–ground and visual discrimination, spatial relations, and position in space. Accurate visual perception requires that all these elements work together. It also must be remembered that most actions and mental processes are a combination of these elements. Perceptual problems can occur in those with cerebral palsy; as well as children with other developmental disabilities, including minimal brain dysfunction, learning disorders, and after head trauma (Fig. 18-1).

Depth perception and *figure–ground discrimination* are needed for accurate reach used in educational, vocational, and daily living tasks. Depth perception has been shown to depend on binocular vision. Figure–ground discrimination is the ability to visually isolate an object or figure from a background pattern. Problems in either of these areas can affect eye–hand coordination.

Visual discrimination is used to differentiate and classify objects by size, shape, and color. The infant begins this process by visually attending to and tracking objects within the visual field. Initial exploration of objects is done by mouthing. As hand function develops, manipulation of objects with the hand and fingers increases. The child relates the tactile sensations received from the object to its visual characteristics. Gradually, these associations develop into abilities to assimilate differences and similarities in objects visually. Visual discrimination is used in most daily, educational, and vocational tasks. Shape differentiation underlies the recognition of numbers and letters, forming a basis for communication and education.

Spatial relations and position in space reflect object perception and how various objects relate to each other in three-dimensional space. The child's ability to reach in different planes provides a sense of distance and direction. Gross motor activities assist in further developing this skill. The child continues to learn about three-dimensional space through rolling and climbing through, under, over, and in between objects. In performing these activities, children learn to orient themselves to objects in space. The sensations received from movement are integrated with visual perceptions and contribute to their accuracy and development.

Visual motor abilities enable the coordination of the eyes and hands in functional activity, e.g. writing.

Auditory perception.   The components of auditory perception include localization, figure–ground discrimination, auditory memory and auditory sequential memory.

Localization of auditory stimuli is noted by the head turning in the direction of the sound. This requires normal hearing and voluntary motor control of head movements.

Figure–ground discrimination is the ability to distinguish meaningful sounds from background noise. This is thought to be due to CNS capacity to screen out irrelevant sounds, allowing attention to be focused without constant distraction.

Auditory memory is the ability to recall and carry out auditory messages accurately. It often involves abilities in receptive and expressive language as well.

Auditory memory is used to follow verbal directions in daily, educational, and vocational tasks. Sequential memory allows an individual to follow three- and four-step commands in the right order.

Motor planning.   Motor planning, or praxis, is defined as the ability to conceive of, organize, and carry out a sequence of unfamiliar actions.[4] A good body scheme is particularly important in this case, as is accurate sensation of proprioception and kinesthesia. Feedback from movement is essential when learning new action sequences. The concept of directionality and established laterality are also important components of motor planning. *Laterality* contibutes to the ability to establish a preferred hand. *Directionality* is the concept of right, left, up, and down. As the new action sequence is repeated, it no longer requires motor planning. Learning a new motor skill of any type, e.g., typing or swimming, requires motor planning at the onset.

An individual with cerebral palsy who has movement difficulties and sensorimotor delay frequently has perceptual problems as well. Assessment and isolation of specific perceptual problems in cerebral palsy can be difficult because of motor overlay on performance. Emphasis is placed on how perception is related to functional tasks rather than on labeling specific deficits.

Treatment

Perceptual status is important when adaptive equipment is being considered. Language or communication boards and motorized wheelchairs for patients with more severe motor problems are examples of types of equipment that require adequate perceptual abilities.

Therapy for children identified as having perceptual problems consists of providing a variety of gross motor, sensorimotor, and upper-extremity activities (Fig. 18-2). The purpose of the activities is to facilitate movement and exploration of the environment, since these facilities are extremely important in the development of perception. A child having difficulty in wheel chair mobilization and continually bumping into corners and furniture may be encouraged in therapy to climb over and through objects of varying sizes.

In cases where the perceptual problem cannot be remedied, the patient is taught to compensate if possible. An adolescent in a prevocational program, for instance, who is having trouble discerning subtle size differences necessary in sorting nuts and bolts,

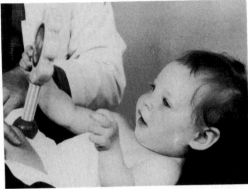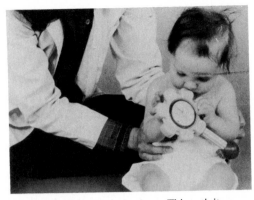

Figure 18-2. (A) Girl aged 11 mo with spasticity regarding her face in a toy mirror. This activity is utilized to increase visual perception, (B) as well as tactile exploration.

could be provided with a sizing template. Parents, educators, vocational counselors, and other relevant staff must be made aware of the problem and its implications on performance.

Upper-Extremity Function

Upper-extremity function includes the development of fine motor skills, hand usage, sensation, strength and movement, and indications for splinting. It develops as the infant acquires proximal stability and control, which allows independent use of the arms and hands for manipulative and purposeful activity. Accurate perception augments the quality of upper-extremity function. As reach and grasp become refined, the hands become the primary means for interaction with the environment and the fundamental vehicle for performing a broad range of life activities.

Fine motor skills. Fine motor skills begin when grasp and reach become refined.[26] Infants are born with a grasp reflex. Stimulation to the palm causes the hand to become fisted automatically. As the grasp reflex is modified, voluntary grasp begins to develop. Initially, grasp consists of the digits' flexing toward the palm and rarely involves the thumb. This is referred to as a *raking* grasp. Grasping is more efficient on the ulnar aspect of the hand at this point. As grasping is refined, the radial protion of the hand develops, rendering thumb opposition to the fingers. With the development of thumb movements there emerges a greater variety of gross grasping patterns, such as the cylindric and spherical grips. Further refinement involves finger differentiation and isolated

finger movements. This enables pinch patterns, which in themselves become refined. The types of patterns are three-point pinch, lateral pinch, and inferior and superior pincer grasp. The release of objects follows a sequential pattern of development as well.[20]

Hand usage. Hand function can be categorized into three types: unilateral, bilateral, and reciprocal. Unilateral hand usage is observed when an activity is performed entirely with one hand. Very few activities within the daily routine are done exclusively with one hand. Stabilization is often needed in situations where refined usage is demanded of the dominant hand. Holding a piece of paper down while writing is one example. Bilateral hand usage includes moving both hands simultaneously in the same pattern, such as in using a rolling pin. Reciprocal movements occur when both hands are moving simultaneously in opposite directions, as in opening containers. Skilled bilateral and reciprocal hand usage partially depends on integration of both sides of the body.

Sensation. The interrelationship of sensation and movement is an important factor. Sensory information is obtained as one manipulates objects and includes proprioception, kinesthesia, light touch, stereognosis, two-point discrimination, and localization of tactile stimuli. The discriminatory functions of the sensory mechanisms in the hand play a major role in activity performance. Other sensations often assessed in hand function are temperature, deep touch, and response to pain.

For many individuals with cerebral palsy, fine motor abilities and reciprocal hand function can be difficult. The predominance of primitive and abnormal reflexes, poor postural reflexes, and abnormal muscle tone limit these skills. Perceptual and cognitive deficits can also limit upper-extremity abilities. The amount of upper-extremity limitation is directly related to the severity of deficits found in the aforementioned areas. The grasping pattern is a motor response and will reflect the person's overall motor characteristics. Therefore, a single grasping pattern typical of cerebral palsy does not exist, since the clinical spectrum varies greatly. Many patients with cerebral palsy lack the variety of grasping patterns seen in the normal population. Individuals may demonstrate more than one pattern but rarely, except in very mild cases, exhibit all types. Manual dexterity, the ability to move an object within the hand, may also be limited or absent. In more severe cases the grasp reflex does not become fully integrated, causing the hand to assume a continual fisted posture. A typical hand deformity is the cortical thumb, in which the thumb rests in the palm of the hand. This may lead to contracture of the thumb in that position over time as well as greatly limit the hand's functional abilities.

Treatment

The focus of treatment is to relate upper-extremity function to the performance of functional tasks and not solely for refinement. When hand function is severely impaired through movement disorders, sensory deficits, or structural deformities, alternative means of interacting with the environment should be considered, such as adaptive equipment.

When structural deformities of the hand require surgical correction, pertinent information on the individual's current level of sensation, fine motor abilities, hand usage, and task performance must be known. The impact of surgery on the individual's emotional status and performance must carefully be taken into account. Because of the complexity of problems often found in the patient who requires hand surgery, the orthopaedist and therapist should work closely both in preoperative assessment and in postoperative therapy.[29] Preoperative splinting may be considered to evaluate the potential effectiveness of surgery. Therapeutic management postoperatively may include serial splinting, active and passive range of motion, and graded activities to facilitate functional usage.

The purposes of splinting include positioning or stabilization of the hand, restorating or improving function, protecting weak muscles, and enhancing correction of deformities.[26] As in any therapeutic intervention, splinting requires evaluation and reas-

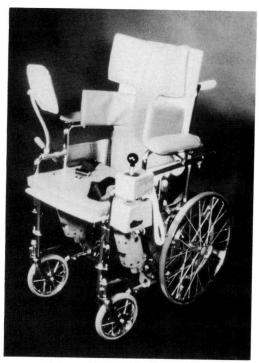

Figure 18-3. Example of a wheelchair adapted to provide better positioning and improve stability. (Designed and fabricated by Alternative Design, Wrentham, Mass).

sessment. The long-term effects of splinting in minimizing deformity when used in patients with abnormal tone and movement disorders have not been thoroughly investigated, and further research is needed.

Activities of Daily Living

Activities of daily living include all those tasks that are performed in self-care and daily hygiene. They can be thought of as a continuum from basic care skills, such as eating and dressing, to more advanced skills that are used to function in the community, such as transportation and shopping. Occupational therapy applies patterns of movement and use of adaptive equipment, including those of environmental design, to enable the individual with cerebral palsy to be as independent as possible (Fig. 18-4). Promoting independence very often increases self-esteem and confidence. In the evaluation, program design, and therapy for these tasks, it is necessary to involve the patient as much as possible.

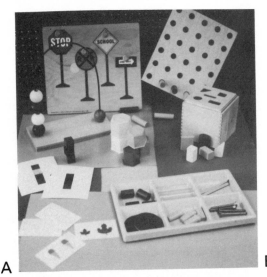
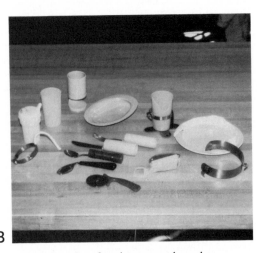

A   B

Figure 18-4. A variety of treatment activities is provided. Examples of equipment used are above. (A) Perceptual motor and (B) feeding.

Often, individuals have devised their own methods for accomplishing these tasks. These should be observed and analyzed to see what type of movement patterns are used, the individual's efficiency at the task, and how task demands fit into the overall management plan (Fig. 18-5).

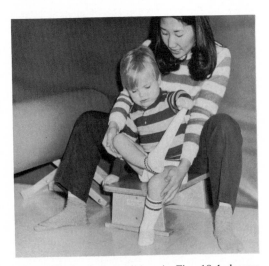

Figure 18-5. Same child as in Fig. 18-1 demonstrating sock removal with proximal stability provided. Supported activities allows improved fine motor skills, increased body awareness, and activities of daily living.

One particular skill that is a vital component of daily living is eating. The eating process includes the oral structures and oral motor control to ingest food and liquids as well as establishment of the hand-to-mouth pattern and utensil use for self-feeding. It should be clearly understood that deficits in sensorimotor function can affect oral motor control as well. Resulting oral motor deficits, such as poorly coordinated lips, tongue, and swallowing movements, can cause eating difficulty. Identification of feeding and eating problems that most commonly occur in cerebral palsy and techniques for facilitating normal oral motor development have been described by Morris.[27,27a] Feeding and eating problems often become intensified with solid foods, which require chewing. An oral motor treatment program usually aims to increase oral motor functioning to facilitate more normal eating patterns so that a variety of food can be ingested for greater nutritional value.

Self-feeding requires good oral motor control, adequate head and trunk control, ability to bring the hand to the mouth, and other perceptual and cognitive skills. The occupational therapist provides an assessment of self-feeding abilities and any necessary equipment and training that would make the patient more independent.

We have found feeding and eating problems with an institutionalized population to be complex, interwoven with behavioral components, nutritional and medical concerns, oral motor, and self-feeding issues. An interdisciplinary feeding team was established at our facility to confront the multifaceted problems of feeding and eating. The feeding team consists of an occupational therapist, a physical therapist, a speech therapist, a nurse, a psychologist, a nutritionist, and direct care providers. Representatives from the medical, dental, and pharmacy staffs are available as consultants. The team attempts to evaluate patients who are referred with feeding problems of such magnitude that they create management problems for direct care providers or parents. Based on joint evaluation, the team develops an integrated plan that can be implemented by the direct care service provider, parent, or particular clinical service. It is important that this specialized team, as well as being well coordinated, clearly identifies its role and function within the patient's overall management plan.

Many daily living tasks require refined hand movements, such as bilateral or reciprocal hand usage, which make accomplishment difficult or impossible for many cerebral palsied patients. In these instances the occupational therapist must look for alternatives to increase independence. Adjustments of task demands, adaptations to the tasks performed, and environmental modifications are frequently used.

Adaptive Equipment

The overall purpose of adaptive equipment is to increase independence in task performance and to provide proper positioning (Fig. 18-3).[7,31] It can be used in tasks of daily living, education, vocation, leisure, and mobility. Adaptive equipment should be regarded as a treatment modality; its need and use should be carefully assessed, monitored, and periodically reassessed.

In prescribing equipment, several factors must be assessed. The patient's intellectual, perceptual, and motor potential to use the equipment effectively are crucial considerations. A training period may be necessary before its initiation. Equipment should also be age appropriate. The patient's reaction to the item and its cosmetic effect are important. It is essential to note the recipient's psychologic and emotional acceptance of special equipment, particularly before its purchase or construction. This point can be easily overlooked by care providers anxious to enhance a person's independence. Sensitivity to parental readiness to accept the need for equipment and its implications is warranted. Occasionally, children and their families feel that special equipment sets them further apart from the normal population and view it as a trademark of their handicap.

Adaptive equipment encompasses a wide variety of devices that can be either simple or complex. Highly complex sophisticated equipment is often difficult to replace and can be cumbersome. Equipment materials and design should be kept as streamlined and simple as possible. A large amount of equipment is available commercially and can be ordered rather than constructed. The durability and cost of the item, particularly in relation to the patient's financial status, should be considered.

A determination should be made on whether the adaptive equipment will be used on a long- or short-term basis. The specific use of the equipment should be explained in detail to all who will be involved with it. Abnormal tone, associated reactions, and abnormal movement patterns can occur with the use of new equipment. The therapist should monitor this and make modifications as needed as well as schedule equipment use based on clinical judgments of the patient's performance. If the patient is unable to monitor the equipment, family or service providers must be identified to ensure its proper usage, cleaning, storage, and replacement when necessary.

Designing and obtaining mobility devices requires an interdisciplinary process. Determining which position or positions are the most functional, maintaining optimal body alignment, and affording the greatest degree of normalized tone should be a joint venture of both disciplines. Proximal stability of head and trunk can be attained through adapted equipment. These are prerequisites for adequate hand function, which will allow the patient to accomplish activities of daily living, school, leisure, and vocation. Factors such as use of the device for transportation to school, family trips, outdoor and indoor use, and accessibility through doorways and to tables must be taken into account. Physical therapy, medical, and orthopaedic aspects must also be considered. Patients with severe physical deformities should be reviewed by an orthopaedist to determine if any surgical intervention would improve positioning and if there are any contraindications to the desired position.[19]

Play and Leisure

Play and leisure experiences serve an important role for everyone and should be considered in the overall management of individuals with cerebral palsy. Throughout the evaluation and treatment process, play and leisure activities are applied and assessed when appropriate. It is often highly desirable to incorporate leisure and play activities into the treatment program as a means of employing treatment objectives. For the school-aged child, play activities assist cognitive and motor development as well as peer group interaction. Interacting and playing with others is essential for the development of social skills. For example, children learn about cooperation and competition when engaged in group activities.

The ability to participate in recreational activities is equally important for the adolescent and the adult. Satisfactory use of unstructured time for pleasurable leisure experiences requires development of specific skills and accessibility to resources.

Availability of community resources for social functions, leisure activities, recreation, and advocacy groups should be explored. The family or the patient may need encouragement and direction to seek out resources that can provide needed assistance and emotional support. Opportunities available will vary depending on community awareness and ability to provide services for the individual with a physical handicap. Architectural barriers are a major consideration when seeking community activities. Transportation, curbs, entrances to buildings, accessibility to bathrooms, telephones, and water fountains should all be taken into account.

Educational and Work Readiness Skills

Occupational therapy services within the realm of educational and vocational training usually include evaluation, on-site consultation, and direct services when motor, perceptual, or organizational abilities influence work performance. Because of the complexities encountered as a result of the broad nature of disabling conditions in cerebral palsy, the occupational therapist, vocational rehabilitation counselor, educator, physician, and social worker should work in close association.

It should be recognized that although some individuals are quite capable of vocational enterprises, not all have this potential. Those with the more severe motor disorders may not possess the motor abilities to perform required job tasks, even with the aid of adaptive equipment and mechanical devices. Some individuals may need to use abnormal or reflexive movement patterns with many associated reactions to accomplish the job. These can affect work endurance and productivity and may cause health problems over time. It should be decided whether it is in the individual's best interests, both psychologically and physically, to continue with such vocational tasks. If vocational training and placement is not feasible, other alternatives, such as adult education or leisure skills, should be sought. In these cases particularly, the management plan demands that serious decisions be made with the individual patient as active a participant as possible.

EDUCATION

One of the primary roles of the occupational therapist is educating the patient, family (including siblings and other care providers). The focus can be individualized or more generalized, i.e., involve teaching small groups about the nature of cerebral palsy and general principles of management.

It is important that the patient and family participate in the development of treatment objectives and understand important principles of the patient's program. The therapist must also understand the nature of the home, school, and work environments in order to use activities routinely performed in these settings.

The therapist must develop rapport with the patient and family in order to successfully provide education. He or she must be sensitive to the readiness of patient and family to absorb specific information and grade their teachings accordingly. It is equally important that the therapist respect the knowledge base of the patient and family and assume the "student" role in the educational process when appropriate. The therapist must allow opportunities for the patient and family to demonstrate their understanding and receive feedback and support for their efforts.

REVIEW OF EFFECTIVENESS OF TREATMENT

It is essential that service providers establish mechanisms for reviewing the quality of their care and the effectiveness of their interventions. Quality assurance is a process by which care can objectively be reviewed. It has been described as the interface between *clinical practice* and *clinical research*.[32] The responsibility for performing quality review should not be taken lightly because of the necessity for receiving feedback about services rendered. Specific methods for performing quality assurance activities are available from the American Occupational Therapy Association.[2,3]

REFERENCES

1. American Occupational Therapy Association: Occupational Therapy: 2001. Rockville, Md., The Association, 1979
2. American Occupational Therapy Association: Patient Care Evaluation in Action: An Audit Manual for Occupational Therapists. Rockville, Md., The Association, 1978
3. American Occupational Therapy Association: Standards of Practice. Rockville, Md., The Association, 1978
4. Ayres J: Sensory Integration and the Child. Los Angeles, Western Psychological Services, 1980
5. Ayres J: Sensory Integration and Learning Disorders. Los Angeles, Western Psychological Services, 1975
6. Banus B: The Developmental Therapist. Thorofare, N.J. Charles B. Slack, 1979
7. Bergen A: Selected Equipment for Pediatric Rehabilitation. Supplement I. Blythedale Childrens Hospital, Valhalla, N.Y., 1974
8. Bobath B: Abnormal Postural Reflex Activity caused by Brain Lesions. William Heinemann, London, 1971
9. Bobath B, Bobath K: Motor Development in the Different Types of Cerebral Palsy. London, William Heinemann, 1975
10. Bobath K: A Nuerophysiological Basis for the Treatment of Cerebral Palsy. London, William Heinemann, 1980
11. Bower TGR: A Primer on Infant Development. San Francisco, W. H. Freeman and Co., 1977
12. Brazelton TB: Infants and Mothers. New York, Delacorte, 1969
13. Brazelton TB: Toddlers and Parents. New York, Delacorte, 1974
14. Capute AJ, Accardo PJ, Vining PG, et al: Primitive Reflex Profile. Baltimore, University Park Press, 1978
15. Colangelo C, Bergan A, Gottleib L: A Normal Baby. The Sensory–Motor Processes of the First Year. Valhalla, N.Y., Blythedale Childrens Hospital, 1976
16. Conner FP, Williamson GG, Siep JM: Program Guide for Infants and Toddlers. New York, Teachers College Press, 1978
17. Ellis E: Physical Management of Developmental Disorder, in Clinics in Developmental Medicine, no. 26. London, Spasticity Society Medical Education, London, 1967
18. Finnie N: Handling the Young Cerebral Palsied Child at Home (ed 2). New York, Dutton, 1975
19. Fiorentino M: A Basis for Sensorimotor Development—Normal and Abnormal. Springfield, Ill., Charles C Thomas, 1981
20. Gesell A: The First Five Years of Life. Hagerstown, Harper & Row, 1940
21. Gilfoyle E: Training, Occupational Therapy, Education, Management in Schools: American Occupation Therapy Association. Dept. of Education, Office of Special Education and Rehabilitation Services, 1980
22. Gilfoyle E, Grady A, Moore J: Children Adapt. Thorofare, N.J., Charles B. Slack, 1981
23. Illingsworth RS: The Development of the Infant and Young Child. Normal and Abnormal. New York, Churchill Livingston, 1975
24. Kopp CB: Fine-motor abilities of infants. Dev Med Child Neurol 14:629, 1974
25. Levitt S: Treatment of Cerebral Palsy and Motor Delay. Oxford, Blackwell, 1977
26. Malick M: Manual on Static Hand Splinting. Pittsburgh, Harmarville Rehabilitation Center, 1979
27. Morris S: The Normal Acquisition of Oral Feeding Skills: Implications for Assessment and Treatment. Therapeutic Media, Inc. 1982
27a. Morris S: Oral-motor function and dysfunction in Children, in Wiseson JM (ed): Chapel Hill, University of North Carolina Press, 1978
28. Pearson P: Physical Therapy Services in Developmental Disabilities. Springfield, Ill., Charels C Thomas, 1972
29. Samilson C: Orthopaedic Aspects of Cerebral Palsy. London, Walter Heinemann, 1975
30. Scott AD, Trombly CA: Occupational Therapy for Physical Dysfunction. Baltimore, Williams & Wilkins, 1977
31. Robinzuelt I: Functional Aids for the Multiply Handicapped. Hagerstown, Harper & Row, 1973
32. Williamson J, Ostrow PC, Braswell H: Health Accounting for Quality Assurance: A Manual for Assessing and Improving Outcomes of Care. Rockville, Md., American Occupational Therapy Association, 1981

Mary Cassidy-Conway
Richard M. Zawacki

19

Physical Therapy

Any attempts to provide physical therapy management for individuals with a developmental disability such as cerebral palsy must be preceded by an assessment of that individual's needs. Such an assessment can have various forms or structures of implementation and can be performed for various purposes. The situation may call for an indepth, complex evaluation or for a screening. It is not the intent of this chapter to present or discuss the various neurodevelopmental and pediatric assessment and rehabilitation techniques described by many authors; instead, it will focus on general concepts in the evaluation and treatment of the musculoskeletal and motor development of the child with cerebral palsy at the various stages of growth and development.[1,3–13,15,16]

MOTOR FUNCTION

In the assessment of motor function, emphasis has long been placed on the quantity of motor achievements, i.e., how many and which motor milestones has a child achieved? It is also important to consider, however, the quality of motor behavior that is exhibited. An individual may have achieved a certain motor skill, but if the balance, stability, or postural symmetry of such a milestone is compromised, functional efficiency will necessarily be diminished. Another important consideration is the overall importance movement makes in an infant's, toddler's, and growing child's world. It is through movement that an infant can first express his or her capacities to interact overtly with the environment. As such interactions continue with further growth and development, the child is able to exert more control over certain aspects of the environment. Realization of the influence that impairment or loss of such control can have on individuals with cerebral palsy is crucial. Such realization brings with it an appreciation of the physical needs, goals, and priorities of each child and family.

In terms of assessment, note that any one aspect of a motor examination rarely gives an accurate picture of an individual's abilities. Total comprehensive and integrated assessment of numerous parameters is necessary. The conclusions of results of such assessments should always be considered in conjunction with evaluations performed by other disciplines.

Certain guidelines or suggestions for motor evaluation in a population with central nervous system (CNS) dysfunction are discussed below. This is not meant to be an all-inclusive discussion but, rather, a background to the physical management of the growing child with cerebral palsy.

Muscle Tone

Muscle tone has classically been understood as resistance to passive stretch. This implies passive manipulation of a muscle or muscle group. The lack of objectivity and generalization of such an assessment should be apparent. By expanding the working definition of muscle tone, more functional and reproducible criteria can be added. Such a definition would depict tone as it affects active movement and functional abilities. One must also be aware of how intrinsic and extrinsic variables such as fatigue, anxiety, and fear can influence the expression of muscle tone. Such an approach to the assessment of tone reflects the realistic influence that tone disorders can have on function and independence.

Muscle Strength

Muscle strength is generally considered as the ability of a muscle or muscle group to build up tension voluntarily in response to a load or resistance. Key words in this definition are *voluntary* and *in response*. *Voluntary* implies that any observed and palpable increase in muscle tension is under the person's control. The importance of the term *in response* lies in the fact that such tension is directly related to the superimposed load and not to any ongoing state of tension in the muscle. These distinctions in definition between muscle tone and muscle strength are important because they allow at least a theoretic difference between the two variables to be appreciated. In clinical practice, such a delineation is frequently difficult to assess clearly. Until knowledge of the interrelationship of these two neuromuscular parameters becomes more sophisticated, qualitifications must be made whenever statements about muscle strength are made in the presence of abnormal muscle tone.

Range of Motion

Assessment of range of motion is an important part of any evaluation of motor performance. Standard testing is performed in positions with universally accepted criteria of measurement.[14] There may be times, however, when such classic testing procedures can only be implemented with modifications in children with cerebral palsy. Certain adaptive positioning or relaxation techniques should be used when one examines joint motion in such patients. These procedural modifications can assist in selecting out the confusing variables of abnormal muscle tone from muscle contractions and real or true joint motion. Although all joint range-of-motion evaluations should be performed passively, knowledge of the active motion possible at a particular joint or a certain arc of motion is frequently helpful.

Reflex Profile

A reflex is a relatively stereotypic motor response to a particular stimuli given under a certain situation. Over the years, the relative importance of the influence of a child's reflexive profile has fluctuated, both in normal development and in the presence of motor dysfunction. The methods of primitive reflex evaluation and categorization of reflexes and postural responses are discussed in Chapter 17. In terms of assessment, the examiner must be aware of how certain repetitious, stereotypic responses can influence motor behavior and functional skills. It then remains for one to judge whether the response has a positive or negative influence on motor function and what approach to treatment is needed.

Movement Patterns

An appraisal of an individual's movement, movement patterns, and functional skills is generally considered the substance of a physical therapy evaluation; however, one cannot separate the influence and interaction of all the previously mentioned evaluation parameters on overall movement. Movement skills and quality must always be assessed with consideration of the child's chronologic skeletal, and gestational age. Many qualities or aspects of observed movement must be addressed. It is important to ascertain whether a movement pattern can be easily reproduced and whether complex or stereotypic patterns are used. Above and beyond noting a child's level of stability, balance, and quality of posture, one must look for that which is frequently lacking in these children, namely, the ability to make smooth positional movements. Assessment of the more classic funtional status is crucial in order to achieve a realistic appraisal of the extent of involvement and degree of physical impairment.

Additional Assessments

Further areas of assessment may best be performed in conjunction with other members of the evaluation team. Collaboration with the occupational therapist, speech pathologist, and nutritionist should occur during examination of oral–motor function and feeding skills. Any needs and plans for special or adaptive equipment should be the joint work of therapists, parents and physicians. When families are included, unnecessary or inappropriate ordering of equipment can frequently be avoided by determining that either the family feels it the item is needed or that the equipment does not fit the patient's or the family's lifestyle.

INTERVENTION STRATEGIES

It is crucial that guidelines and strategies be formulated for the delivery of appropriate, quality physical therapy intervention to individuals with cerebral palsy. Perhaps a primary question to pose is when an under what circumstances should a physical therapist become involved with a particular child. Whenever there is a concern about motor skills or when abnormal neurologic signs are present, assessment by a physical therapist with experience in child development and developmental delays that vary from normal should also be evaluated. Some of these children may not require any direct therapeutic intervention and may need only periodic reevaluation of developmental progress. Children in whom intervenion is usually necessary includes those with overt pathology of the neuromotor system, e.g., the presence of abnormal muscle tone, persistent primitive reflexes, and postural responses or deviant movement patterns.

There are obviously various forms of physical therapy intervention. The appropriateness of any particular form lies in the interaction between numerous variables surrounding the handicapped person, the family, the available health care delivery system, and financial considerations. In general, the forms of intervention would include (1) consultation, (2) evaluation with recommendations, and (3) direct service in either individual or group settings. Whatever the form of intervention, services should not be duplicated, should be appropriate to the patient's prioritized needs, and should consider social and psychologic factors.

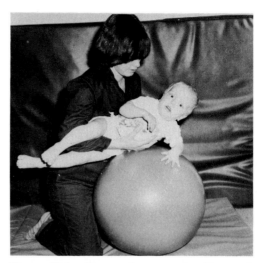

Figure 19-1. Boy aged two years with spastic quadriplegia receiving early neurodevelopmental intervention. Gymnastic ball is used to facilitate trunk rotation and weightbearing on the upper extremities to improve rolling and upper-extremity stability.

Maturational Issues

Infant and Toddler Years

One of the more important issues during treatment is the working relationship the physical therapist has with the child and the family. Most families learn during this period that something is different about their child, whether it relates to the child's potential physical, mental, or social development. Parents need support and honesty particularly during this time. Since the majority of interactions during this time occur within the home setting, therapists often share in many personal aspects of the child's family life. In most cases this can facilitate acceptance of the therapist and of program suggestions from the evaluation team. Therapist must be aware of the need to maintain a professional relationship with these families, however, in order to maintain objectivity in managing the child's physical development and advocating for his or her needs.

A therapist, along with other members of an evaluation team, must assist parents in understanding the meaning and implications of the child's diagnosis and disability. Initial discussion and establishment of realistic short- and long-term goals along with treatment suggestions can often help give parents who are overwhelmed something concrete to focus on and do for their child's benefit. The implementation of therapeutic programming is often crucial at this time, especially for children with overt motor dysfunction

(Fig. 19-1). Such programming should always be kept within a realistic framework in attempts to facilitate compliance. Often during this time a child undergoes a first hospitalization, which may include a surgical procedure. After consultation with the physician and other members of the hospital team, the therapist can often review with the family what to expect during the hospital stay. When this is done in the home, as opposed to in a busy clinic or physician's office, families often have a better understanding of what will happen to their child. Another service that a therapist can provide during this period is to educate and guide the family in how to be appropriate consumers of medical and educational services for their child, who, in many cases, will need these services through adulthood.

Preschool Years

The implementation of therapeutic services during the preschool years has been largely influenced by Public Law 94–142. This law requires the delivery of publically funded education with supportive services to all children with developmental disabilities who are three years of age or older (see Chapters 30 and 31). Many children with cerebral palsy thus become introduced to specialized educational programming at an early age. It is often beneficial to work with parents before the transition to public schooling.

They can be educated on the statutes of Public Law 94–142, on how the system functions in their particular town or state, and on how they can effectively advocate for their child.

This is often the beginning of parents' having to deal with governmental agencies when attempting to procure services for their child. Such procedures are usually necessary, however, and they assist in providing parents with formal lines of comunication giving them a strong voice in the planning of their child's educational needs. For children with physical disabilities, the physical therapist plays a crucial role in assisting the educational team in determining optimal placement and programming. It is crucial that the child's current needs be prioritized toward areas of principal strength. The therapist must objectively determine where the need for physical therapy services fits in with a particular child's other needs. If it is determined that physical therapy is needed, what form of intervention should be used? What level of professional should provide the service (registered physical therapist, physical therapist assistant, aid)? In what setting should the service be provided, and what should its duration and frequency be? These questions present complex issues. The parents' ability to advocate effectively for their child, the availability of community resources, and the fiscal integrity of the special education budget are only a few of the factors that influence service delivery. The physical therapist must always strive to make mature, responsible recommendations for a child's educational plan, considering his or her needs and the capacity of the school system to meet those needs. An additional and sometimes underestimated role of the therapist during

these and any school years is to facilitate communication between the educational and the medical professionals. It is often crucial that a regular exchange of information occur between these parties. The physical therapist, having knowledge of both systems, can fulfill this role quite well.

Another issue that generally has become quite apparent by this stage of development is the need for adaptive equipment. By this age, a child's physical limitations have often become clear. Knowledge of the school setting also provides information about the kind of activities or functional skills that a child may benefit from if provided with proper external support. The child's needs for mobility, i.e., getting from one place to another, and stability, i.e., staying in one place, can often be assisted with specialized equipment (Fig. 19-2). Any difficulties encountered in feeding, dressing, or toileting can often be diminished with the use of some assistive device. Therapists may only become involved with the recommendations for such equipment, which would be procured, fitted, and maintained by the family, orthotist, or teacher, but therapist should be prepared to participate in the actual fabrication and modification of equipment. It is important to remember that educational personnel are, in most cases, unfamiliar with the appropriate use or fit of such devices. Training and ongoing supervision in this area is always warranted.

Elementary School Years

Although the disabled child and the family may have been acquainted with public education during the preschool years, for most children the elementary school environment brings about many changes. It

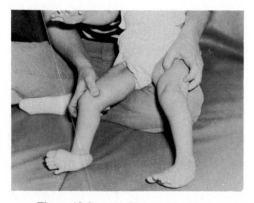 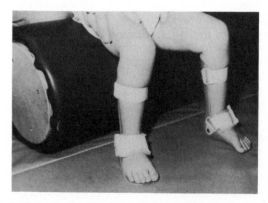

Figure 19-2. (A) Girl aged three years with spastic diplegia who does not ambulate and has poor lower-extremity muscle control. (B) After application of total contact ankle–foot orthoses (AFO), there is improved position of the feet and lower extremities. The child was subsequently able to pull to standing and ambulate with external support while wearing her orthoses.

may be a child's first actual dealing with a public school setting, since many preschool children are frequently placed in a "special" environment. As is the case with all children, physically disabled or not, this is the first contact with a standard classroom environment.

Assessment of the physical environment of the school is best done before classes begin. Both obvious and obscure barriers to physical accessibility must be determined. Any and all areas that the child may need to get to and from should be examined. This includes ramps, curbs, stairs, bathrooms, cafeteria, gym, playground; in the classroom this includes the size of desks, width of aisles, and height of blackboard. The availability of certain audiovisual components e.g., typewriters, communication boards (Fig. 19-3), and tape recorders, for more disabled children should be examined as necessary aids to the learning process. Another area that may be frequently overlooked is a plan of exit in case of fire, particularly for the more physically disabled child. Individuals using a wheelchair, a walker, or orthotic devices will need prearranged plans that coordinate with other evacuation procedures.

It is important for all pediatric health care providers to understand the unique relationship between therapy services and the schools. It must be remembered that a therapist is a medical professional working in the structure and framework of an educational model. The primary goal of the educational system is education. In keeping with this, physical therapy may be placed at various leels of priorities, depending both on the child's overall performance and needs and on the system's ability to meet those needs.

When introducing physical therapy into the classroom setting, one must anticipate the impact it will have on overall classroom functioning. If it has been determined that classroom personnel will assist in implementating certain aspects of the therapy program, certain questions must be addressed. For example, are these personnel willing to perform these services? Were they part of the decision-making process? Is there time available within the classroom schedule to allow for implementation? Can arrangements be made for ongoing instruction of staff and supervision by the therapist? Another point to consider is that for some children, physical therapy services can best be provided in an out-of-school setting. Some children who need only periodic follow-up care and who cannot afford to have their class schedule interrupted might be better suited for therapy provided at home or in an outpatient facility (Fig. 19-4). One must consider alternatives such as this so that optimum services can be provided to children in the most cost-effective manner and in a way that best meets the child's needs.

Therapists working in an educational setting must also understand how they fit into the organization within the system. A therapist's location within the organizational flow of the school system is generally not as clear as in a medical setting. The line of responsibility is generally even more unclear. Therapists should consider themselves ethically responsible for the related actions of any individual who has been instructed to carry out any part or portion of the therapy program, however. The question of liability for the therapist and for those whom the therapist supervises remains unanswered. If these and similar issues can be addressed early in a school year, the quality of the child's school experience and the therapist's overall effectiveness can be better ensured.

Junior High and High School Years

The preadolescent and adolescent school years are difficult times for any individual. It appears obvious that the additional variable of a physical disability can only serve to compound these difficulties. In terms of physical functioning, many children with cerebral palsy have reached or have come close to their optimal level of independence and motor skills (Fig. 19-5). In addition, it is likely that they have been performing, or have been requested to perform, some kind of therapeutic home programming for many years. This, combined with the lack of progress in their motor skills and their frequent desire to decrease special services that call further attention to their differences, results in a decrease in the desired and actual need for physical therapy services.

Any therapeutic programs designed for this age group should be formulated by a joint patient–therapist effort. Determination of special areas of interest, such as sports, hobbies, and future occupation, is necessary to formulate a realistic program. Such a program should not be extensive and should preferably be carried out personally by the patient and require little intervention by parents and families. This is an important consideration, since the added stress of parental supervision is not needed during adolescence, when many adolescent–parent problems may already exist. In addition to the smaller amount of actual direct therapeutic service that may now be needed, a therapist's consultation role may actually increase. Strategies may be discussed with the family or school staff on ways to compensate for certain areas of dysfunction or to formulate prevocational and vocational programs. It is often helpful

100 VOCABULARY (December 1975)

Blissymbolics Communication Foundation
862 Eglinton Avenue East,
Toronto, Ontario, Canada M4G 2L1

	a	b	c	d	e	f	g	h	i	j
1	0	1	2	3	4	5	6	7	8	9
2	hello good-bye	question	I, me (my)	like	happy	make action	food	pen, pencil	friend	animal
3	please	why	you (your)	want	angry	mouth	drink	paper, page	GOD	bird
4	thanks	how	man	come	afraid	eye	sleep	book	house	flower
5	I'm sorry	who	woman	give	funny	legs	toilet	table	school	water
6	opposite	what thing	father	make	good	hand	pain	television	hospital	sun
7	much, many	which	mother	help	big	ear	clothing	news	store	weather
8	music	where	brother	think	young, new	nose	outing	word	show	day
9		when	sister	know	difficult	head	car	light	room	week-end
10		how many	teacher	wash	hot	name	wheelchair	game, toy	street	birthday

A

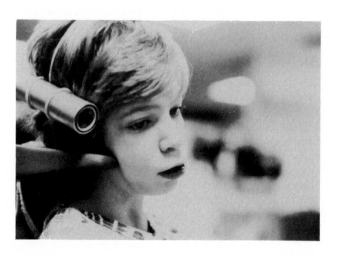

B

198

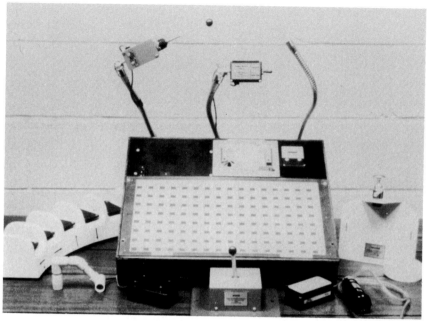

C

Figure 19-3. (A) Bliss Symbol board used as an aid in communciation for non-verbal children. (Courtesy Blissymbolics Communication Foundation, Toronto, Ontario, Canada.) (B) Illuminated head-controlled pointing stick for use with a symbol board in severely disabled nonverbal children with poor extremity control. (Courtesy Prentke-Romich-Beery Co., Shreve, Ohio.) (C) Electronic Communication scanner board with various switches that can be specifically adapted to meet nonverbal children's individual communication requirements. (Courtesy Prentke-Romich-Beery Co., Shreve, Ohio.)

for an individual with cerebral palsy to have yearly physical therapy consultation to ensure that any issues concerning physical functioning, independence, and posture can be addressed. For individuals who are more severely disabled, different strategies of therapeutic intervention may be needed. For bed-ridden or wheelchair-bound patients, a therapist may need to supervise a daily program for the maintenance of certain skills. Such a program can be implemented by family, roommates, or a home health aide.

College and Adult Years

Much of the intervention needed in the adult population with cerebral palsy is not all that dissimilar from that needed during the adolescent years. If other variables remain equal, physical functioning often remains stable. Certainly, periodic reassessment should be performed, but the focus of therapeutic interactions change as priorities become concerned with obtaining employment and adequate housing. Educational pursuits and career opportunities must be systematically evaluated by the patient and the med-

ical–educational–vocational team. Physical therapists can provide valuable input to these discussions by helping to coordinate the patient's physical needs with the demands of the proposed environment.

Surgical Management

Because of the complexity of the CNS, any single solution will not alleviate the myriad of problems faced by the patient with cerebral palsy. Developmental therapists frequently have a negative attitude toward surgicalintervetion for their patients. They feel that early application of appropriate neurodevelopmental therapy will result in significant developmental and functional gains that preclude the need for surgery. Conversely, orthopaedic surgeons suggest early surgical intervention for those patients who are predisposed to musculoskeletal deformity.[18,19] Soft-tissue release is usually used at an early age, whereas osteotomy may be necessary later in life if a deformity is allowed to progress.

Surgical intervention frequently becomes the treatment of choice in the individual with cerebral

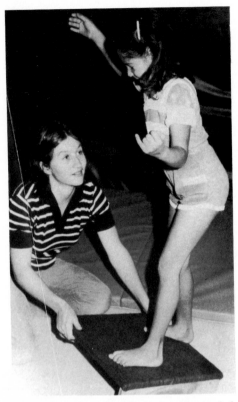

Figure 19-4. Girl aged eight years with spastic left hemiplegia improving equilibrium reaction on a vestibular board. This technique allows the child to improve balance, weight shifting, coordination, and muscle tone.

palsy. Communication between clinicians and orthopaedic surgeons is essential to ensure that treatment goals are understood and integrated into the patient's habilitation program. The physical therapist's evaluative skills can be an important factor in establishing a functional prognosis for a patient after surgery. With the establishment of these parameters, surgical intervention and postoperative rehabilitation succeed.

Preoperative Instruction

Because of postoperative discomfort, patients have difficulty concentrating on and attempting unfamiliar tasks. Successful rehabilitation can be greatly enhanced through preoperative sessions in which the patient is instructed in the remedial measures that will be used in the rehabilitation process. At this time, exercises, assistive devices, and gait patterns, e.g.,

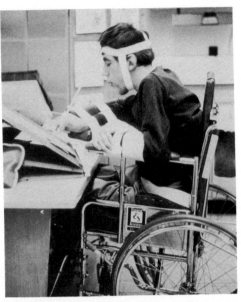

Figure 19-5. Youth aged 18 years with spastic quadriplegia and athetosis uses this customized seating and upper-extremity support system to provide a stable posture and thus allow him to use a head pointer to facilitate his education.

non-weight-bearing, two-point, and four-point, may be taught.

The preoperative evaluation may also be used to allay patient's fears and concerns about surgery. The physical therapist should openly discuss the rationale and components of the rehabilitation process. The importance of postsurgical management should be stressed. Patients and families should thoroughly comprehend their future interactions with the physical therapist.

Postoperative Care

Postoperative rehabilitation may take many forms, depending on the type of surgery, e.g., soft tissue or bone, the location of surgery, and the patient's functional status. It is not the intent of this chapter to provide the specifics of physical therapy interventions for each possible surgical intervention, but, rather, the general guidelines of physical therapy management used in most medical centers.

Foremost in the mind of the physical therapist treating a patient postoperatively should be (1) maintaining the surgical correction and (2) enhancing the functional skills possible as a result of surgery. With appropriate communication between therapist and orthopaedic surgeon before surgery, the goals of the surgery should be apparent to the clinician and allow him or her to develop an appropriate plan of care.

The specifics of physical therapy intervention depend on the goals of the surgery. Soft-tissue surgery is a common procedure particularly in the younger patient, e.g., if adductor tenotomy is used to prevent adduction contracture, the goal of therapy should be to maintain the range of motion provided by the surgical procedure. Range of motion may be active or passive, depending on the patient's capabilities. It is also encumbent on the therapist to ensure that appropriate positioning is used to maintain the surgical correction outside of the therapy sessions. Use of positioning devices varies according to the surgeon involved. Some may use bivalved spica casts; others may use an abductor wedge. In any event, whatever the positioning device, the physical therapist should train staff in appropriate positioning should a situation exist where skilled nursing staff are unavailable.

Should adductor tenotomy be used to alleviate a "scissoring" gait, the goals of therapeutic intervention are twofold: (1) maintaining the surgical correction and (2) developing an improved functional gait pattern. The child who has been ambulating for a prolonged time with a "scissoring" gait will need intensive rehabilitation to develop an improved gait pattern.

Osteotomies usually require prolonged immobilization. During the period of immobilization, attention should be directed to the uninvolved extremities for passive or active exercises. Once sufficient healing has occurred to eliminate the need for immobilization, therapeutic goals depend on the initial intent of the surgery.

The extent of hospitalization will vary according to type of surgery and the patient's condition. After discharge, therapeutic intervention may only occur on a periodic basis, e.g., biweekly or monthly. Progress at home and school is of prime importance at this stage. Family and school personnel should be instructed in those aspects of care that would be appropriate for them to participate in. Positioning becomes an important aspect of care in both the home and school. Family members are frequently reliable in implementing exercise programs as needed. The physical therapist at this stage functions as a monitor for postoperative care and should implement modifications in the treatment plan as the patient's condition warrants. Communication with the orthopaedic surgeon remains of prime importance throughout the rehabilitative process, because it is through physician, therapist, patient, family, and school personnel interaction that success is generated.

Institutional Services

Historically, medical services in residential facilities for mentally retarded persons, especially allied health services such as physical therapy, have been nonexistent or minimal at best. In the last decade, with mandated standards of care through Title XIX of the Social Security Act, the health care professions have been challenged to serve a population that has long been neglected and for which information on treatment is minimal.

Residents of the institutions have varied profiles. Intellectual levels vary from mild to profound mental retardation. Physical characteristics range from absence of any motor dysfunction to total-care major physical disabilities. Age may range from childhood to the geriatric population. Yet with many states developing a community-based residential and program service delivery system and restricting admissions to institutions, institutional populations will be primarily composed of adults in the future.

Physical therapists face a particularly unique challenge with the institutionalized adult with cerebral palsy who may also be mentally retarded. Prolonged institutionalized and inadequate medical services have left many of these individuals with minimal functional skills and major physical disabilities. The effect of muscle tone disorders on maturing musculoskeletal systems, in the absence of treatment, has left many individuals with multiple soft-tissue contractures, spinal deformities, and hip dislocations. Because of the progression of the deformities, many individuals have lost the ability to sit and are relegated to a bed or a stretcher. Some have lost ambulatory skills and are wheelchair-bound. The more severely involved patients may have oral–motor problems that make feeding difficult. Consequently, the nutritional status of these patients is poor, affecting their overall medical condition. Respiratory problems, both acute and chronic, are abundant. Poor pulmonary ventilation due to spinal deformity and overall immobility predispose this population to such problems as recurrent pneumonia, bronchitis, and chronic pulmonary congestion. Aspiration pneumonia is frequent because of the oral–motor difficulties.

The overall magnitude of the problems physical therapists encounter in institutions can be overwhelming. Many therapists might question their ability to improve the situation, yet the physical therapist is an integral part of any treatment regimen for the institutionalized patient with cerebral palsy. The knowledge and skills of a physical therapist, integrated into a total care plan, can have a profound effect on each patient's quality of life.

Service Delivery

Acute care. In developing a physical therapy service delivery system within the institution, one should give priority to providing acute care. Although the problems may be magnified, the medical problems that occur in the institutionalized population are compatible with those of the general public. Of particular interest to the physical therapist are orthopaedic surgeries, fractures, and respiratory problems.

Treatment protocol for acute physical therapy services need not vary from accepted methods. Our experience has shown that occasionally modifications in treatment plans are necessitated by the patient's intellectual level, yet the therapist can meet the established treatment goals with ingenuity. Therapists who are treating patients with behavior problems can use the services of a psychologist in developing the treatment plan. Use of staff, both physical therapy and direct care, familiar to the patient is beneficial to treatment success. We have found it helpful to have a physical therapist develop a working relationship with a patient who has a behavior problem before admission for elective orthopaedic surgery.

Since acute care is a priority, provisions should be made for seven-day coverage if at all possible. This is especially essential for acute respiratory problems, particularly if help from other medical personnel is unavailable, such as nursing and respiratory therapy. A rotating on-call system has proved beneficial for weekend coverage.

Chronic care. The issue of chronic care service delivery can be perplexing. Whom do you treat? What do you do? How much treatment do you give? When do you stop? All the above questions focus on one central theme: direct service. Physical therapists in institutions must remove themselves from the traditional clinical role of providing treatment for a particular problem. The role of the physical therapist in the institution must be an integration of the clinical role into the total spectrum of service delivery for a given patient. Once the physical therapist is able to function in a teaching capacity as well as in the traditional clinical role, profound effects can be generated on basic quality of life issues in this population.

As previously mentioned, the majority of patients seen by physical therapy staff will be adult. In reality, the potential for developmental gains is poor. Yet within their varied functional levels, there is the potential for an improved status. The physical therapist must work to enhance the functional skills that exist in each individual and should begin to think in terms of promoting *experience* rather than just exercise.

Physical therapy services for a chronically disabled population should take a threefold approach: direct service, indirect service, and training. All developmentally disabled patients with cerebral palsy warrant a thorough physical therapy evaluation. Of particular importance in the adult is the functional assessment towards prognosis for functional gains.

1. *Direct Care.* Direct physical therapy intervention in adults is warranted when potential for developmental or functional improvement exists. It is evident from a comprehensive assessment that some patients will not benefit from direct service. For those patients who leave the therapist in doubt, a trial program of three to six months is appropriate to ascertain the efficacy of treatment. Direct treatment should continue for as long as the patient progresses toward established goals. Successful treatment depends on consistent service delivery (five times a week), preferably with a therapist who has developed a working relationship with the patient.

   Physical therapists should be cautioned against providing maintenance services within the institution. Too frequently, excessive maintenance service leads to discrete service delivery by the physical therapist rather than integration into the patient's daily routine. Range of motion can be effectively provided by nursing and direct care staff during periods of bathing and dressing and through proper positioning. Ambulation for its own sake is merely an exercise and can best be managed throughout the day by residential and program area staff. Therapists should scrutinize their service delivery, and therapy that can be effectively accomplished by other staff should be appropriately delegated.

2. *Indirect Care.* Once a patient has been discharged from direct service, the role of the physical therapist continues in an indirect manner. Patients who have acquired functional skills, such as ambulation, transfers, wheelchair propulsion, and other skills should be allowed to use their skills throughout their day. This frequently requires facilitation

of the activity by all staff involved with the patient. It is incumbent on the physical therapist to (1) instruct all concerned in appropriate techniques of skill facilitation and management, including guarding techniques during ambulation, and (2) maintain a monitoring responsibility of the skill until it becomes a routine within the patient's daily life.

3. *Training*. A prime responsibility of the physical therapist within the institutional setting lies in staff training relating to quality basic care. Physical therapists should ensure that all staff involved in the management of patients with cerebral palsy have been trained in appropriate handling and positioning techniques, appropriate feeding interventions for those with oral–motor problems, and appropriate lifting techniques. Training in these areas is best accomplished in the work situation itself. Physical therapy staff should spend time in residential and program areas and serve as models in the training context. Modeling for the staff has proved to be an effective method of training within the institution.

Related Areas

Orthopaedic clinic. The role of the orthopaedic surgeon within the institutional setting is of prime importance.[18,19] Many patients reach a stage whereby progress is precluded by their existing deformities. Surgical intervention is frequently warranted to enhance function and prevent further deformity. The physical therapist plays a key role in successful surgical intervention. The orthopaedic surgeon requires a comprehensive patient profile, including functional status and potential for functional gains, in order to make an accurate decision on any surgical intervention. Because the majority of patients referred to the orthopaedic surgeon have cerebral palsy, the physical therapy department should be the coordinating body for the orthopaedic clinic and the delivery of orthopaedic services.

Adaptive equipment. The use of adaptive equipment is an integral part of a service delivery plan for patients in the institution.[2,17] Customized seating inserts, including total support systems, are a major focus. Positioning devices, such as side-lying and prone standers, are also important.

An institution should allocate resources to develop an adaptive equipment workshop. The workshop should be staffed by individuals with expertise in design and fabrication. Clinical input into the design process is mandatory. Input from an orthotist is required for patients with severe deformities who present with major positioning problems.

Feeding teams. Oral–motor problems are common and may compromise patients' nutritional status. An interdisciplinary approach through an institutional feeding team consisting of physical therapy, occupational therapy, speech therapy, nursing, psychology, and medical staff is an effective means of addressing feeding problems. Comprehensive evaluations, program development, and staff training can be generated through the use of team members appropriate to specific problems. One goal of the feeding team's intervention, for example, is to ensure that appropriate feeding techniques are used three times a day, seven days a week.

Adapted physical education. Adapted physical education is a diversified program of developmental activities, games, perceptual–motor skills, sports, aquatics, and dance. Physical therapists are frequently requested to work with individuals who ambulate independently yet demonstrate delays in motor development, physical fitness, and perceptual motor skills. Adapted physical education instructors (see below) can effectively meet the needs of these individuals. They would be provided with selected modified exercises activities, and skills that are adapted according to individual needs, interests, and capabilities.[9]

REFERENCES

1. Barnes M, Cruthfield C, Geriza C: The Neurophysiological Basis of Patient Treatment, vol. 2. Reflexes in Motor Development. Wheeling, W. Va., Stokesville Publishing, 1978

2. Bergen A: Selected Equipment for Pediatric Rehabilitation, supplement 1., Valhalla, N.Y., Blythedale Children's Hospital, 1975

3. Bobath B, Bobath K: Motor Development in the Different Types of Cerebral Palsy. London, Whitefriars Press, 1975

4. Bower TGR: A Primer of Infant Development. San Francisco, W.H. Freeman and Co., 1977

5. Brazelton TB: Infants and Mothers. New York, Delacorte, 1969

6. Brazelton TB: Toddlers and Parents. New York, Delacorte, 1974

7. Colangelo C, Bergen A, Gottlieb L: A Normal Baby. The Sensory–Motor Process of the First Year. Valhalla, N.Y., Blythedale Children's Hospital, 1976

8. Connor FP, Williamson GG, Siep JM: Program Guide for Infants and Toddlers. New York, Teachers College Press, 1978

9. Curriculum Handbook: Adapted Physical Education Department. Wrentham, Mass., Wrentham State School–Children's Hospital Medical Center, 1980

10. Finnie N: Handling the Young Cerebral Palsied Child at Home (ed 2). New York, Dutton, 1975

11. Illingsworth RS: The Development of the Infant and Young Child: Normal and Abnormal. New York, Churchill Livingstone, 1975

12. Kopp CB: Fine-motor abilities of infants. Dev Med Child Neurol 14:629, 1974

13. Levy J: The Baby Exercise Book for the First Fifteen Months. New York, Random House, 1973

14. The American Orthopaedic Association: Manual of Orthopaedic Surgery. Chicago, The Association, 1979

15. Morris S: in Wiseson JM (ed): Oral Motor Function and Dysfuction in Chldren. Chapel Hill, University of North Carolina Press, 1978

16. Pearson P, Williams C: Physical Therapy Services in the Developmental Disabilities. Springfield, Ill., Charles C Thomas, 1980

17. Robinwelt I: Functional Aids for the Multiply Handicapped. Hagerstown, Harper & Row, 1973

18. Samilson RL (ed): Orthopaedic Aspects of Cerebral Palsy. Philadelphia, Lippincott, 1975

19. Wilson G: Orthopedic Aspects of Developmental Disabilities. Chapel Hill, University of North Carolina Press, 1979

James C. Drennan
James R. Gage

20

Orthotics in Cerebral Palsy

An *orthosis* is an assistive, substitutive, or corrective external device designed to improve the quality of a patient's functioning. Winthrop Phelps was one of the first to develop a system of bracing for cerebral palsy.[10] In this system, bracing was used "to prevent and correct deformities; to control unwanted motions; to assist in training and strengthening wanted motions; and to determine the possible effect of surgery." Considerable advances in the design and use of orthoses have occurred in the ensuing 50 yr. This progress has resulted from the introduction of engineering principles and new materials that permit reduction in the size, weight, and rigidity of orthoses.

Appropriate use of orthotics in neuromuscular disease requires an understanding of both the principles of bracing and the pathophysiology of cerebral palsy.

GENERAL PRINCIPLES IN ORTHOTIC PRESCRIPTION

Orthoses are prescribed to (1) protect a body segment or joint, (2) prevent deformity, (3) provide stability, or (4) enhance function. Failure to recognize that orthoses cannot correct a fixed deformity is the major reason for brace failure. In cerebral palsy, dynamic joint contractures, the necessity for trunk mobility to maintain balance, and the need to use primitive reflexes in ambulation may present relative contraindications to orthotic use.

There is always a functional cost–benefit "trade-off" when an orthosis is prescribed. The major costs are weight, thermal discomfort, bulk, restriction of mobility, cosmesis, and skin irritation. With the introduction of lightweight plastics, the major benefits have been a decrease in weight and bulk as well as improved cosmetic appearance. A polypropylene knee–ankle–foot orthosis (KAFO) worn in a regular shoe demonstrates these advantages (Fig. 20-1). Ankle-joint rigidity can be modified by adjusting the ankle trim line to allow some mobility within a functional range. Since plastics are worn in intimate contact with the skin and are nonporous, skin irritation and thermal discomfort remain as deficits.

Currently, the speciality of orthotics describes an orthosis by the combination of the joints it encompasses.[5] The first initial of each joint is used in the description. Thus, a short leg brace is an ankle–foot orthosis (AFO), whereas a long leg brace with a pelvic band is a hip–knee–ankle–foot orthosis (HKAFO).

PATHOPHYSIOLOGY OF CEREBRAL PALSY

The functional deficits in cerebral palsy that limit or preclude ambulation are

(1) impaired or absent selective control of muscle function, (2) primitive midbrain locomotor patterns that may be only under partial voluntary control,

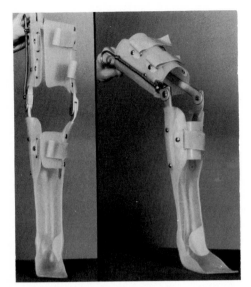

Figure 20-1. KAFO constructed of thermoform plastic offers several advantages over the conventional metal and leather orthoses. It is lightweight, cosmetically more acceptable, and can be worn with a variety of footwear.

(3) primitive reflexes or movements including abnormal stretch reflexes, body position tone, and vestibular tone, (4) dysequilibrium, and (5) sensation or body image deficits.

Classification of Cerebral Palsy for Orthotic Treatment

Hoffer's classification of cerebral palsy is useful in prescribing orthoses (Table 20-1).[6,7] The type of cerebral palsy is determined and then further subclassified by geographic distribution. Once this is accomplished, however, further objective assessment and problem identification are necessary to obtain consistent treatment results.

Types of Cerebral Palsy

Spastic. Spastic cerebral palsy is characterized by increased muscle tone, hyperactive reflexes, and the propensity to develop joint contractures with growth. There is loss of voluntary control of individual muscles. Ambulation is accomplished through a midbrain locomotor center. The gait is characterized by reciprocal mass limb patterning in flexion or extension. Ambulation is further compromised by the

Table 20-1

Simplified Classification of Cerebral Palsy for Orthotic Treatment

Type	Neonatal reflexes
Spastic	Balance reactions
Motion disorder	Tonic neck reflexes
Mixed	*Limb examination*
Geographic distribution	Control
Hemiplegic	Sensation
Diplegic	*Communication*
Total body involve-ment	*Cognition*

(From Hoffer MM: Basic considerations and classifications of cerebral palsy, in Instructional Course Lectures, The American Academy of Orthopaedic Surgeons. St. Louis, CV Mosby, 1976. Reproduced with permission.)

interference of the primitive stretch reflexes, inconsistency of tone (which varies with body position), balance deficiencies, and abnormal sensory feedback.[9] It is thus not surprising that a severely disabled child cannot walk and that no amount of orthotic intervention will enable walking. Inappropriately applied orthoses would do nothing but compound the problem by further restricting mobility and interfering with the gait patterns emanating from the primitive locomotor center.

Motion disorder. Athetosis is characterized by dancelike movements. Damage to the basal ganglia results in abnormal or dystonic muscle tone. These children generally do not develop fixed joint contracture with growth. Positioning in space for nonambulators becomes a major orthotic goal in this group.

Mixed type. Mixed-type cerebral palsy combines spasticity with motion disorders and forms one of the most difficult groups to manage orthotically.

Geographic Distribution

Hemiplegic. Most hemiplegic children will achieve ambulation. Voluntary control of the lower extremity is better than in the upper. All these patients have sensory deprivation on the affected side and show strong hand preference for the normal extremity, even if they retain good voluntary control of the affected limb. An active occupational therapy program to maximize function may be useful in the younger child. We have not found daytime functional bracing of the upper limb helpful in these children. In spastic hemiplegia, however, a night splint that maintains the wrist and hand in a functional position may help prevent progressive growth deformity.

Diplegic. Diplegia is the most common form of cerebral palsy. These patients lack normal selective control in both lower extremities. The upper extremities are minimally involved. In spastic diplegia, ambulation is generally achieved but is delayed. The average age at which walking begins is three and one half years. Specific requirements for nonambulatory and ambulatory patients will be discussed later.

Total body involvement. Patients with total body involvement are totally neurologically involved in all aspects of cerebral function, and their functional goals may be extremely limited. Root has reported that 78 percent of these patients are confined to a wheelchair.[11] Ambulation is thus generally not a realistic goal. It is imperative to prevent fixed deformity so that emphasis can be placed on independent sitting, head control, transfer, and wheelchair mobility.

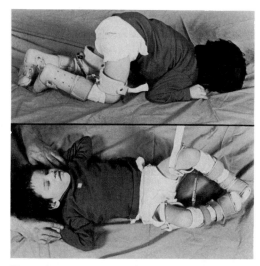

Figure 20-2. A hip abduction bar and bilateral AFOs are well tolerated for prophylactic night splinting of dynamic contractures of the triceps surae and hip adductors in this child with spastic quadriplegia.

SPECIFIC FORMS OF ORTHOTIC MANAGEMENT

Night Splinting

Muscles grow by repetitive stretching as joints are carried through a full range of motion during daily activity. With spasticity, muscle imbalance interferes with this mechanism, and there is a tendency for progressive loss of joint motion during growth. Also, during sleep the more severely involved joints remain in a position of deformity, e.g., the ankle in plantar flexion and the hip in adduction. Night splinting takes advantage of the reduction of tone that occurs during sleep to keep the overactive musculature under mild stretch and to remove stretch from the weaker antagonists.

Children will not sleep "like a clam in a half shell" with full extremity and trunk bracing. The child must be sufficiently unencumbered to allow some mobility in bed. At Newington, we have found that a child will accept a combination of AFOs and hip abduction orthoses provided free flexion and extension of the hips and knees are allowed (Fig. 20-2). A separate knee extension orthosis can be fabricated when an isolated knee flexion contracture requires treatment. When all three joints require night maintenance, alternate night use of the knee orthosis or the combination of AFOs and hip abduction orthoses are used. To ensure compliance, parents must be made aware of the reasons for splinting.

Surgically corrected deformities have a strong tendency to recur in a growing child. Therefore, surgical correction, once obtained, should be maintained with night splinting. We recommend night splinting for growing children with all forms of spastic cerebral palsy who demonstrate progressive deformities. Children with pure athetosis generally do not develop fixed joint contractures, and therefore night splinting is rarely indicated. The amount of spasticity determines whether patients with a mixed type of cerebral palsy would benefit from treatment.

Lower-Extremity Bracing: AFO

Hemiplegic patients develop a dynamic equinovarus that requires orthotic management. Mild cases may be appropriately handled by nighttime use of an AFO, with the patient not using a brace during the day. Night splinting can be discontinued when skeletal growth is complete. Daytime orthotic use may be needed when a child or adult walks with a functional drop foot or to control dynamic varus prepositioning during the swing phase of gait. In addition to providing a better cosmetic gait in adulthood, the AFO may also partially substitute for ankle dorsiflexors during the deceleration phase of gait imme-

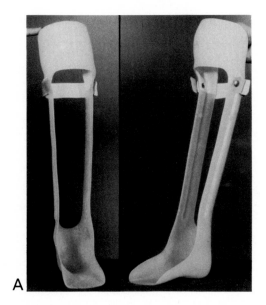

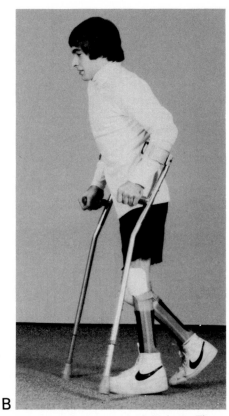

Figure 20-3. (A and B) The Saltiel orthosis uses ground reaction forces to extend the knee. The rigid ankle creates an extension moment, which is transmitted to the knee through the prepatellar pad.

diately following heel-strike to provide shock absorption for the ankle.

AFOs are used in the postoperative management of hindfoot surgery in all forms of spastic cerebral palsy. In spastic diplegia the position of the foot is important in controlling the knee and hip. AFOs may be used to prevent dynamic equinus. Patients with a crouch gait may use an anterior shell or Saltiel-type AFO (Fig. 20-3) to provide an extension moment to the knee.[13] The more rigid the ankle component of the orthosis, the greater the extension moment applied to the knee during the stance phase of gait. The use of the Saltiel AFO is contraindicated in the presence of a fixed knee or hip flexion contracture. Serial casts or surgery may be required to establish the prerequisites of full knee or hip extension.

Daytime orthoses should be prescribed for functional needs or to prevent deformity. The advantage of controlling motion must be weighed against the limitation of either trunk or joint mobility. Long leg

braces with pelvic bands (HKAFOs) generally hamper ambulation in the spastic diplegic patient, since they interfere with the primitive reflex patterns used in gait.[8] Torsional abnormalities, particularly femoral anteversion, are not amenable to orthotic management and may require surgical correction if severe.

Additional Orthotic Requirements

Patients with spastic diplegia generally have poor posterior equilibrium but usually do not require a balance-assisting device.[1] More severely disabled individuals also may be deficient in lateral (side-to-side) balance and thus require an upper-extremity balance assist such as crutches or a walker. Crutches or even a cane may suffice for children with minimal loss of lateral balance. The standard pick-up walker requires momentary independent standing balance. The standard walker with wheels, which requires limited use

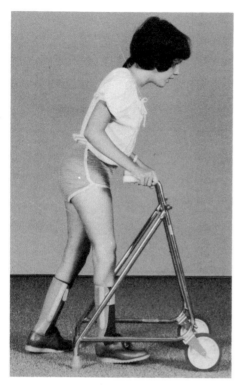

Figure 20-4. This child has adequate strength for ambulation but requires a wheel walker for balance. AFOs are used to protect recent arthrodeses of the subtalar joints and to control dynamic equinus.

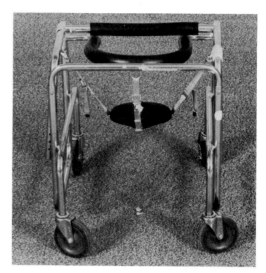

Figure 20-5. A ring walker provides maximum balance assistance for a child with cerebral palsy.

of the upper extremities and trunk for balance substitution, offers slightly more stability to the youngster (Fig. 20-4). The young child with severely deficient lateral balance may require a ring walker (Fig. 20-5).

Sitting Devices

Sitting can be divided into three subclasses: independent, self-propped, and propped. Although independent sitters do not require orthoses for sitting, careful attention should be paid to their wheelchairs. These chairs can be subdivided into two major types: hand driven and power driven. The wheelchair should be specifically ordered for the patient after careful consideration of sitting and mobility needs. Measurements of sitting height and lengths of the thigh, leg, foot, and arm are required. Additional components include armrests, headrest, and footrests (and whether they are to be removable) and special inserts such as abduction wedges and lateral trunk pads to

control position and spinal deformity. Seating cushions may have to be fabricated to prevent pressure sores. Removable hard seats may be necessary to avoid functional pelvic obliquity resulting from hammock seats found in collapsible, portable wheelchairs. The feet should be maintained in a plantigrade position, and footrests should be adjusted to the correct height to allow proper distribution of weight between the buttocks and thighs.

A special chair such as the Mulholland Growth Guidance Chair (Mulholland Associates), the Safety/Travel Chair (Safety Travel Chair Inc.) or the Cushion Lift Travel Chair (Ortho-Kinetics) (Fig. 20-6) is required for the self-propped sitter. Propped patients include those with total body involvement or severe motion disorders. They may require a reclining type of quadriplegic chair with considerable individual modification. Their spinal deformity can usually be controlled by a thoracolumbosacral orthosis (TLSO) (Fig. 20-7). When there is an absence of balance or in the presence of severe extensor thrust, upright positioning can be accomplished by flexing the hips and knees beyond a right angle to reduce extensor tone. This can be combined with the use of a thoracic suspension orthosis (TSO) (Fig. 20-8) to control the position of the trunk in space.[2] Head control often improves once adequate trunk control has been provided. The use of a custom-made headrest or sling can also position the head and neck and thereby be used to reduce tonic neck reflexes.

Special wheelchair-seating devices may have to

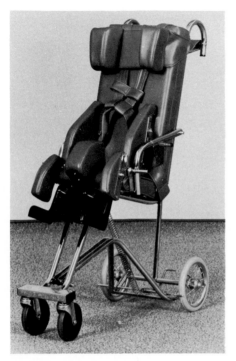

Figure 20-6. Travel chairs, such as the Ortho-Kinetics chair pictured here, are very useful for children severely affected with cerebral palsy. Various combinations of pads are available to support the head and spine or to provide sitting balance. By maintaining the hips and knees in flexion, the extensor thrust can be minimized. When the chair is lowered to its frame, it serves as a car seat so the child can travel in an automobile in the chair.

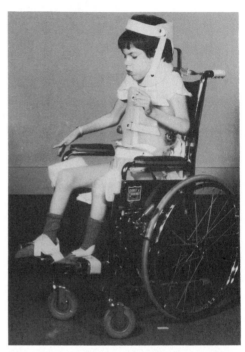

Figure 20-8. A head support and a thoracic suspension orthosis enable this child to sit. Grooved metal dowels attached to the suspension jacket are held in supporting hooks attached to the wheelchair.

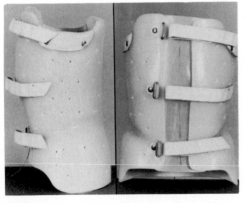

Figure 20-7. TLSO can control spinal deformity while providing trunk support for sitting.

be ordered or fabricated for the child. A unilateral drive chair may be ordered for the patient who has control of only one upper limb, although electric-drive chairs are usually far easier for these children to control. Innovative control devices (Fig. 20-9) have been designed for children and adults who are unable to use the standard joystick. Community activity may require the combination of an electric-drive chair plus a van equipped with hydraulic elevators or ramps.

Transfer Devices

Transfers become increasingly important as the growing child becomes heavier. Inability to transfer taxes the family's capability to maintain the handicapped child in the home. The ability to use a KAFO with a bail-lock or drop-lock knee (Fig. 20-10) may provide sufficient stability to allow assisted transfer and offer physical relief to the parents. Transfer techniques should be practiced before they are actually needed so that both the patient and family are comfortable with their use. Transfer boards and Hoyer lifts (Everest & Jennings) are examples of devices

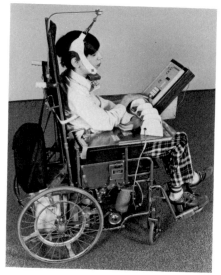

A

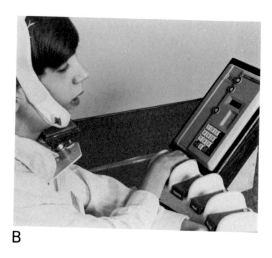

B

Figure 20-9. This child has athetoid cerebral palsy with total body involvement. His intelligence is normal. (A) Mobility is achieved with an electric wheelchair with Stanford slot control switches. This control system was designed for patients who do not have sufficient control of their upper extremities to use a conventional joystick. Five slots are used: forward, backward, right, left, and rest. (B) The child communicates with a computer voice synthesizer by tapping a code into the synthesizer with his chin.

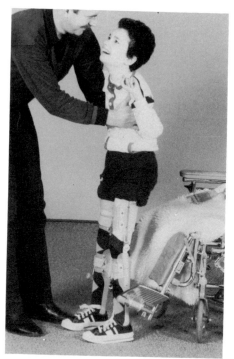

Figure 20-10. This severely handicapped child is able to perform assisted transfers with the aid of polypropylene KAFOs. The knee joints of the orthoses lock automatically in full extension and release easily when the patient is returned to the sitting position.

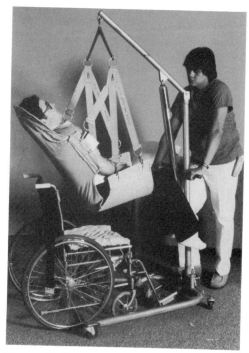

Figure 20-11. A child being transferred to his wheelchair by means of a Hoyer lift.

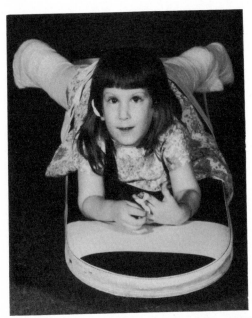

Figure 20-12. A creeper or "bug" enables a child who cannot crawl to have some independent mobility.

that may be required for the severely involved patient (Fig. 20-11).

A young child with sufficient limb control may be able to use a creeper or "bug" (Fig. 20-12) to substitute for crawling. Caster carts or modified walkers also can be used as mobility devices, provided the child has sufficient limb control. Considerable research in bioengineering is presently directed toward providing better mobility devices for the nonambulatory patient. Several federally designated rehabilitative engineering centers are specifically working in this area.

Damping Orthoses

Recent work suggests that purposeful movement lies buried in athetoid movements.[4,12] Present damping devices that permit functional volitional movement are too bulky and cumbersome for practical application.

THE FUTURE

Tremendous strides have been made in orthotics in the past decade. Increased professionalization has resulted in training programs now requiring a bachelor's degree with a strong engineering emphasis. The advent of biomedical engineering and the technologic spillover of space-age engineering advances into orthotics has led to major advances in materials and microcircuitry. Functional electrical stimulation of paretic musculature also holds promise. Peroneal nerve stimulators are already used to control drop-foot posturing in adult hemiplegics. Peripheral pacers of this type may eventually replace some conventional AFOs in cerebral palsy, while feedback devices to substitute partially for missing sensation and proprioception are also well within the practical realm of modern electronics.

The introduction of sophisticated gait laboratories has led to a more precise definition of gait analysis that will assist in decision making. Better definition of the functional problem will decrease the orthotic prescription errors that now occur. Biomechanical analysis of muscle and joint function should result in more functional orthoses. Polycentric knee hinges (Fig. 20-13), which allow the knee joint to move through its functional range without a static instant center of rotation, are just one example.[3] These

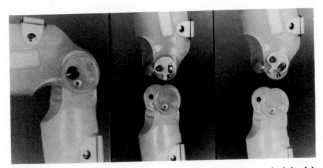

Figure 20-13. Genucentric knee joint. The slotted disk sandwiched between thigh and calf sections permits the instant center of the joint to move through a variety of paths. This allows the joint to follow the path of the individual anatomic knee while providing the necessary support.

innovative joints allow intimate fit, support, and stability of the limb segments through the full range of motion.

Communication is the greatest need for orally handicapped persons. Computer-synthesized speech devices used by patients with communication disorders allow bright minds to establish communication with the world around them. These speech devices should be considered orthoses that replace or augment lost verbal function.

Robots, already used in industry, may soon be used for rehabilitation. Although these programmed machines may not look like mechanical men, they will be functional robots in the sense that under user control they will perform specific tasks that the handicapped person cannot do alone.

It can be seen that the brightest light on the horizon for the person handicapped by cerebral palsy lies in the combined field of orthotics and rehabilitative engineering. The extent of its contribution may challenge the most futuristic dreams of our time.

REFERENCES

1. Bleck EE: Orthopaedic Management of Cerebral Palsy. Philadelphia, Saunders, 1979
2. Drennan JC, Renshaw TS, Curtis BH: The thoracic suspension orthosis. Clin Orthop 139:33, 1979
3. Foster F, Milani J: The genucentric knee orthosis—a new concept. Orthot Pros 33:31, 1979
4. Garrett AL: New concepts in bracing for cerebral palsy. Phys Ther 46:728, 1966
5. Harris EE: A new orthotic terminology. A guide to its use for prescription and fee schedules. Orthot Pros 27:6, 1973
6. Hoffer MM: Basic considerations and classifications of cerebral palsy, in Instructional Course Lectures, The American Academy of Orthopaedic Surgeons, vol. 25. St. Louis, Mosby, 1976, pp 96–106
7. Hoffer MM, Garrett A, Koffman M, et al: New concepts in orthotics for cerebral palsy. Clin Orthop 102:100, 1974
8. Perry J: Kinesiology of lower extremity bracing. Clin Orthop 102:18, 1974
9. Perry J: Pathologic gait, in Atlas of Orthotics: Biomechanical Principles and Application, The American Academy of Orthopaedic Surgeons. St. Louis, Mosby, 1975, pp 144–168
10. Phelps WM: Bracing in the cerebral palsies, in Orthopaedic Appliances Atlas, vol. 1. Ann Arbor, J. W. Edwards, 1952, pp 521–536
11. Root L: The totally involved cerebral palsy patient. Instructional course lectures, the 44th annual meeting, American Academy of Orthopaedic Surgeons, Las Vegas, 1977
12. Rosen M: Technology in the management of cerebral palsy. Presented at the 34th annual meeting of the American Academy for Cerebral Palsy and Developmental Medicine, Boston, 1980
13. Saltiel, J: A one-piece laminated knee locking short leg brace. Orthot Pros 23:69, 1969

Estelle M. Argie

21

Child Life Specialist

A poem by Lewis succinctly expresses the feelings of children who enter the hospital for medical or surgical procedures.

> When the doctors give the shots
> They don't know how it feels
> They say it's not gonna hurt
> Only because it doesn't hurt them.[7]

The issue that arises in the last line may suggest more than the fact that the physician cannot appreciate the child's physical pain. Issues of separation, confinement, discomfort, and, more important, fear of the unknown are embodied in this poem.

When children enter the hospital, they leave behind all that is familiar and predictable, e.g., family, friends, home, and school, and enter an unfamiliar and often frightening environment. They will be required to comply with various expectations, yield to painful and stressful procedures, and be surrounded by unfamiliar faces. Their daily activities such as eating, sleeping, toileting, communication, and schooling may well be altered, and some may possibly be neglected for more important aspects of care.[9,10]

The appreciation of these feelings and reactions have resulted in most children's hospitals allowing unlimited visiting by parents and even allowing parents to sleep over (room in) with their children if possible. More important, the approach to the hospitalized child has been studied, analyzed, and systematized to provide a meaningful intervention program that will convert a potentially negative emotional experience into a positive one. This program has come to be known as child life and education, and the persons who staff these programs are referred to as child life specialists or child life workers.

CHILD LIFE AND EDUCATION

The "Child Life Activity Study Section Position," published by the Association of the Care of Children's Health, has stated that the first essential goal is minimizing stress and anxiety for the child and adolescent.[2] For this reason, the child life specialist is an integral part of each child's hospital stay. Some of the specific activities and intervention techniques as listed by Thompson and Sanford include (1) providing materials and guidance for play, (2) preparing children for hospitalization, surgery, and medical procedures, (3) lending emotional support to parents and siblings, (4) advocating the child's point of view to hospital personnel, and (5) maintaining a receptive environment for children and their families.[13] I would like to add one more item to the list that relates specifically to children with cerebral palsy, i.e., promoting the attainment of each child's potential for growth and development. To these ends, the child life specialist understand both the effects of hospitalization and child development.

Finally, at the center of these activities must be close professional relationships with physicians, on the one hand, and with the patient, on the other, thereby providing the all-important link for the child from the outside world to the world within the hospital. Issues involving timing of surgery, explanations of procedures, preparation for postoperative management, and eventual discharge can then be dealt with appropriately and, if necessary, repetitively to help ensure optimal outcome of the surgical procedure.[5]

PREPARATION AFTER HOSPITALIZATION

Preparation after hospitalization should not merely be seen as a temporal sequence of events; it is a complex ongoing process. Plank has stated that "the age of the child, his personality, and family relationships, his previous medical experiences, and the nature of the impending procedure, all make a difference."[12]

Assessment

Before any intervention is undertaken, a full assessment is required for each child. Additional variables must be considered in children with developmental disabilities or multiple handicaps.[8]

Developmental Level of Function

The assessment of what a child can understand and how he or she can communicate is basic to the determination of how to share information. With disabled children, level of understanding may not correlate with chronologic age and there may be special problems in communication. The system in which the information is shared must therefore be tailored accordingly.

With each hospitalization, each child, developmentally disabled or not, is at a different stage of development. At each stage of development there are new fears and expectations that alter a child's functional level.[14] Anna Freud has stated that "the surgical procedure is interpreted by the child in terms of the level of development. What the experience means to the child does not depend on the type and seriousness of the operation, but on the types and depths of the fantasies aroused by it."[2] Therefore, the child life specialist must assess the child's present behavior and intellectual functioning in order to prepare each child adequately. For example, although adults regard the electroencephalogram (EEG) as a relatively benign and noninvasive procedure, the impact it might have on each child must be carefully considered.

Nature, Effects, and Limitations of Disability

In assessing the child's present level of development and behavior, the child life specialist must also consider behavior before hospitalization and illness, family relationships, prior medical experience, and obvious reactions to hospitalization and procedures. It is also imperative, when assessing developmentally disabled children, that the child life specialist have a working knowledge of the child's disability. This knowledge will enable the specialist to distinguish between the limitations of the disability, the child's stage of development, and the child's reactions to hospitalization.

Kessler emphasizes seven factors in distinguishing the limitations of the disability and its psychologic effects as follows:[6]

1. Age of onset
2. Deprivation of experience
3. Organic effects on intelligence and personality (especially in patients with central nervous system [CNS] deficits)
4. Parental attitudes
5. Traumatic events
6. Effects of treatments prescribed
7. Child's fantasies and self-concept

Consider the following case study.

Jeff, aged 16 yr, has cerebral palsy in both upper and lower extremities and has been confined to a wheelchair for the past several years. He has been admitted to the hospital for orthopaedic surgery. He was placed in a hip spica cast, and the projected outcome of the surgery is *walking*. The preparation surrounding Jeff's surgery was predominantly to define and redefine the outcomes of surgery (walking), maintain his independence and privacy, help him cope with a confining hip spica cast, stabilize his emotional environment during months of hospitalization, and give Jeff the opportunity to have some control over decisions concerning his own body. During his hospitalization, Jeff stated very emphatically: "I'm 16 yr old, and I've had 18 surgeries. I'm not having any more!" It is this kind of communication and trust that the child life specialist strives for. This statement enabled the staff to focus on and work toward the important issues stated above. The seven factors Kessler describes were considered carefully. Jeff's disability from birth, his limited experiences, his difficulties with learning and with a special school, his medical treatments and numerous hospitalizations, and his fantasies about his body and its capabilities were just fragments of the factors that child life specialists address.

Repeated Hospitalization

Repeated hospitalization for surgical procedures is another problem children with cerebral palsy face.

The presence of a child life specialist on the health care team helps to provide continuity and to turn the situation to advantage. The relationship that develops between the patient and the child life specialist becomes diagnostic as well as therapeutic in terms of behavioral and emotional issues concerning hospitalization and surgery.[11]

Procedure

Once an assessment is made and treatment programs are outlined, the child life specialist can begin to present the child with concrete information. To approach the child on his or her own level, one must consider communication skills, interaction with peers and staff, and the child's ability to play. All levels use the following basic techniques:

1. Simple illustrations and statements in concrete terms (Figs. 21-1 and 21-2).
2. A sequential step-by-step approach to surgery and postoperative care emphasizing the procedure (Fig. 21-3), injections, diet, anesthesia, intravenous (IV) fluids, casts (Fig. 21-4), confinement, and postoperative treatment
3. The opportunity, with supervision, to play with medical equipment such as anesthesia masks, hypodermic needles (Fig. 21-5), and IV equipment

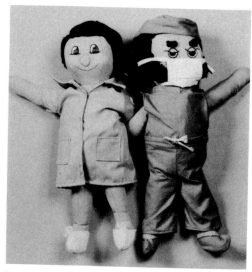

Figure 21-2. Dolls can be useful to demonstrate the dress and appearance of nurses and surgeons, thus reassuring the child.

4. Constant reassurance that all procedures will be explained and that the child life staff will be available to provide support and information

Factors to be considered in applying the basic preparatory techniques are the timing of the proce-

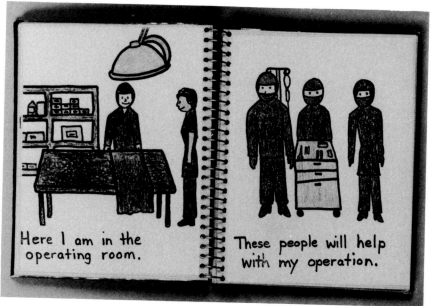

Figure 21-1. Illustration manual demonstrating, in simple terms and drawings, the preparation process for surgery as well as for various radiographic and medical procedures.

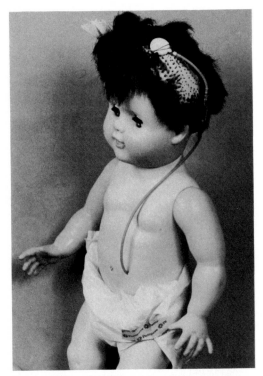

Figure 21-3. Procedures such as ventriculoperitoneal shunts can be simply illustrated with dolls.

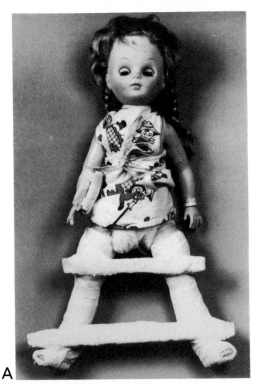

A

Figure 21-4. Various postoperative casts can be demonstrated with dolls. (A) A-frame casts after soft-tissue releases about the hips. (B) One and one half hip spica cast, frequently used after osseous hip procedures. (C) Risser cast after spinal fusion for scoliosis.

dures, other ongoing processes, communication, considering the unexpected, and, finally, the child's fantasies.

Timing

Some children may want to be told only small parts of what will happen ahead of time. Other children may want to be told more than once about surgery; they may be unable to adequately understand because of anxiety, lower intellectual functioning, or both. Retarded children frequently do best if they are given information shortly before the scheduled procedure. It is difficult for them to appreciate time, and information given too early may only confuse them.

Ongoing Process

No matter how many hospitalizations or surgeries the child has had, it is necessary to discuss what will take place this time. The number of medical experiences does not necessarily alleviate fear. The opportunity for questions and expressions of feelings is necessary.[1]

Communication

It is important to involve parents as much as possible. Developmentally disabled children are often very dependent, and sometimes communication occurs solely through the parents. If the parents have a good understanding of upcoming procedures, it can alleviate anxiety; often, they can ask questions the child is unable to ask. The information that is communicated to the child and parents is then communicated to staff. Physicians, nurses, physical therapists, child life specialists, and other pediatric health care providers can reinforce factual data.[3]

The Unexpected

Professionals must be able to explain unavoidable delays or cancellations or why the child cannot

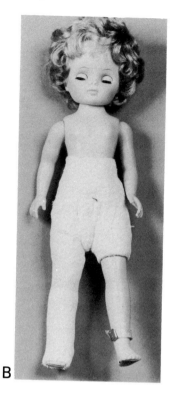

B

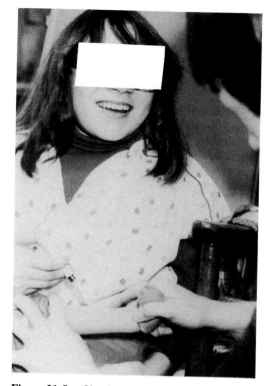

Figure 21-5. Simulated injection with an actual syringe.

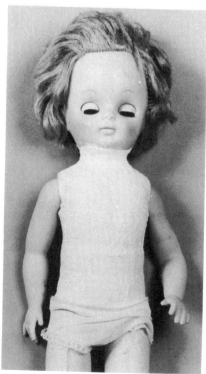

C

eat or drink before a test without alienating the child or increasing anxiety.

Child Fantasies

As Freud has stated, "The child is unable to distinguish between feelings of suffering caused by the disease inside the body and suffering imposed on him from outside for the sake of curing the disease. He has to submit uncomprehendingly, helplessly, and passively to both sets of experiences. . . . Factors of the latter kind . . . may even be the decisive ones in causing the child's psychological breakdown during illness or in determining the aftereffects."[4] This inability to distinguish the cause of suffering is a paramount problem for the developmentally disabled child. Often the outcome of a surgical procedure is a gain in minimal correction or a degree of comfort in positioning rather than an enhanced degree of mobility, but the child's suffering and fantasies may nonetheless be great. These recurrent situations must take priority in the surgical preparation of the developmentally disabled child.

REFERENCES

1. Bullard D: The response of the child to chronic physical disability. J Amer Phys Ther Assoc 48:592–601, 1968
2. Child Life Activity Study Section Position Paper: Association for the Care of Children's Health, 1979
3. Cline K, Rothenberg M: Preparation of a child for major surgery. J Amer Acad Child Psychiat 13:78–94, 1974
4. Freud A: The role of bodily illness in the mental life of children. Psychoanal Study Child 7:69, 1952
5. Geist A: Onset of chronic illness in children and adolescents: psychotherapeutic and consultative intervention. Amer J Orthopsychiatry 49:4–23, 1978
6. Kessler J: The impact of the disability on the child. J Am Phys Ther Assoc 50:153, 1966
7. Lewis N: The needle is like an animal: How Children view injections. Children Today January 1978, pp 18–21
8. Mattsson A: Long term illness in childhood. Pediatrics 50:801–805, 1972
9. O'Connor A: Nursing of children and adolescents. Amer J of Nursing Co New York, N.Y., 1975
10. Petrillo M, Sanger S: Emotional Care of Hospitalized Children. J.B. Lippincott, Philadelphia, 1980
11. Plank E: Working with Children in Hospitals. Case Western Reserve University Press, Cleveland, 1962
12. Plank E: Preparing children for surgery. Ohio State Med J :809, 1963
13. Thompson R, Stanford G: Child Life in Hospitals: Theory and Practice. Springfield, Ill., Charles C. Thomas, 1981
14. Whitt J, Weiss D, Taylor C: Children's conceptions of illness and cognitive development. Clinical Pediatrics 18:327–339, 1979

John W. Shaffer

22

Hand and Upper Extremities

The upper extremities of the child who has cerebral palsy and, in particular, spastic hemiparesis can be improved in appearance and function by a combination of operative and nonoperative techniques. The typical deformity of shoulder internal rotation, elbow flexion, forearm pronation, wrist flexion, finger flexion, and thumb-in-palm deformity produces striking alteration in appearance (Fig. 22-1 and extreme difficulty in using the involved limb as a helper for activities of daily living. It is extremely difficult for the patient to perform basic hand functions of gross grasp and release, pinch, and reach. The abnormalities of hand function and deformities from brain damage are difficult to diagnose in the neonatal period, and a review of the development of hand function in the early years of life will help to emphasize the altered development of the child with cerebral palsy.

PRIMITIVE REFLEXES AND
UPPER EXTREMITY FUNCTION

In the nursery, the characteristic posturing of the newborn upper extremity is just as described above for the child with cerebral palsy. If one attempts to passively extend the limb rapidly, a Moro reflex can be triggered. Arm positioning does not appear to be affected by head positioning in the newborn, however. The asymmetric tonic neck reflex (ATNR) (Fig. 22-2) develops and persists up to six months. When this ATNR persists beyond six months of age, it is abnormal and will be an adverse factor in upper-extremity function. Emphasis must be directed toward keeping the head postured in the midline of the ATNR, thus minimizing reflex activity of the extremities.

A child aged four months can usually hold his head in the midline and appears to develop hand–eye coordination. He can usually get his hand to the mouth. Very often, when placed prone, he can support his trunk with the use of a forearm. Diminution of the tonic labyrinthine reflex (TLR) after six months of age is necessary for stable sitting and is a necessary adjunct to upper-extremity development. In addition, the parachute reaction usually develops shortly after six months of age and remains as a protective response. Just as in the persistence of the ATNR, the failure of the parachute reaction to develop is a poor prognostic sign when evaluating hand function (Fig. 22-3). By 18 mo of age, the child has developed a grasp pattern, and by 2 yr of age, the child can usually grab objects with the fingers rather than with the whole hand.

This very brief overview of some upper-extremity developmental milestones in a normal child is a striking contrast to the findings in the cerebral palsied child. Cerebral palsy results in the preservation of primitive reflex patterns (see Chap. 17) and the delay or absence of developmental milestones. Consequently, these children very often have a total flexion

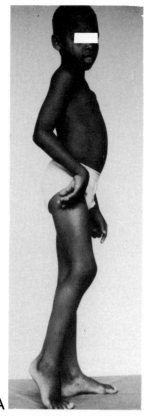 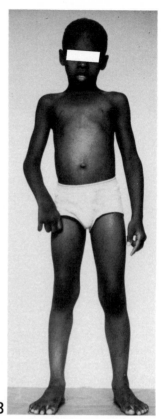

A   B

Figure 22-1. (A) Photograph of a child with a right spastic hemiplegia demonstrating the typical deformity of shoulder adduction and internal rotation, elbow flexion, forearm pronation, wrist flexion, finger flexion, and thumb-in-palm deformity. (B) Front view of child in (A).

pattern in their upper extremity with shoulder internal rotation, elbow flexion, forearm pronation, wrist flexion, finger flexion, and thumb-in-palm deformity.

EVALUATION

The evaluation of the upper extremity requires several examinations and is best done by both an experienced hand surgeon and a hand therapist. The hand therapist has an advantage in that he or she can probably reproduce a play setting for the patient that will permit observation of hand function during activities that the patient enjoys. This complements the examination of the hand surgeon, who assesses joint deformities and contractures, stability, and strength of deforming muscle groups and their antagonists. It is important to identify the dominant pattern, i.e., spasticity, athetosis, or mixed with spasticity domi-

nating. Any consideration of reconstructive surgery should be directed toward those patients with spasticity alone or the mixed pattern with spasticity dominating. The presence of a stretch reflex in those patients who have mixed spasticity and athetosis is a reliable indication that surgical procedures may be considered for improved function. Surgery should not be seriously considered in patients with extrapyramidal disorders with pure athetosis. Very often, joint deformity may change to the opposite deformity in these patients, and the likely outcome after soft-tissue procedures is uncertain.

Evaluation of the upper extremity includes many modalities that permit more accurate assessment of functional deficits and potential surgical treatments. Samilson feels that use of motion pictures, braces, splints, casts, local nerve blocks, electromyography (EMG), detailed hand evaluation with written summaries, and electrical stimulation constitutes a com-

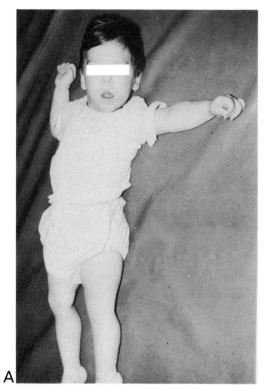 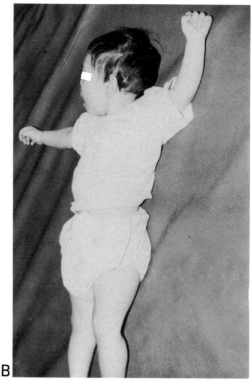

A   B

Figure 22-2. (A) Boy aged nine months with cerebral palsy demonstrating a persistent tonic neck reflex. Impaired hand function can therefore be anticipated during growth, development, and later life. (B) Turning the head to the opposite side results in an obligatory extension of the arm on the ipsilateral side and flexion of the contralateral limb.

plete evaluation; this can then be followed by an accurate treatment plan.[12]

In contrast to photography, which shows the hand posed in different positions of function, serial motion picture recordings demonstrate the hand at rest and with attempted function. One can observe a patient's gross grasp and release, pinch, and reach on film. The patient can be asked to perform simple activities of daily living so that the pattern of crutch walking, wheelchair mobilization and transfer, shoelace tying, and eating can be observed. This permits retrospective analysis as well as prospective analysis if a serious consideration of surgery is entertained.

The judicious use of braces, splints, and casts, especially at night, helps to improve the evaluation of the spastic muscles as well as the very often nonspastic antagonists. Very often a wrist that has a flexion deformity may not have spontaneous wrist extensor function. By applying a wrist extension splint or serial casts to stretch out a wrist flexion contracture, one may subsequently be able to observe spon-

taneous function in the wrist extensors. Several weeks of cast treatment helps to resolve this uncertainty. Similarly, when considering a wrist arthrodesis, it is important not to fuse the wrist when finger flexor and extensor function depends in part on the synergistic action of the wrist. Wrist flexion facilitates finger extension, and wrist extension facilitates finger flexion. This pattern must be recognized; if an immobilized wrist prevents spontaneous finger flexion and extension, in all likelihood arthrodesis would not be recommended. Immobilization is generally preferred when the patient is asleep. If the hand function needed for performance of daytime activities can be preserved without splint or orthosis, patient compliance is often improved. Because of the muscle imbalance at the wrist, however, nonoperative treatment may require that a patient wear a wrist splint for functional activities.

To assist in the evaluation of nonspastic, overstretched, and weak antagonist muscle groups, local anesthetic block of nerves innervating spastic mus-

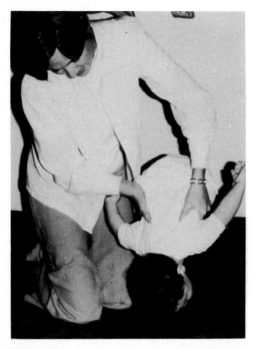

Figure 22-3. When the parachute protective response fails to appear by six months of age, as in this child aged two years, impaired hand function can be anticipated.

culature permits more accurate assessment of non-spastic antagonist muscles. When this is successful, long-acting local anesthetics permit the observation of hand function over a more extended period.

The EMG assessment of the upper extremity has been emphasized but not universally used. Samilson has pointed out that normal muscles are silent at rest and that the cortralateral limb activity does not produce electrical activity in the resting limb.[12] In the child with cerebral palsy, however, continuous electrical activity of spastic muscles is seen even at rest, and the amplitude of electrical activity seems to increase if the contralateral limb moves actively. The use of the EMG to evaluate a muscle activity as a prelude to possible tendon transfer helps to determine whether a potential muscle tendon transfer will be synchronous with the new muscle function that will be required after transfer. This information may make it more likely for the tendon transfer to give a predictable excursion rather than just acting as a tenodesis, as has been seen quite often.

The emergence of hand centers with skilled hand therapists has permitted even better documentation of hand function on serial examinations. Detailed hand-evaluation sheets are completed by the hand therapist, and the findings are available for critical review by the hand surgeon. Differences in findings can be discussed and lead to repeat examination so as to come up with the most accurate assessment of hand dynamics before any decision making regarding possible surgery.

Electrical stimulation may be used to help in diagnosis when muscles appear to be nonfunctional. For example, the overstretched wrist extensors may not appear to be contracting; electrical stimulation, however, may elicit a response. In addition, electrical stimulation may help in teaching a patient to use wrist and finger extensors that very often are under voluntary control. It appears that splints, serial casts, and nerve blocks have been more reliable than electrical stimulation, however.

The muscle examination of the spastic limb requires observation of active motion and palpation of the muscle when assessing contraction. The patient can be asked to pass objects back and forth and can be observed during play activities. Sensory examination usually shows abnormalities in stereognosis, two-point discrimination, and position sense in over 75 percent of patients.[5,15] This is an adverse factor when evaluating functional activities, but with good eye–hand coordination the visual cues can very often substitute for the impaired sensation. Patients can either be blindfolded or have the head turned to the side, and they can be asked to grasp objects of different configurations and consistencies. Identification can be recorded and repeated several times.

Zancolli has described a surgical classification of the spastic hand that will be emphasized here in moderate detail.[17] It includes an extrinsic and intrinsic dominant spasticity. The more common extrinsic dominant spastic hand is represented by the typical forearm pronation—wrist flexion deformity. Extrinsic dominant spasticity can be broken down into three groups, with the grouping dependent on the severity of the flexion contracture of the wrist and finger flexors and the weakness or paralysis of the antagonist extensors. Group I spasticity is mild and is usually localized to the wrist flexors (Fig. 22-4). These patients can usually completely extend their fingers when the wrist is close to neutral position. They lack ability to actively extend beyond the neutral position. Group II spasticity permits fingers to be actively extended but only when the wrist is postured in flexion (Fig. 22-5). This spasticity occurs predominantly in the wrist and fingers flexors. Group II deformities are felt by Zancolli to be ideal for reconstructive surgery. By reducing spasticity, one can accomplish better muscular balance and improve extension of the fingers and wrists. Group II patients are either classified

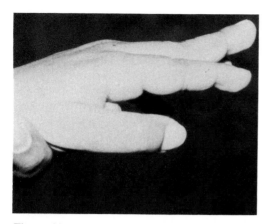

Figure 22-4. Zancolli group I hand. The fingers can usually be extended completely even when the wrist is close to neutral position. However, usually the fingers cannot be extended beyond the neutral position.

as being able to actively extend the wrist, which can be determined by having the patient with a clenched fist actively attempt to extend, or as having wrist extensor weakness. The latter group of patients requires not only reduction of the deforming finger and wrist flexors but also augmentation of the wrist extensors by a tendon transfer. Group III is associated with spasticity of the flexor, pronator musculature, and paralysis of the extensor musculature, and it is so marked that it is not possible to extend the digits actively even when the wrist is held in maximum flexion (Fig. 22-6). These patients are poor surgical candidates for improved function. When surgery is considered, it is purely for cosmetic purposes and to cut down on intertriginous skin irritation.

In Zancolli's intrinsic type of spastic hand deformities, the spasticity is seen in the interosseous and lumbrical muscles. The fingers are postured in the intrinsic position, and the deformity is such that the metacarpal–phalangeal joints are flexed and the interphalangeal joints are extended.

SURGERY

Prerequisites

Reasons for considering surgery include attempts to improve a child's performance in activities of daily living, increase the speed of hand and forearm movement, improve cosmetic appearance, and im-

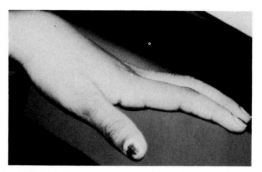

Figure 22-5. Zancolli group II hand. The volar musculature spasticity permits fingers to be actively extended only when the wrist is postured in flexion. This spasticity is predominantly seen in the wrist and finger flexors.

prove personal hygiene. The Intellectual quotient (IQ) is a consideration in evaluating patients for possible surgery. If the IQ is less than 65–70, Mital and Sakellarides emphasize that one cannot count on the patient to be able to cooperate in a postoperative rehabilitation program.[9] Therefore, surgery should be tailored to a program that will not require complicated postoperative therapy. An important goal in a low-IQ patient is improvement in hygiene and the prevention of intertriginous dermatitis and skin macer-

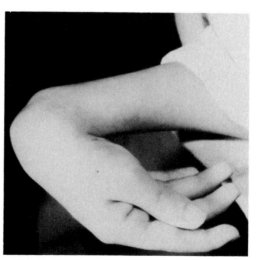

Figure 22-6. Zancolli group III hand. Spasticity is seen in the flexor–pronator musculature and paralysis of the extensor–supinator musculature. The muscle imbalance is so marked that it is not possible to actively extend the digits even when the wrist is held in maximum flexion.

ation. In the child who has an IQ over 65–70, surgery goals can include improved function. Goals of surgery include making the involved limb more of a helper so that it will assist the normal contralateral limb in functional activities. It is unreasonable for the patient, family, and physician to anticipate that the limb will become normal after surgery. It is reasonable to anticipate improved grasp, pinch, release, and reach by appropriately conceived and indicated procedures.

In summary, the prerequisites for surgery should include reasonable expectations, patient motivation, absence of primitive reflexes, voluntary control of the shoulder and elbow for hand placement, and good sensation or at least good visual acuity.

General Principles

Tendon transfers should not be considered in patients who have joint contractures. Most deformities should be evaluated for several weeks before surgery by serial casts or splints to evaluate the functional potential of antagonist musculature. When considering tendon transfers, one should be aware of the capabilities of the potential muscle tendon units for transfer. For example, the brachioradialis and the flexor carpi ulnaris are felt by Boyes to have the greatest work capacity in the forearm; the flexor digitorum sublimis and flexor digitorum profundus, the greatest work capacity in the hand.[1] Weak muscles become weaker when transferred. If tendon transfers are done, the transfers should be anchored into bone when possible. They should also be directed in a straight direction of pull toward their new insertion whenever possible. Tendon transfers should be put in with appropriate tension, which is subjective. Attempts should be made to avoid putting the transfer in too tightly, leading to reverse deformity, or too loosely, leading to inadequate function of the transfer.

Useful comprehensive reviews of surgical techniques and specific operations available for upper-extremity surgery in cerebral palsy have been reported by Goldner, Swanson, Sakellarides, and Samilson.[3,4,9,11,14]

Shoulder and Elbow

For the hand to be functional in grasp, release, and pinch, the patient must be able to place the hand without restriction of movement caused by shoulder and elbow deformity. The typical shoulder deformity is one of adduction and internal rotation. When the patient has a contracture, surgical improvement of the patient's placement potential can be gained by

release of the subscapularis and pectoralis major. This can be accomplished without great difficulty through a deltopectoral approach to the anterior shoulder. The subscapularis can be released at its insertion into the lesser tuberosity, and the pectoralis major can be released by an oblique transection, which will then permit improved passive mobility about the shoulder. For the first four to six weeks after surgery, the extremity can be immobilized with a long-arm cast connected to a plaster pelvic band that maintains the limb in 30 degrees abduction and 20 degrees external rotation. Upon removal of the cast, the patient works with a therapist to regain active mobility of the shoulder, and the therapist performs range-of-motion exercises on the shoulder.

When elbow flexion contracture exceeds 45 degrees, many patients experience difficulty placing the hand in purposeful positions of function. Very often these patients have dynamic flexion deformities that are significantly greater. Mital has documented improved function by a release of the elbow flexion deformity through an anterior incision that crosses the cubital region obliquely.[8] The lacertus fibrosus is released, and the median nerve and brachial artery are identified and protected. The biceps tendon is Z-lengthened, and the aponeurosis of the brachialis muscle is incised. Often a partial brachialis myotomy is necessary, as is anterior elbow-joint capsulotomy. Postoperatively, the extremity is immobilized in extension in a long-arm cast; after four to six weeks of immobilization, the patient begins a therapy program of passive motion performed by the therapist and attempts to regain active elbow flexion as well. After the initial long-arm cast is removed, these patients require several months of night bivalve cast immobilization of the elbow in extension.

Forearm and Wrist

The surgical treatment of the forearm pronation and wrist flexion deformities varies among surgeons. Treatment options for these deformities include stretching by brace or cast during the several weeks before surgery, tendon lengthening, tendon transfer, wrist arthrodesis, and, in the postoperative period, bracing as an adjunct. The preoperative stretching of the spastic wrist flexors is extremely important to permit more efficient assessment of the antagonist extensor musculature. Treatment depends in part on the function of the antagonist extensor muscle group. Nerve blocks, nerve stimulation, and preoperative casts are all intended to permit more accurate assessment of the wrist extensors, which very often are not functioning at the time of initial assessment.

Zancolli varies his treatment depending on the

severity of the deformity.[17] In group I patients, treatment often is not necessary, but if there is mild wrist flexion deformity, he will treat these patients by flexor carpi ulnaris tenotomy and treat the thumb deformity according to techniques mentioned below. Group II patients with functioning wrist extensor musculature can be treated by a release of the volar forearm musculature aponeurosis, flexor carpi ulnaris tenotomy, and treatment of the thumb deformity, if present. Those patients in group II whose wrist extensor musculature are not functioning are treated by a release of the volar forearm musculature aponeurosis and transfer of the flexor carpi ulnaris through the interosseous membrane to the extensor carpi radialis brevis; the thumb deformity is treated when present as necessary. In group III patients whose surgical indications may only be for better cosmesis and to prevent intertriginous dermatitis, Zancolli performs release of the contracted muscle tendon units as necessary to permit passive mobility of the wrist and digits such that extension passively can be accomplished.

In contrast, Sakellarides has had his greatest success in dealing with the wrist and forearm deformities proximally at the muscle origins.[9] In his series, lengthening of the muscle tendon units in the forearm and wrist has led to binding of all tendons into a homogeneous scar. His proximal release may well require dissection into the middle third of the forearm to detach the wrist and finger flexors completely from the ulna in addition to the medial epicondyle. If passive mobility is not accomplished completely, deformities will probably recur.

Sakellarides has also recently published the results of transfer of the insertion of the pronator teres in the management of pronation contractures.[10] The insertion is changed, thus making the pronator teres a supinator and thereby correcting the existing contracture and allowing more functional motion.

Goldner has emphasized tendon lengthening distally of the wrist and finger flexion deformity in conjunction with tendon transfers as necessary.[3] He has favored the use of the extensor carpi ulnaris as an adjunct rather than the sole use of the Green procedure (flexor carpi ulnaris transfer to the extensor carpi radialis brevis).[6] It is felt that the transferred extensor carpi ulnaris becomes more biomechanically efficient when its potential for ulnar deviation is lessened, and it also becomes a more efficient dorsiflexor. In his experience, the flexor carpi ulnaris is often spastic, and therefore results of this transfer may be harder to predict. Often there is a problem of phase shift with the flexor carpi ulnaris; by making it a spastic wrist extensor, the transfer does not function actively.

When there is no active wrist extensor transfer

available, passive realignment of the wrist by fusion into the function position may be considered if the finger flexors and extensors are under voluntary control. If the patient can grasp and release with the wrist in a fixed position, both function and appearance will be improved. Any consideration of wrist arthrodesis should be preceded by a trial of short-arm cast and the observation of active finger flexion and extension. If finger mobility depends on the synergistic action of the wrist, such that finger flexion is assisted by wrist extension and finger extension is assisted by wrist flexion, one cannot improve function in these patients by wrist arthrodesis.

Fingers

Finger flexion deformity may well occur in association with wrist flexion deformity. Treatment includes preoperative splinting to permit more accurate assessment of antagonist extensor muscle function, proximal release of the common flexor origin from the medial epicondyle and the proximal ulna, lengthening of individual muscle tendon units in the forearm and wrist, and occasionally tendon transfers.[3,4,16] Postoperative bracing is used as an adjunct to treatment for an extended period, especially at night. During the day the hand is left free for exercise and functional activities. For improved finger extension, Goldner has used the extensor carpi radialis longus, the flexor carpi ulnaris, the extensor carpi ulnaris, and the brachioradialis as tendon transfers in selected patients.[3] These tendon transfers are usually performed along with lengthening of the spastic flexor digitorum sublimis to the fingers when voluntary strong finger extension has not been demonstrated after a prolonged preoperative period of splinting. Active excursion of tendon transfers to the finger extensors is facilitated by the synergistic action of the wrist flexion.

A fairly common finger deformity is the hyperextension deformity of the proximal interphalangeal (PIP) joints of the fingers. This swan neck deformity is felt to be due to overaction of the extensor digitorum. It can be best demonstrated by passively flexing the wrist, which will accentuate the hyperextension deformity of the PIP joint. To even further emphasize the deformity, passively flex the wrist and the metacarpal–phalangeal joints and note the increasing hyperextension deformity of the PIP joints in digits manifesting the swan neck deformity. Mild deformities improve with correction of the wrist flexion contracture; more severe deformities improve after surgical treatment of the wrist flexion deformity. In addition, Swanson's technique of tenodesis of the flexor digitorum sublimis to the middle phalanx with the proximal interphalangeal joint secured at 20–40 degrees flexion works quite well to eliminate the swan neck deformity.[14] Additional treatments include a proximal volar plate advancement at the proximal interphalangeal joint and intrinsic release.

Thumb

Thumb-in-palm deformity can be treated by several surgical options, including thumb intrinsic muscle origin release, capsulorraphy of the metacarpal–phalangeal joint of the thumb, metacarpal–phalangeal joint arthrodesis, and tendon transfers. Mital and Sakellarides have classified thumb deformities into four types.[9] Type I thumb deformities are caused by a weak or paralyzed extensor pollicis longus. The metacarpal–phalangeal joint may be unstable. Type II thumb deformities are caused by spastic or contracted adductor pollicis, abductor pollicis brevis, and flexor pollicis brevis muscles. Type III thumb deformities are caused by a weak or paralyzed abductor pollicis longus. The carpal–metacarpal joint may well be subluxed. Type IV thumb deformities are caused by flexor pollicis longus spasticity with or without contracture. Treatment varies with each group. In Type I, if the metacarpal–phalangeal joint is stable, the extensor pollicis longus can be rerouted to the radial side of Lister's tubercle. If it is very weak, its function can be augmented by a motor that can include the palmaris longus, flexor carpi radialis, flexor carpi ulnaris, or extensor carpi ulnaris. If the metacarpal–phalangeal joint is unstable and the patient is over 13 yr of age, arthrodesis can be performed without concern about the epiphysis. With appropriate surgical care, arthrodesis can be performed in the patient under 13 yr and the epiphysis can remain open. As an alternative to a metacarpal–phalangeal joint arthrodesis in the patient under 13, some have advocated plication of the volar capsule for improved thumb stability.[2]

Type II thumb deformities can be treated by the appropriate release of the contracted muscle, with most favoring the release being done at the muscle origin.[7,13] In type III thumb deformities, if the abductor pollicis longus is weak, this can be plicated for improved mechanical advantage. If the abductor pollicus longus is paralyzed, its function can be augmented by transfer of an appropriate motor including the palmaris longus, flexor carpi radialis, or brachioradialis. For carpal–metacarpal joint instability, one may well require capsular reefing. In type IV thumb deformities, the flexor pollicis longus can be lengthened. In all patients, postoperative immobilization is

accomplished by four to six weeks of immobilization in a thumb spica cast or a bulky dressing with appropriate splinting. After removal of the cast, rehabilitation (which includes mobilization of the stiff joints), training of appropriate tendon transfers, and strengthening of the lengthened muscle tendon units is accomplished by a program supervised by the hand therapist.

Results

Green and Banks described a functional rating system to evaluate their patients who underwent the Green transfer of the flexor carpi ulnaris to the extensor carpi radialis brevis.[6] This rating system has been applied to all surgical results in children with cerebral palsy. The goal is not to produce a normal extremity, but to produce an improved extremity for more efficient helping-hand activities. Poor results are seen in patients who have retained an absent grasp and relase, poor control, and the use of the hand only as a paperweight. Fair results are seen when the hand functions as a helper but without effectual use in dressing and when only moderate grasp and release and only fair control are demonstrated. Good results are seen when the hand assists in dressing and eating with effective grasp and release and good control. Excellent results are seen when the hand is active in dressing, eating, and general activities with effective grasp and release and excellent control. Samilson and Morris refined the rating system to evaluate 128 operative procedures that were performed on the upper limbs of 40 patients from 1937–1963.[15] In evaluating results, they emphasized function, which included grasp, release, thumb pinch, and wrist extension. They also emphasized cosmetic effect, which included the absence of contractures of the wrist, fingers, elbow, and forearm. They emphasized environmental use, which included the use of the treated extremity for eating, the ability to tie shoelaces, the use of the hand to move a wheelchair or to walk with a crutch or to lift heavy objects, and the patient's overall satisfaction. Using the classification described above before surgery, 31 patients rated poor, 12 rated fair, and 3 rated good. After operation, 11 rated poor, 13 rated fair, 10 rated good, and 11 rated excellent. These authors were encouraged by the improved function and favorable results of their surgical endeavor in dealing with the spastic upper extremity. The hand did not regain normal function but was improved in function as a helper. In general, patients were extremely happy with the results.

REFERENCES

1. Boyes JH: Selection of a donor muscle for tendon transfer. J Hosp Joint Dis 23:1, 1962
2. Filler BC, Stark HH, Boyes JH: Capsulodesis of the metacarpo–phalangeal joint of the thumb in children with cerebral palsy. J Bone Joint Surg 58A:667, 1976
3. Goldner JL: The upper extremity in cerebral palsy, in Samilson RL (ed): Orthopaedic Aspects of Cerebral Palsy. Philadelphia, Lippincott, 1975
4. Goldner JL: Upper extremity surgical procedures for patients with cerebral palsy, in American Academy of Orthopaedic Surgeons Instructional Course Lectures, vol. 28. St. Louis, Mosby, 1979, p 37
5. Goldner JL, Ferlic DC: Sensory status of the hand as related to reconstructive surgery of the upper extremity in cerebral palsy. Clin Orthop 47:87, 1966
6. Green WT, Banks HH: Flexor Carpi Ulnaris Transplant and Its Use in Cerebral Palsy. J Bone Joint Surg 44A:1343, 1962
7. Matev I: Surgical treatment of spastic "thumb-in-palm" deformity. J Bone Joint Surg 47A:274, 1963
8. Mital MA: Lengthening of the elbow flexors in cerebral palsy. J Bone Joint Surg 61A:515, 1979
9. Mital MA, Sakellarides HT: Surgery of the upper extremity in the retarded individual with spastic cerebral palsy. Orthop Clin North Am 12:127, 1981
10. Sakellarides HT, Mital MA, Lenzi WD: Treatment of pronation contractures of the forearm in cerebral palsy by changing the insertion of the pronator radii teres. J Bone Joint Surg 63A:645, 1981
11. Samilson RL, Morris JM: Surgical improvement of the cerebral-palsied upper limb. J Bone Joint Surg 46A:1203, 1964
12. Samilson RL: Principles of assessment of the upper limb in cerebral palsy. Clin Orthop 47:105, 1966
13. Silver CM, Simon SD, Litchman HM, et al: Surgical correction of spastic thumb-in-palm deformity. Dev Med Child Neurol 18:632, 1976
14. Swanson AB: Surgery of the hand in cerebral palsy, in Flynn JE (ed): Hand Surgery (ed 2). Baltimore, Williams & Wilkins, 1975
15. Tachdjian MO, Minear WL: Sensory disturbances in the hands of children with cerebral palsy. J Bone Joint Surg 40A:85, 1958
16. White WF: Flexor muscle slide in the spastic hand. The Max Page operation. J Bone Joint Surg 54B:453, 1972
17. Zancolli EA: Structural and Dynamic Basis of Hand Surgery (ed 2). Philadelphia, Lippincott, 1979

George H. Thompson

23

Hip and Knee Deformities

Muscle imbalance and spasticity in the lower extremities in cerebral palsy can have a profound effect on gait, balance, and the ability to sit. This imbalance can eventually result in soft-tissue contractures, which further impair musculoskeletal function and ultimately produce secondary osseous changes that require extensive surgery for correction. There is a close interrelationship between hip and knee disorders in spastic cerebral palsy, and the assessment and management of these joints is considered together.

HIP DISORDERS

Muscle imbalance, soft-tissue contractures, and osseous deformities adversely affect hip function and can result in spastic subluxation and dislocation with resultant painful, degenerative osteoarthritis that can preclude ambulation and even impair the ability to sit comfortably. Since these changes are progressive, they can be altered or reversed by awareness of potential hip-at-risk factors and appropriate early surgical intervention. Treatment of spastic hip disorders is therefore directed foremost at prevention of contractures that can produce the secondary osseous changes in the proximal femur and acetabulum.[25,28,32]

Assessment of Hip Function in Cerebral Palsy

Evaluation of hip function in spastic children is difficult and must be repeated on several occasions before accurate assessment of the range of motion and the extent of impairment can be made. Unfamiliar surroundings, anxiety, fatigue, and other factors can produce significant alterations in spasticity, and repeated clinical examination is therefore necessary. The methods of assessment include physical examination, gait analysis including movies, dynamic electromyography (EMG), and roentgenographic studies.

Physical Examination

The range of motion of the hips and knees must be carefully measured and recorded and compared serially. The best motion recorded is regarded as the functioning level. Evaluation for contractures of individual muscles must be performed, with particular attention directed at the adductors, iliopsoas, rectus femoris, and medial hamstrings, since these are the muscles or muscle groups most commonly involved in spastic hip deformities.

Gait Analysis

Children with cerebral palsy who ambulate, regardless of the need for orthoses or external support, frequently show a crouched, scissoring type of gait. This is primarily due to muscle imbalance about the hip with secondary muscle imbalance about the knee and ankle. Spasticity of the hip flexors, adductors, and internal rotators (medial hamstrings) overpowers their antagonists, resulting in the abnormal gait. This imbalance can be even more pronounced in severely retarded nonambulatory patients and can eventually result in an early spastic dislocation.

Gait movies give an accurate method of assessing gait preoperatively and postoperatively and can be useful in periodic documentation of the child's neuromuscular development.

231

Dynamic EMG

Bleck has performed dynamic EMG analysis on the major muscle groups of the hip during the gait cycle both in normal children and in those with spastic diplegia.[6–8] He found three types of muscle responses in cerebral palsy: (1) dysphasic, in which the muscle is active out of phase, (2) prolonged phasic contractions, and (3) phasic contractions with exaggerated normal intermittent muscle activity during the gait cycle.

Adductors. The hip adductors, primarily the adductor longus and gracilis, in spastic cerebral palsy tend to be dysphasic and thus active during the swing phase of gait, producing the scissoring of the lower extremities commonly seen during ambulation.

Abductors. The gluteus medius was found to contract phasically but with activity prolonged beyond normal. This contributes to some of the internal rotation of the lower extremities as well as trunk sway due to the loss of pelvic and trunk stability.

Flexors. The iliopsoas muscle, the major hip flexor, was found to be phasic in some children and dysphasic in others. The rectus femoris, however, was consistently dysphasic and contracted concomitantly with the vastus muscle groups.

Perry and associates have evaluated children with spastic hip deformities both preoperatively and postoperatively.[24] They found that gait analysis with EMG telemetry gave the most accurate assessment when planning operative procedures. Static EMG performed during stretch tests was less helpful. Chong and associates made similar observations in their assessment of the mechanics of the internal rotation gait in cerebral palsy.[11]

Radiographic Assessment

Every child with spastic cerebral palsy should have periodic radiographs taken of the hips, since the development of secondary osseous changes, especially acetabular dysplasia and subluxation, cannot always be determined by physical examination. An anteroposterior radiograph with the patella pointing forward and a Lauenstein (frog) lateral radiograph are used for routine assessment. The direct lateral and the abduction–internal rotation radiographs can be useful when evaluating femoral anteversion or internal femoral torsion and coxa valga.

Pathogenesis of Hip Deformity and Dislocation

Incidence

The incidence of spastic dislocation of the hip is affected by several factors: the extent of the neurologic lesion, the patient's ambulatory status, the presence or absence of pelvic obliquity, the severity of spasticity, and the magnitude of contractures of the hip muscles, especially the adductors and iliopsoas. Ambulatory or less severely disabled children have an incidence of dislocation of approximately 4 percent, while in the more severely disabled nonambulatory child the incidence is approximately 25 percent.[25] The average age of dislocation is 7 yr, but the range can vary from 2–10 yr. Beals documented that age and duration of ambulation were more important factors in the development of osseous changes than the severity of the cerebral lesion alone.[3]

Contributing Factors

It is important that pediatric health care providers involved in the care of children with cerebral palsy be aware of the sequential events in the pathogenesis of spastic dislocation of the hip (Fig. 23-1).

Since most children who develop spastic cerebral palsy had normal intrauterine growth and development, it is reasonable to assume that their hips were relatively normal at birth. As the initial flaccidity resolves, spasticity and muscle imbalance ensue, with the hip flexors and adductors overpowering the extensor and abductor muscles. Untreated muscle imbalance eventually results in soft-tissue contractures and an alteration in hip biomechanics. The presence of hip flexion and adductor imbalance produces a change in the axis of hip rotation from the center of the femoral head to the lesser trochanter. Hip motion thus changes to an anteromedial-to-posterolateral direction around this abnormal lower axis of rotation.[13,25] The femoral head becomes progressively uncovered as the hip capsule and ligamentum teres stretch, and pressure erosion occurs along the superior and posterolateral aspects of the acetabulum from the excessive compressive force exerted in these areas, resulting in acetabular dysplasia and subluxation.

Secondary changes also occur in the proximal femur as a result of contractures and the shift in the hip axis of rotation. Femoral anteversion or, more appropriately, internal femoral torsion and coxa valga occur or are allowed to persist, since the abnormal forces prevent spontaneous resolution of the normal physiologic femoral torsion and coxa valga that would

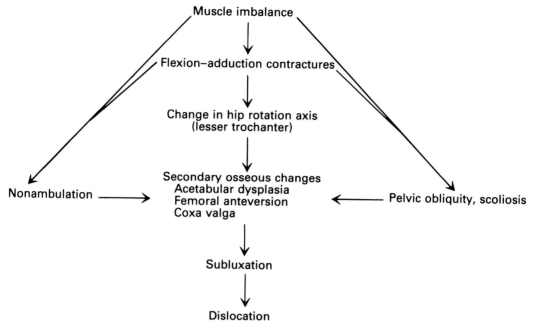

Figure 23-1. Pathogenesis of spastic hip deformities and dislocation. (Modified from Drummond DS, Rogala EJ, Cruess R, et al: The paralytic hip and pelvic obliquity in cerebral palsy and myelomeningocele, in American Academy of Orthopaedic Surgeons Instructional Course Lectures, vol. 28. St. Louis, Mosby, 1979, pp 7–36.)

occur in an otherwise normal child.[3] Lamb and Pollock and Baker and associates also feel that weakness in the hip abductors (gluteus medius) can cause progression of coxa valga by lack of appropriate greater trochanteric apophyseal stimulation.[1,20] Jones, however, feels that adductor spasm and contractures are responsible for progressive valgus.[19] Whatever the precise mechanism of coxa valga, the combination of muscle imbalance, contractures, and abnormal hip axis and the secondary osseous deformities of acetabular dysplasia, femoral torsion, and coxa valga all result in a noncontrentric reduction of the hip and deficient stimulation to provide for adequate growth and development of the hip joint. If the subluxation progresses, a spastic hip dislocation can occur. Dislocations are either posterosuperior or posterior depending on tbe magnitude of the flexion deformity. Adduction contractures alone are usually not sufficient to produce a spastic dislocation.

Relationship with Pelvic Obliquity and Scoliosis

Coexistent pelvic obliquity increases the portion of the femoral head that is uncovered on the elevated or high side of the pelvis, and this enhances the development of acetabular dysplasia and potential instability. Pelvic obliquity thus can be a major factor in the development of a dislocation. Obliquity can be produced by muscle imbalance and contractures above (spinopelvic) or below (femoropelvic) the pelvis. Scoliosis or spinopelvic factors are the major cause of a fixed oblique pelvis. Treatment of the scoliosis and associated pelvic obliquity must be undertaken before considering treatment of the hip deformities, since otherwise the deformity will recur or worsen, and dislocation again becomes a possibility. Conversely, pelvic obliquity secondary to femoropelvic contractures can produce a compensatory scoliosis that may later become a structural spinal deformity.

The incidence of scoliosis and pelvic obliquity tends to parallel the incidence of spastic dislocation in children with cerebral palsy, since they have a cause-and-effect relationship. Scoliosis is found in approximately 7 percent of ambulatory children with spastic cerebral palsy and in 35 percent of children who are not ambulatory.[13] Careful clinical examination of the spine is required in the routine evaluation of a disabled child.

*Natural History of Spastic Dislocation of
the Hip*

Moreau and associates recently evaluated 88 institutionalized adult cerebral palsy patients to determine the incidence and natural history of untreated spastic dislocations.[23] They found that 24 percent of the hips were dislocated, 10 percent subluxated, and 13 percent dysplastic. Half the patients with dislocated or subluxated hips had significant pain. The presence of pain was noted to be more frequent in patients with moderate intellectual function and when athetosis coexisted with spasticity. The more severely disabled, mentally retarded, nonambulatory patients had a lower incidence of pain. They concluded that every effort should be made to prevent spastic dislocations or subluxations but that extensive procedures to relocate and stabilize existing dislocations be reserved for those children with enough neurologic maturity and intelligence to benefit from the surgery and who otherwise would be predisposed to precarious sitting balance and painful hips as adults.

Since pain associated with degenerative osteoarthritis is the major sequel of severe contractures, subluxation, or dislocation, any child demonstrating pain during a routine hip examination, no matter how retarded or spastic he or she may be, should be considered a candidate for surgery. Hoffer and associates have documented relief of pain, better sitting balance, and improved perineal care after soft-tissue releases supplemented, on occasions, with osseous procedures.[17]

Prevention of Spastic Hip
Deformities and Dislocation

Clinical and radiographic hip-at-risk factors exist that allow physicians to recognize those hips developing secondary osseous deformities that have the potential for a spastic dislocation.[25,28,32] These factors are (1) hip abduction less than 45 degrees on each side, (2) hip flexion contractures greater than 20 degrees, especially when occurring in combination with limited hip abduction, (3) uncoverage of one third or more of the femoral head, (4) a break in Shenton's line, and (5) pelvic obliquity.

Sharrard and associates compared the clinical and radiographic findings of hips in children with cerebral palsy who were managed conservatively (physical therapy and orthoses) and those in whom soft-tissue surgical procedures (open adductor myotomy and occasional iliopsoas release) were performed to correct the adduction and flexion deform-

ities.[28] In the conservative group, 11 percent of the hips were dislocated, 28 percent were subluxated, 46 percent were dysplastic, and only 15 percent were normal. In the surgical group, no hips were dislocated, 13 percent were subluxated, 35 percent were dysplastic, and 52 percent were normal. These results emphasize that the pathogenesis of spastic hip deformities can be significantly altered and the incidence of dislocation minimized or eliminated by being cognizant of hip-at-risk factors and the importance of early treatment. Thompson and Rang recently emphasized the preventive aspect of spastic dislocation and have a poster (Fig. 23-2) available for use in outpatient clinics to serve as a constant reminder to be alert for risk factors, especially limited hip abduction.[33]

Treatment

Treatment of spastic hip deformities is primarily surgical. Bleck has stated there are no objective reports that correction of spastic hip flexion, adduction, or internal rotation deformities can be achieved by physiotherapeutic or orthotic methods.[8] These latter methods are beneficial in the prevention of recurrent deformities after corrective surgery, however. Conservative treatment is therefore recognition of the hip-at-risk factors and appropriate early surgical intervention using soft-tissue release to prevent the ultimate sequelae of spastic dislocation.

Hip Adduction Deformities

Limitation of hip abduction to less than 45 degrees on each side has been shown to be a major hip-at-risk factor.[28] Treatment is indicated in any child despite age, intelligence, or ambulatory potential. Current methods include percutaneous tenotomy of the adductor longus and gracilis tendons at their origin, open adductor myotomy with or without a neurectomy of the anterior branch of the obturator nerve, and transfer of the origins of the adductor longus and gracilis to the ischial tuberosity.[2,12,13,15,26,28,29,31]

Personal experience with both the percutaneous adductor tenotomy and the open adductor myotomy with a neurectomy of the anterior branch of the obturator nerve has shown very little difference in long-term results. As a consequence, the percutaneous technique is preferred, since it is safe, simple, and has negligible complications. The hips are maintained in 90 degrees of abduction for 2 wk postoperatively in an A-frame plaster cast (long-leg casts with double cross bars). One week postoperatively the casts are bivalved, and passive range-of-motion exercises are instituted. Ambulation is resumed 2 weeks later, but nighttime splinting in the bivalved casts is continued for 3 to 4 months.

Other authors feel that the remaining medial hamstrings (the semitendinosus and semimembranosus) in addition to the gracilis contribute to hip adduction deformities and that lengthening of these muscles at the knee should be performed simultaneously in severe cases.[1,16] This was confirmed by Perry and associates when they performed dynamic EMG analysis on patients with adduction contractures.[24]

Root and Spero has recently compared the results of hip adductor transfer to adductor tenotomy with and without anterior branch obturator neurectomy and reports improved functional class, pelvic stability, gait, sitting balance, radiographic appearance, and a decreased hip flexion contracture with the transfer.[26] There was a significant increase in postoperative complications, however, as 22 percent of patients had wound drainage. I have limited experience with this procedure at this time and recommend a cautious approach, since it is a technically a more difficult procedure with a high complication rate.

Flexion Deformities

Careful attention to the presence of hip flexion contractures must be made when performing release of existing adduction deformities. It has been shown by Samilson et al. and Sharrard et al. that release of the adductors alone is insufficient in preventing progression of osseous changes when a significant hip flexion contracture is present.[27,28] Flexion contractures greater than 20 degrees as measured either by the Thomas test or by the prone extension test described by Staheli require surgical intervention if concommitant adduction contractures are present.[30] The iliopsoas is the single major cause of hip flexion deformities and is also a major contributor to the development of internal femoral torsion or anteversion, coxa valga, and acetabular dysplasia. Because it exerts an external rotation force, it causes the head of the femur to face anteriorly while the adductors and medial hamstrings inwardly rotate the distal femur. These forces do not allow a concentric reduction of the head of the femur into the acetabulum; therefore, the normal stimulation for growth and development is deficient, resulting in a predisposition to the secondary osseous deformities.

Procedures to correct hip-flexion deformities include iliopsoas recession, lengthening, and tenotomy at the level of the hip joint.[4,5] The preferred technique

EVERY CHILD WITH RETARDATION OR CEREBRAL PALSY SHOULD HAVE A HIP EXAMINATION

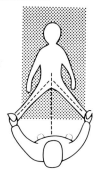

1. LAY THE CHILD DOWN.
2. ABDUCT HIPS WITH HIPS AND KNEES EXTENDED.
3. IF EACH HIP DOES NOT ABDUCT 45 (90 COMBINED) THE HIPS ARE TIGHT.
4. AN X-RAY AND ORTHOPEDIC CONSULTATION ARE REQUIRED.
5. TIGHT HIPS ALWAYS LEAD TO DISLOCATION AND SCOLIOSIS, DIFFICULT NURSING AND POOR SITTING.

DISLOCATED HIPS AND SCOLIOSIS ARE PREVENTABLE

Produced by the P.S.I. Foundation and the Hospital for Sick Children Toronto

Figure 23-2. Poster indicating the importance of the hip examination and limited hip abduction in children with cerebral palsy. (Courtesy of The Hospital for Sick Children and Ontario Crippled Children's Centre, Orthopaedic Division, Toronto, Ontario.)

at Cleveland Metropolitan General Hospital, Cleveland, Ohio, is the intrapelvic iliopsoas recession coupled either with the percutaneous adductor tenotomy when indicated. The intrapelvic recession is favored because of the ease of accessibility to the iliopsoas tendon, the cosmetic aspects of the incision, and the effectiveness of the procedure itself, since it maintains the iliopsoas in continuity. A Z-lengthening of the distal iliopsoas tendon is difficult, and tenotomy with suturing of the proximal segment of the tendon to the hip capsule has not seemed logical or warranted. Postoperatively, patients are maintained in the A-frame, long-leg plaster cast with double bars between them, thus maintaining 90 degrees of hip abduction. Lying prone is encouraged as soon as the patient is comfortable enough to stretch the iliopsoas further. Long-term results have shown good correction of the deformities with minimal tendency for recurrence. The accentuated lumbar lordosis typical in the preoperative period is usually completely corrected. During the first six months postoperatively the patients may show weakness of hip-flexion power of approximately one grade less than their preoperative state. At 6–12 mo postoperatively, however, the hip-flexion power is usually normal.

The rectus femoris can also be a source of significant hip-flexion deformity. Dynamic EMG analysis is occasionally necessary in distinguishing between the iliopsoas and the rectus femoris as a cause of deformity. When treatment is necessary, a release of both the direct and reflected origins is usually sufficient to provide adequate correction. If the tenotomy of the rectus femoris muscle is the only procedure performed, no postoperative casting is necessary and ambulation can be started when the patient is comfortable.

Spastic Subluxation

Management of spastic subluxation of the hip is usually age dependent. The first priority, despite the patient's age, is correction of any existing pelvic obliquity and restoration of muscle balance by performing the percutaneous adductor tenotomy and iliopsoas recession.

Young children. In children under eight years of age, the soft-tissue releases to restore muscle balance are all that is usually necessary to prevent progression of the subluxation and allow for a concentric reduction of the hip. Eilert and MacEwen have documented adequate remodeling of the acetabulum after a concentric realignment of the hip in children under age eight.[14]

Older children. In children older than eight years, adequate remodeling does not uniformly occur because of inadequate remaining growth, and these children frequently require osseous procedures to correct coexistent acetabular dysplasia, internal femoral torsion, and coxa valga. It has been our experience, and that of others, that spastic internal femoral torsion is the major abnormality of the proximal femur in older children, not coxa valga.[22,56] Radiographs taken preoperatively with the hips in extension, 15 degrees of abduction, and enough internal rotation to bring the greater trochanter to a direct lateral position allows an accurate method of assessing the femoral neck angle. If this is normal (less than 150 degrees), then a distal femoral rotational osteotomy is performed to correct the existing femoral torsion (Fig. 23-3). This is performed percutaneously, similar to the technique described by Hoffer and associates.[18] Lateral, transcutaneous, threaded Steinmann pins maintain position in a spica or long-leg cast until

satisfactory union has been obtained in six to eight weeks.

When coxa valga is documented by femoral neck angle greater than 150 degrees in the older child and there is minimal to mild acetabular dysplasia, a proximal femoral varus derotational osteotomy is required. It is important that the osteotomy allow for 90–115 degrees of varus angulation of the femoral neck.[14,19,21,27,34] The Sampson Pediatric Fluted Nail System* is preferred because of its ease of insertion and because it allows precise varus angulation of 115 degrees (Fig. 23-4). The varus derotational osteotomy, as well as the soft-tissue procedures to restore muscle balance, are usually performed simultaneously, and the child is maintained in a double hip spica cast for approximately 8 weeks until a solid union is present. In most instances, the double hip spica cast is used as a nighttime splint for an additional two or three months while the child undergoes extensive physical therapy.

When acetabular dysplasia is advanced, with an acetabular index greater than 30 degrees, staged pelvic and femoral osteotomies are indicated. Two types of displacement pelvic osteotomies have been performed: a Chiari osteotomy and a modified Chiari osteotomy for older children or adolescents with marked acetabular dysplasia (Fig. 23-5).[10] The latter consists of separating the articular cartilage of the superior margin of the acetabulum from the ilium and then performing the Chiari osteotomy 4–5 mm medial to the labrum at the approximate level of the true dome of the acetabulum. When the distal fragment is displaced medially and posteriorly, the proximal fragment will slide downward and laterally, thereby folding the articular cartilage over the femoral head and obviating the need for a capsular interposition that occurs with the standard Chiari osteotomy. Less postoperative stiffness has been observed with this procedure, but the long-term results have yet to be determined, since the longest follow-up study is only 3 years. However, any procedure that preserves the physiologic hyaline articular cartilage should result in significant longevity of the hip as compared to those in which articular fibrocartilage metaplasia has occurred. It must be emphasized that rotational pelvic osteotomies, such as those described by Salter, are contraindicated in neuromuscular disorders because they result in decreased coverage posteriorly and predispose to a posterior dislocation.

---

*3M Company, 20-01 Pollitt Drive, Fair Lawn, N.J. 07410

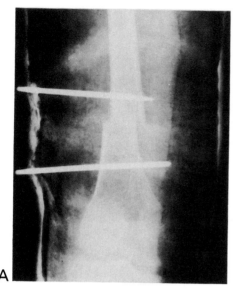
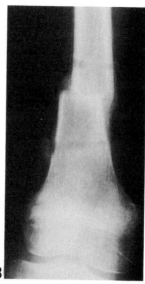

A　　　　　　　　　　　　　　　　B

Figure 23-3. (A) Postoperative radiograph of a girl aged 15 yr with radiation-induced spastic paraplegia demonstrating the percutaneous distal femoral or supracondylar derotation osteotomy. The two threaded Steinmann pins are incorporated in the plaster cast to maintain position. (B) Radiograph weeks postoperatively, demonstrating maintenance of alignment of the proximal and distal segments and a satisfactory union.

Coexistent severe acetabular dysplasia and internal femoral torsion need combined staged pelvic and femoral osteotomies for correction. The soft-tissue procedures and pelvic osteotomy are performed first and followed in two weeks by the femoral osteotomy. Again, the distal femoral or supracondylar derotational osteotomy is used when there is no significant coxa valga, and a proximal femoral varus derotational osteotomy is used when the true femoral neck angle exceeds 150 degrees.

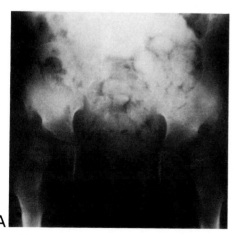
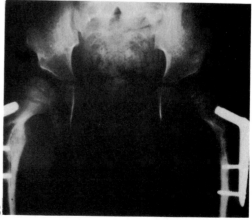

A　　　　　　　　　　　　　　　　B

Figure 23-4. (A) Preoperative radiograph of girl aged eight years with spastic diplegia demonstrating acetabular dysplasia with uncoverage of the femoral head, disruption of Shenton's line, and coxa valga. (B) One year after a proximal femur varus derotational osteotomy using the Sampson Pediatric Nail Plate. There is improved coverage of the femoral head, restoration of Shenton's line, and correction of the coxa valga.

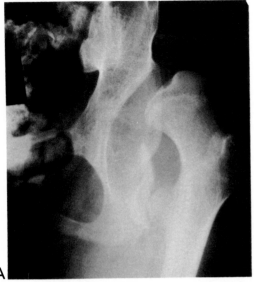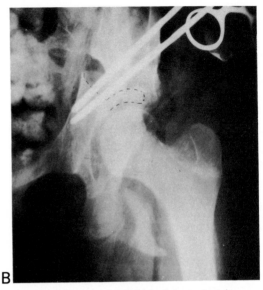

A   B

Figure 23-5. (A) Severe acetabular dysplasia and subluxation of the left hip of the patient in Figure 23-2. This hip is moderately painful, and ambulatory ability is limited. An iliopsoas tenotomy at the lesser trochanter had been performed previously. (B) Correction of the acetabular dysplasia and subluxation has been accomplished after a modified Chiari pelvic osteotomy. Note the turned-down articular surface and subchondral bone, allowing interposition of hyaline cartilage instead of the hip capsule. Shenton's line is also restored, and with internal rotation of the proximal femur there is no associated coxa valga. The percutaneous distal femoral supracondylar derotation osteotomy was performed two weeks later to complete the realignment of the hip.

Spastic Dislocation

In recent years, the principles of the natural history of spastic dislocation set forth by Moreau and associates have been followed.[23] Existing unilateral or bilateral dislocations in children who are extremely intellectually impaired, nonambulators, bedridden, or institutionalized are generally not treated since these patients are usually not aware of pain and the benefits of surgery are negligible when compared to the risks involved. In children who have moderate intelligence and walking or sitting potential, however, the benefits to be derived from reduction are significant and the procedures are warranted.

Again, the first principle involved is the correction of any existing pelvic obliquity, especially of the spinopelvic form with scoliosis. Once this is accomplished, then the spastic dislocation can be treated. These patients require release of existing contractures and restoration of muscle balance through appropriate soft-tissue releases followed by open reduction of the dislocation and combined pelvic and femoral osteotomies to correct the existing acetabular dysplasia and deformities of the proximal femur. Skeletal traction

is usually not well tolerated by these patients, and shortening of the proximal femur is used to obviate the necessity for traction in those children with a very high dislocation. Frequently, the femoral head lies just lateral to the superior margin of the acetabulum, and, as a consequence, femoral shortening is not necessary, since these hips can be adequately reduced after extensive soft-tissue releases.

The open reduction technique in a spastic dislocation consists initially of a percutaneous adductor tenotomy followed by an anterior iliofemoral (Salter) approach to the hip. The intrapelvic iliopsoas recession is performed, followed by an extensive capsulotomy of the hip joint and resection of the ligamentum teres. If a gentle reduction of the femoral head into the acetabulum cannot be accomplished, then a proximal femoral-shortening derotational osteotomy with or without varus angulation is performed through a direct lateral incision. A single Smith–Petersen skin incision can be used instead, but the postoperative scar is excessive. Two incisions are more cosmetic, and the procedure is facilitated through better exposure. After reducing the femoral head and appropriately realigning the proximal femur, a Chiari or modified Chiari osteotomy is performed with a domed biplane osteotomy of the ilium using a Gigli saw. The distal fragment is displaced medially and posteriorly, thereby providing superior and posterior coverage of the femoral head. Usually two threaded Steinmann pins transfix the proximal and distal segments. There is a bare area of hip capsule medially between the displaced segments, and this is grafted with bone from the anterior superior iliac spine. If a proximal femoral osteotomy is not required, then the ideal position for the proximal femur is chosen after the pelvic osteotomy and maintained during the closure of the hip capsule and wound and while a one-and-one-half or double hip spica cast is applied. Intraoperative radiographs are obtained to assess the status of the coverage of the femoral head and the position of the proximal femur. Two to three weeks after the open reduction and pelvic osteotomy, the femoral osteotomy is performed. If the femoral neck angle is less than 150 degrees, the supracondylar percutaneous distal femoral derotation osteotomy is performed, maintaining the ideal position of the proximal femur while rotating the distal or supracondylar segment to the neutral position with the patella pointing forward. The pins are incorporated into a new hip spica cast. If there is coxa valga in excess of 150 degrees, a proximal femoral varus derotational osteotomy with a 115-degree nail plate is performed. It is advantageous to be able to use two separate procedures in order to accomplish the open reduction and reconstruction of the hip because of the instability in trying to adequately align and maintain both the pelvic and femoral segments.

Both procedures require immobilization of the patient in a spica cast for approximately eight weeks. When there is satisfactory union of both osteotomy sites, motion and physical therapy are resumed. The spica cast is occasionally maintained for use as a nighttime orthosis, but since these procedures are usually performed in older children, this is not always necessary. The nail plate and threaded Steinmann pins from the pelvic osteotomy are usually removed 12–18 mo postoperatively.

The chronically dislocated, deformed, painful hip in a severely retarded nonambulatory adolescent or young adult is usually not a candidate for open reduction and stabilization, and serious consideration should be given to proximal femoral resection and soft-tissue interposition, as recently described by Castle and Schneider.[9] This affords pain relief, improved perineal hygiene and nursing care, and improved sitting balance.

KNEE DISORDERS

Spasticity and contractures about the knee can also result in alterations of stance, gait, and sitting balance. Hip and ankle contractures, however, can produce similar functional aberrations that appear to be of knee origin; therefore, careful detailed assessment of the lower extremities is necessary to determine the true source of the problem.

Knee disorders encountered in spastic cerebral palsy include flexion contractures, recurvatum, genu valgum, chondromalacia, and patella alta.

Assessment of Knee Function in Cerebral Palsy

The methods of assessment of knee function are similar to those of any other musculoskeletal examination in spastic children. The examination should be repeated on several occasions to ensure an accurate evaluation.

Physical Examination

The major deforming muscles about the knee are the quadriceps femoris and hamstring muscles, in particular the rectus femoris and the medial hamstrings (gracilis, semitendenosis, and semimembranosus). The prone rectus femoris test is useful in determining the extent of contractures in the quadriceps muscles while the hamstrings are tested, with the child lying supine with the hips flexed to 90 degrees followed by gentle knee extension. The lack of full extension is recorded in degrees and indicates the magnitude of the hamstring knee-flexion contracture.[51]

It must be remembered that the rectus femoris and the hamstrings are two joint muscles and therefore can act both at the hip and at the knee. The gastrocnemius, likewise, is a two-joint muscle that can have an effect at the knee as well as at the ankle. Careful assessment of these muscles is necessary before undertaking any form of treatment.

Gait Analysis

A crouched, internally rotated gait usually indicates spastic hamstrings, but crouching can also be due to hip-flexion deformities (iliopsoas, rectus femoris) as well as gastrocnemius contractures. This again emphasizes the importance of a careful musculoskeletal examination to determine the source of crouching before any consideration is given to treatment.

Dynamic EMG

Csongradi and associates have performed dynamic EMG analysis of the quadriceps femoris and medial hamstrings in children with spastic cerebral palsy to determine the alterations from normal as well as the relationship between these two interrelated muscles.[38]

Quadriceps femoris. There is increased activity beyond normal in the rectus femoris and vastus medialis muscles. Normally they are active at heel-strike and in the early portion of stance phase, with the duration of activity approximately 31 percent of the gait cycle. In spastic cerebral palsy, these muscles were found to be either dysphasic or to have a prolonged phasic activity, with the duration of activity being increased to approximately 78 percent of the gait cycle.

Hamstrings. Medial hamstrings are activated late in the swing phase, with continued activity up to mid-stance. This results in a deceleration of the limb and stabilization of the knee from heel-strike to the foot-flat position. A second phase of activity is occasionally encountered just before toe-off. The duration of normal activity is approximately 39 percent of the gait cycle. In spastic cerebral palsy the duration of activity is prolonged to approximately 71 percent of the gait cycle, and there is primarily a prolonged phasic activity of the muscle, although a dysphasic pattern has also been seen.

The results of this study indicate that the rectus femoris and medial hamstrings are quite similar and that a spastic quadriceps muscle usually accompanies a spastic hamstring, with the latter producing the more significant deforming force. Care must therefore be taken when treating a crouched gait to prevent an iatrogenic genu recurvatum deformity.

Radiographic Evaluation

Radiographic evaluation of the knee in cerebral palsy is important to determine the state of development of the femoral condyles and the tibial plateau. Flexion contractures may produce secondary osseous changes in the articular surfaces that may affect any form of soft-tissue surgery.[45] The status of the patella is also important, since patella alta, fragmentation of the distal pole of the patella, and patella malalignment are all common radiographic findings in the spastic knee.

Treatment

Flexion Deformities

A functional flexion deformity about the knee in spastic cerebral palsy can be primary or secondary. A primary deformity is characterized by hamstring contractures and the inability to extend the knee fully during stance or gait. Secondary deformities may be due to hip flexion or ankle equinus contractures. Careful examination will distinguish between primary and secondary knee-flexion deformities.

Hamstring contractures of 30–40 degrees generally allow full knee extension during walking but result in a flattening of the lumbar lordosis ("tucked-tail" position), while contractures greater than 40 degrees result in a clinically obvious knee-flexion deformity during stance and gait. Knee-flexion contractures also result in a shortened stride length and difficulty in lifting the feet off the ground during walking. Sitting balance becomes compromised as the contracture progresses because of the loss of lumbar lordosis and the development of lumbar kyphosis.

The treatment of knee-flexion deformities can be conservative or surgical. Conservative methods involve serial casting of mild contractures; surgical techniques include recession, lengthening, or transfer of the hamstrings or combinations thereof.

Serial plaster casts. Flexion contractures of 40 degrees or less can frequently be managed by serial plaster casts, especially in younger children.[58] Cylinder casts are applied and changed at one- or two-week intervals. Hamstring stretching exercises (sit-ups, straight-leg raising) are performed daily. Once complete correction has been obtained, the casts are bivalved for nighttime use. This is continued for three to six months. If orthoses are necessary during the daytime, a total-contact polypropylene ankle–foot orthosis (AFO) is recommended. A floor-reaction AFO with 5 degrees of plantar flexion (Fig. 23-6) to provide a mild knee extension thrust during stance phase with good clinical results can be used.

Surgical procedures. Transfer of the hamstrings to the femoral condyles was advocated by Eggers but is rarely performed today because of the problems of genu recurvatum, decreased posterior pelvic support, increased lumbar lordosis, and loss of knee flexion.[40] Various modification of this procedure have been used to minimize these complications.[35,36,41–44,48,49,51,56] Release of the proximal hamstrings from the ischial tuberosity was recommended by Seymour and Sharrard, but Drummond and associates found increased lumbar lordosis, especially when a coexistent hip-flexion deformity was present, as well as an increased incidence of genu recurvatum.[39,54] Ray and Ehrlich have reported good correction of flexion deformities and spastic internal rotation with improved function by transferring the semitendinosus to the lateral intermuscular septum and the semimembranosus to the biceps femoris.[50] The transfer of the medial hamstrings laterally has the advantage of maintaining knee-flexion power while eliminating any internal rotation deformity. There was only one patient in their series with genu recurvatum, and apparently no patient had an increase in lumbar lordosis.

At Cleveland Metropolitan General Hospital a combination of release and recession have been utilized with good success. The gracilis and semitendinosus tendons are simply divided and allowed to retract, while the semimembranosus and biceps femoris are recessed by incising their investing aponeurosis 4–5 cm above the knee joint (Fig. 23-7). The peroneal nerve is usually exposed and protected while the knee is extended. If complete correction cannot be obtained or if the peroneal nerve becomes taut, no further surgery, such as a posterior capsulotomy of the knee, is performed but, rather, the remaining portion of the contracture is corrected with serial plaster casts.

The usual postoperative regimen consists of two weeks of long-leg cast immobilization, and then the casts are bivalved to allow active knee flexion. Ambulation is resumed, as tolerated, and nighttime bivalved casts are used for three to six months. Only one patient of the 85 who have undergone this procedure has had any significant long-term genu recurvatum; however, it is not unusual to see mild genu recurvatum for the first two to three months after ambulation is resumed because of hamstring weakness. Once strength is regained, this is no longer a problem, and, in fact, palpation in the popliteal fossa indicates there has been reconstitution of the released gracilis and semitendinosus tendons. Increased lumbar lordosis has not been a problem in any patient, and functional abilities have significantly improved. Persistent internal rotation gait is usually not significant, since soft-tissue releases about the hip are performed simultaneously. As stated previously, all indicated surgery is performed at one operation to minimize hospitalization and allow maximum rehabilitation.

If postoperative bracing is necessary, a AFO

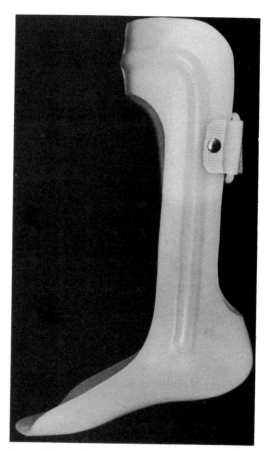

Figure 23-6. Floor-reaction AFO with the ankle in 5 degrees of equinus to provide a knee-extension thrust during stance phase.

floor-reaction orthosis to provide a knee-extension thrust is used. However, every child is given the opportunity to ambulate without orthoses before making this decision.

Genu Recurvatum

Genu recurvatum is characterized by failure of forward tibial motion during stance phase.[55] This can be due to several causes: overcorrected knee flexion deformities (most common), tendo-Achilles contracture, excessive or insufficient calf muscle activity, and excessive quadriceps (rectus femoris) spasticity.[37,46] A lack of progression of forward rotation of the tibia allows the femur to rotate over the stationary tibia with a resultant knee-extension thrust and genu recurvatum.

Appropriate treatment requires precise identifi-

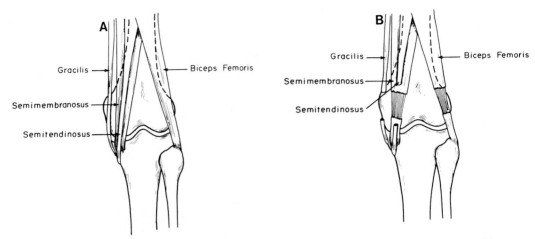

Figure 23-7. (A) Diagram illustrating the posterior aspect of the knee and the normal relationship of the medial and lateral hamstring muscles. (B) Diagram of the combination hamstring release and recession for knee-flexion contractures. The gracilis and semitendinosus muscles are released while the semimembranosus and biceps femoris are recessed in continuity.

cation of the etiologic factors of the deformity. Tendo-Achilles lengthening when contracted or overactive calf muscles are present will result in improvement, as will release of the pelvic origin of the rectus femoris when contracted. Recurvatum secondary to lengthened hamstrings or insufficient calf muscle activity is best managed orthotically. A floor-reaction total-contact polypropylene AFO similar to that described by Rosenthal is preferred.[53] The orthosis maintains the ankle in 5 degrees of dorsiflexion, thereby providing a knee-flexion thrust during stance phase (Fig. 23-8). The design by Rosenthal has been modified so that the upper polypropylene section is posterior instead of anterior; the flexion thrust is thus constant and cannot be modified by the tension on the Velcro strap. A variable-axis trial orthosis can also be beneficial in determining the precise amount of dorsiflexion that produces the optimal gait before the orthosis is manufactured.

Genu Valgum

Older children with significant internal femoral torsion may develop a compensatory external tibial torsion, resulting in genu valgum. Spasticity in the calf muscle with a subsequent valgus hindfoot and pronated mid-foot and forefoot are commonly associated with the development of this condition. Appropriate soft-tissue releases are indicated to restore muscle balance, followed by derotation of the distal femur and, occasionally, the proximal tibia to restore normal knee alignment and improve function.

Patella Alta and Chondromalacia

Knee-flexion deformity results in the patella being positioned more proximally than normal. Attentuation or lengthening of the patella tendon occurs over time with development of patella alta.[35] It has been shown that in patella alta there is a short moment arm in extension that can weaken terminal extension and thereby enhance maintenance of the knee-flexion deformity.[47] Ambulation in a crouch position results in increased compressive forces between the patella and patellofemoral groove that eventually can cause fragmentation of the distal pole of the patella and fibrillation of articular cartilage with the development of chondromalacia and pain.[35,52] Patella subluxation and dislocation can also occur in older children with coexistant genu valgum.

Treatment of patella alta and chondromalacia in spastic cerebral palsy does not require realignment of the patella but, rather, correction of the knee-flexion deformity by either hamstring or rectus femoris recession, tendo-Achilles lengthening, or a combination thereof.[52,57] Genu valgum should also be corrected, if present, to allow for normal patellofemoral biomechanics.

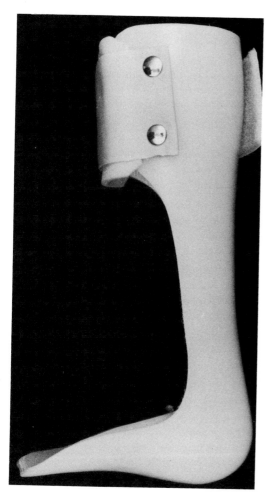

Figure 23-8. Floor-reaction AFO with the ankle in 5 degrees of dorsiflexion to provide a mild knee-flexion thrust during stance phase. This orthosis is used primarily for genu recurvatum deformities.

REFERENCES

Hip Deformities

1. Baker LD, Dodelin R, Bassett F: Pathological changes in the hip in cerebral palsy: Pathogenesis and treatment—a preliminary report. J Bone Joint Surg 44A:1331, 1962
2. Banks HH, Green WT: Adductor tenotomy and obturator neurectomy for the correction of adduction contractures of the hip in cerebral palsy. J Bone Joint Surg 42A:111, 1960
3. Beals RK: Developmental changes in the femur and acetabulum in spastic paraplegia and diplegia. Dev Med Child Neurol 11:303, 1969
4. Bleck EE: Surgical management of spastic flexion deformities of the hip with special reference to iliopsoas recession. J Bone Joint Surg 53A:1408, 1971
5. Bleck EE: Hip deformities in cerebral palsy, in American Academy of Orthopaedic Surgeons Instructional Course Lectures, vol. 20. St. Louis, Mosby, 1971, p 54
6. Bleck EE, Ford F, Sterik HC, et al: EMG telemetry study of spastic gait patterns in cerebral palsy (abstr). Dev Med Child Neurol 17:307, 1975
7. Bleck EE: Orthopaedic Management in Cerebral Palsy. Philadelphia, Saunders, 1979
8. Bleck EE: The hip in cerebral palsy. Orthop Clin North Am 11:79, 1980
9. Castle ME, Schneider C: Proximal femoral resection-intraposition arthroplasty. J Bone Joint Surg 60A:1051, 1978
10. Chiari K: Medial displacement osteotomy of the pelvis. Clin Orthop 98:55, 1974
11. Chong KC, Vojnic CD, Quanbury AO, et al: The assessment of the internal rotation gait in cerebral palsy. Clin Orthop 132:145, 1978
12. Couch WH, DeRosa GP, Throop FB: Thigh adductor transfer for spastic cerebral palsy. Dev Med Child Neurol 19:343, 1977
13. Drummond DS, Rogala EJ, Cruess R, et al: The paralytic hip and pelvic obliquity in cerebral palsy and myelomeningocele, in American Academy of Orthopaedic Surgeons Instructional Course Lectures, vol. 28. St. Louis, Mosby, 1979, p 7
14. Eilert RE, MacEwen GD: Varus derotation osteotomy of the femur in cerebral palsy. Clin Orthop 125:168, 1977
15. Griffin PP, Wheelhouse WW, Shiavi R: Adductor transfer for adductor spasticity: Clinical and electromyographic gait analysis. Dev Med Child Neurol 19:783, 1979
16. Hiroshima K, Ono K: Correlation between muscle shortening and derangement of the hip joint in children with spastic cerebral palsy. Clin Orthop 144:186, 1979
17. Hoffer MM, Abraham E, Nickel V: Salvage surgery at the hip to improve sitting posture of mentally retarded severely disabled children with cerebral palsy. Dev Med Child Neurol 14:51, 1972
18. Hoffer MM, Prietto CA, Koffman M: Supracondylar derotational osteotomy of the femur for internal rotation of the thigh in the cerebral palsied child. J Bone Joint Surg 63A:389, 1981
19. Jones GB: Paralytic dislocation of the hip. J Bone Joint Surg 44B:573, 1962
20. Lamb DW, Pollock GA: Hip deformities in cerebral palsy and their treatment. Dev Med Child Neurol 4:488, 1962
21. Lewis FR, Samilson RL, Lucas DD: Femoral torsion and coxa valga in cerebral palsy— a preliminary report. Dev Med Child Neurol 6:591, 1964

22. Majestro TC, Frost HM: Cerebral palsy—spastic internal femoral torsion. Clin Orthop 79:44, 1971

23. Moreau M, Drummond DS, Rogala E, et al: Natural history of the dislocated hip in spastic cerebral palsy. Dev Med Child Neurol 21:749, 1979

24. Perry J, Hoffer MM, Antonelli D, et al: Electromyography before and after surgery for hip deformity in children with cerebral palsy. J Bone Joint Surg 58A:201, 1976

25. Phelps WM: Prevention of acquired dislocation of the hip in cerebral palsy. J Bone Joint Surg 41A:440, 1959

26. Root L, Spero CR: Hip adductor transfer compared with adductor tenotomy in cerebral palsy. J Bone Joint Surg 63A:767, 1981

27. Samilson RL, Tsou P, Aamoth G, et al: Dislocation and subluxation of the hip in cerebral palsy. Pathogenesis, natural history, and management. J Bone Joint Surg 54A:863, 1972

28. Sharrard WJW, Allen JMH, Heaney JH, et al: Surgical prophylaxis of subluxation and dislocation of the hip in cerebral palsy. J Bone Joint Surg 57B:160, 1975

29. Smith ET: Hip dislocation in cerebral palsy. Dev Med Child Neurol 11:291, 1969

30. Staheli LT: The prone hip extension test. Clin Orthop 123:1215, 1977

31. Stephenson CT, Donovan MM: Transfer of the hip adductor origins to the ischium in spastic cerebral palsy. Dev Med Child Neurol 13:247, 1971

32. Tachjian MO, Minear WL: Hip dislocation in cerebral palsy. J Bone Joint Surg 38A:1358, 1956

33. Thompson GH, Rang M: Preventive pediatric orthopaedics. Orthopaedics 3:522, 1980

34. Tylkowski CM, Rosenthal RK, Simon SR: Proximal femoral osteotomy in cerebral palsy. Clin Orthop 151:183, 1980

Knee Deformities

35. Banks HH: The knee in cerebral palsy. Orthop Clin North Am 3:113, 1972

36. Beals RK: Spastic paraplegia and diplegia. An evaluation of nonsurgical and surgical factors influencing the prognosis for ambulation. J Bone Joint Surg 48A:827, 1966

37. Cottrell GW: Role of the rectus femoris in spastic children. J Bone Joint Surg 45A:1556, 1963

38. Csongradi J, Bleck E, Ford WF: Gait electromyography in normal and spastic children with special reference to quadriceps femoris and hamstring muscles. Dev Med Child Neurol 21:738, 1979

39. Drummond DS, Rogala E, Templeton J, et al: Proximal hamstring release for knee flexion and crouched posture in cerebral palsy. J Bone Joint Surg 56A:1598, 1974

40. Eggers GWN: Transplantation of hamstring tendons to femoral condyles in order to improve hip extension and decrease knee flexion in cerebral spastic paralysis. J Bone Joint Surg 34A:827, 1952

41. Eggers GWN, Evans EB: Surgery in cerebral palsy. J Bone Joint Surg 45A:1275, 1963

42. Evans EB, Julian JD: Modification of the hamstring transfer. Dev Med Child Neurol 8:539, 1966

43. Evans EB: The knee in cerebral palsy, in Samilson RL (ed): Orthopaedic Aspects of Cerebral Palsy. Philadelphia, Lippincott, 1975, pp 173–194

44. Evans EB: Knee flexion deformity in cerebral palsy, in American Academy of Orthopaedic Surgeons Instructional Course Lectures, vol. 20. St. Louis, Mosby, 1971, p 42

45. Gagenheim JJ, Rosenthal RS, Simon SR: Knee flexion deformities and genu recurvatum in cerebral palsy. Roentgenographic findings. Dev Med Child Neurol 21:563, 1979

46. Holt SK: Assessment of Cerebral Palsy. I. Muscle Function, Locomotion and Hand Function. London, Lloyd-Duke, 1965

47. Lotman DB: Knee flexion deformity and patella alta in spastic cerebral palsy. Dev Med Child Neurol 18:315, 1976

48. Masse P, Audie B: Critical evaluation of the Eggers' procedure for relief of knee flexion spasticity. Dev Med Child Neurol 10:159, 1968

49. Pollack GA, English TA: Transplantation of the hamstring muscles in cerebral palsy. J Bone Joint Surg 49B:30, 1967

50. Ray RL, Ehrlich MG: Lateral hamstring transfer and gait improvement in the cerebral palsy patient. J Bone Joint Surg 61A:719, 1979

51. Reimers J: Contractures of the hamstrings in spastic cerebral palsy. J Bone Joint Surg 56B:102, 1974.

52. Rosenthal RK, Levine DB: Fragmentation of the distal pole of the patella in spastic cerebral palsy. J Bone Joint Surg 59A:934, 1977

53. Rosenthal RK, Deutsch SD, Miller W, et al: A fixed-ankle, below-the-knee orthoses for the management of genu recurvatum in spastic cerebral palsy. J Bone Joint Surg 57A:545, 1975

54. Seymour N, Sharrard WJW: Bilateral proximal release of the hamstrings in cerebral palsy. J Bone Joint Surg 50B:274, 1968

55. Simon SR, Deutsch SD, Nuzzo RM, et al: Genu recurvatum in spastic cerebral palsy. J Bone Joint Surg 60A:882, 1978

56. Sutherland DH, Schottstaedt ER, Larsen LJ, et al: Clinical and electromyographic study of seven spastic children with internal rotation gait. J Bone Joint Surg 51A:1070, 1969

57. Sutherland DH, Larsen LJ, Mann R: Rectus femoris release in selected patients with cerebral palsy: A preliminary report. Dev Med Child Neurol 17:26, 1975

58. Westin GW: Personal communication, 1980

John T. Makley
William C. Kim

24

Spastic Equinus Deformities

Cerebral palsy can produce alterations in the function of the foot and ankle. The most common, and usually most difficult, problem is the spastic equinus deformity. Other problems include equinovalgus, equinovarus, and calcaneus deformities as well as hallux valgus and toe deformities. This chapter will focus on the pathophysiology and management of spastic equinus deformities.

Plantar Flexion or Equinus

Plantar-flexed deformity at the ankle–foot complex is a common manifestation of spastic cerebral palsy and may be a significant determinant of the ability to stand and ambulate. A smooth ambulatory pattern depends on a stable base of support, full and free range of motion for all the joints, adequate and balanced motor power, and a normal sensory input. In the cerebral palsied patient with spastic equinus deformity, the base of support is compromised.[9] These patients frequently have joint contractures at various levels as well as imbalance of motor power in the extremities. Another frequently overlooked problem in these children is the fact that there may well be a persistence of primitive reflexes as well as significant impairment of sensory input such as proprioception. Therefore, the significance of equinus deformity in the ability to stand and ambulate must be assessed in relation to other associated central and peripheral abnormalities. Optimal management of equinus deformity depends on accurate diagnosis, which itself must be based on a complete understanding of pathophysiology and pathoanatomy.

PATHOPHYSIOLOGY

A normal ankle–foot complex is structurally and dynamically balanced. Structural balance is conferred by bones and articulations aligned in the line of gravity and also by passive support of ligaments and capsules. Muscle–tendon units crossing these joints provide dynamic balance, which is mediated by voluntary and reflex motor centers within the brain. In a normal growing child, structural and dynamic balance occur in the setting of time-dependent growth and development curve. As such, the various bones, articulations, muscles, and connective tissues of the ankle–foot complex, grow and develop in a parallel fashion. The adaptive forces at play in these tissues are summarized in Wolff's law for bones and the Heuter–Volkmann principle for cartilage.

Spastic equinus deformity occurs in the setting of nonprogressive lesions of the brain. Muscle imbalance, growth and development differences, ipsilateral joint contractures, and gravity can all affect the ankle–foot complex singly or in combination, causing this deformity (Fig. 24-1).

Muscle Imbalance

Muscle imbalance may not only be voluntary but may be due to primitive extensor posturing reflex, in which the gastrocnemius and soleus muscles tend to be stronger than the dorsiflexors. It should be noted that the extensor synergy of the gastrocnemius and the soleus may not be equal in effect because these muscles are really two different muscles with differ

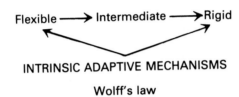

Muscle Imbalance

(voluntary, reflex–local spasm, extensor synergy)

Imbalance of growth and development

Compensatory posture

DEFORMING FORCES

EQUINUS DEFORMITY

Flexible ⟶ Intermediate ⟶ Rigid

INTRINSIC ADAPTIVE MECHANISMS

Wolff's law

Heuter–Volkmann principle

Figure 24-1. Pathophysiology of spastic equinus deformities.

ent innervations and origins, although their insertions are the common tendo Achilles. This may explain their differences in degrees of spasm and contracture.

Growth and Development Differences

In the setting of cerebral palsy, the growth and development curves for various tissues may diverge or progress at a different rate. An interesting observation in this regard is the evidence presented by Tardieu and associates that in a subgroup of cerebral palsy patients, muscles are not able to keep up with the longitudinal growth of its associated long bone.[22] In normal individuals, muscles keep up with skeletal growth by serial addition of sarcomere units, which permits optimal length–tension relationships between the muscle motor and bone lever–arm. In this group of cerebral palsy patients, this adaptive mechanism does not appear to exist. The result is that the muscle progressively shortens in relation to the bone, tethering the ankle–foot complex in a progressive equinus direction as the bone continues to grow.

Ipsilateral Joint Contractures

Spastic equinus deformity may also be due to contractures of the ipsilateral knee or the hip. In this

situation, equinus deformity is a compensatory posture to keep the patient balanced. Conversely, it is also possible for knee and hip contractures to be secondary to spastic equinus deformity at the ankle–foot complex (Chapter 23).

Gravity

Although the previously mentioned deforming forces are of much greater magnitude than gravity, it must be kept in mind that gravity has a power of one grade. It can be a significant addition to equinus-directed vectors, especially in patients who are bedridden and assume equinus posture chronically.

PATHOANATOMY

The pathologic anatomy of equinus deformity in cerebral palsy is secondary to the pathophysiologic forces discussed above. It is important to emphasize that although cerebral palsy is defined by static lesions of the brain due to ongoing pathophysiologic forces, the effects of those lesions, including equinus deformity, can progress with time. The pathoanatomy of equinus deformity can be divided into three stages of progression: flexible, intermediate, and rigid.

Flexible Stage

The flexible stage occurs from the time cerebral palsy begins until soft-tissue contractures and secondary osseous adaptations take place. This stage is therefore characterized by relatively normal anatomy. If the pathophysiologic forces are overcome during this stage, the equinus can be totally prevented or corrected, since no significant structural factors impede correction at this time.

Intermediate Stage

If the pathophysiologic forces of the equinus deformity continue unabated over a prolonged period, the severity of equinus may increase, and secondary structural changes in various soft–tissues and bones may occur. These adaptations to the equinus posture occur simultaneously in all tissues but first become clinically evident in soft tissues. Equinus posture results in a shortened distance between origin and insertion of all structures plantar to the ankle axis of rotation, and the soft tissues therefore adapt to the shortened state by formation of contractures. Contractures take place in the skin, fascia, neurovascular bundles, ligaments, capsules, and muscle–tendon units. The muscles involved include the long-toe flexors, posterior tibialis, peroneals, and triceps surae. Because the triceps surae is composed of two separate muscles that may differ in degrees of spasm, the degrees of contracture may differ between the gastrocnemius and the soleus components.

The differences in the degree of contracture of the soleus and gastrocnemius can be determined by the Silfverskiöld test.[17] This test is based on the anatomic fact that the soleus and gastrocnemius have different sites of origin with respect to the knee (gastrocnemius above and soleus below), although they are conjoined distally and cross the ankle joint together. If dorsiflexion is significantly limited with knee flexed, the soleus is contracted. If dorsiflexion is limited with the knee extended but not with the knee flexed, the gastrocnemius is contracted. (This constitutes a positive Silfverskiöld test.) If dorsiflexion is limited in both knee flexion and extension, either the soleus or both the soleus and the gastrocnemius are contracted significantly.

Rigid Stage

Soft-tissue contractures produce rigidity at the ankle–foot complex, and this produces osseous and articular changes in accordance with Wolff's law and the Heuter–Volkmann principle, respectively. Chronic equinus posture results in modeling of bone and cartilage into an abnormal shape and size. The anterior dome of the talus may enlarge and can become a bony block to dorsiflexion. It must be emphasized that even with rigidity, the primary pathophysiologic deforming forces are still active but masked clinically by the constraints of motion imposed by secondary structural changes in the tissues at the ankle–foot complex.

ELECTROMYOGRAPHY

From the preceding considerations, a situation is imaginable in which dynamic forces can mimic static contractures during routine examination because both can cause limitation of dorsiflexion under the same examining conditions. Perry and associates have shown that such an overlapping situation exists, but it is possible to distinguish dynamic posturing from static contracture with electromyography (EMG).[14] EMG was used during clinical evaluation that included the Silfverskiöld test and gait analysis. Eight of 17 cerebral palsy patients with spastic equinus deformity had a positive Silfverskiöld test. This was initially interpreted to be due to the mechanical effect of contracture of gastrocnemius, but when these same patients were examined under general anesthesia with all reflexes and electrical activities abolished, the Silfverskiöld test became negative. This implied that there was a dynamic neural mechanism that imitated gastrocnemius contracture when the patient was examined awake but was abolished when examination occurred under general anesthesia. EMG of the gastrocnemius and soleus and a quick stretch test of the triceps surae while the patient was awake revealed that with the knee extended, a tonic neural imbalance (primitive extensor reflex) was activated both in the soleus and in the gastrocnemius. The limitation of dorsiflexion with the patient awake hence was not due to gastrocnemius contracture of local gastrocnemius spasm but to triggering of this primitive extensor reflex involving the whole of triceps surae.

In addition, dynamic EMG of the gastrocnemius and soleus during gait revealed that in all patients with cerebral palsy and spastic equinus deformity tested, there was activity in the soleus, gastrocnemius, or triceps surae during the swing phase of gait. Normal individuals have no activity of these muscles during the swing phase. Even in gait in these cerebral palsy patients, the primitive extensor reflex occurred and resulted in phasic distortion. A spastic muscle also, when contracted, tends to activate earlier in the gait cycle, with resultant distortion of phase. Therefore, premature plantar flexion at the ankle during swing phase may be due to local premature activation of an already contracted triceps surae or to participation of the primitive extensor reflex. These two possibilities may be distinguished with gait EMG, and this distinction is important in order to plan proper treatment.

ASSESSMENT

It has been emphasized that spastic equinus deformity in cerebral palsy is characterized by dynamic and static properties. Diagnostic goals thus include defining the primary equinus-directed forces as well as secondary structural changes. The primary deforming forces may include imbalance of muscles (voluntary and reflex), absence of adaptation of muscle to skeletal growth, and imposed compensatory posture. Structural constraints to dorsiflexion may be soft-tissue, osseous, or both and must be distinguished.

Deforming Forces

Muscle Imbalance (Voluntary and Reflex)

Equinus deformity due to muscle imbalance may be due to one of the following mechanisms:[11]

1. Spastic triceps versus spastic dorsiflexors
2. Spastic triceps versus normal dorsiflexors
3. Spastic triceps versus flaccid dorsiflexors
4. Normal triceps versus flaccid dorsiflexors
5. Flaccid triceps versus flaccid dorsiflexors

It is important to determine which of the above categories of muscle imbalance applies for a given equinus deformity, because treatment applied to one situation might be inappropriate for another, and the equinus deformity might be aggravated rather than corrected.

Static clinical testing of triceps and dorsiflexors may not be accurate. Inability to dorsiflex may not be due to absence of motor power but to the fact that the triceps overpowers the dorsiflexors so much that dorsiflexor activity is not clinically detectable. EMG activity of the apparently flaccid dorsiflexor signifies intact motor function, and treatment would be appropriately altered. One clinical test that can be of value is the "confusion test." This is done by sitting the patient on the edge of the table with hips and

knees flexed 90 degrees. The patient is then asked to further flex the hip on the side of equinus deformity against resistance. With a positive response the patient will automatically dorsiflex the affected ankle–foot complex, indicating that the dorsiflexors are not flaccid.

Discrepancies between clinical and EMG activity at rest and during gait are evidence that physical examination alone is frequently inadequate for determining muscle activity. It has been shown that clinical EMG activity of dorsiflexors at rest may become silent during the swing phase of the gait cycle. Treatment based on the static findings may not result in an improved gait pattern.

Absence of Trophic Muscle Regulation During Skeletal Growth

There is evidence that in normal animals, a regulatory mechanism exists in muscles whereby sarcomere units are serially added or deleted depending on whether the muscle is kept in a lengthened or shortened state for a prolonged period. Also, in normal muscles, sarcomere units are added as related bones grow longitudinally to maintain an optimal length–tension relationship.[21] This trophic regulatory mechanism appears to take place whether the imposed shortening or lengthening of the muscle occurs actively or passively. Plaster immobilization of normal muscle in the shortened or lengthened state results in a decrease or increase in sarcomere numbers, respectively.

Based on experimental data and evidence that cerebral palsied children with clinical hypoextensibility show a decrease in sarcomere number, Tardieu and associates hypothesized that there are two groups of cerebral palsied children: those with a normal trophic regulatory mechanism in the hypoextensile muscle and those without this mechanism.[22] Those children with this mechanism would respond to plaster or surgical treatment and also would be able to keep up with bone growth. Those children without this mechanism do not have the ability to keep up with bone growth and therefore tend to have recurrence of their deformity. This hypothesis was confirmed by studying the tibia–calcaneum angular displacement as a function of passive torque applied to the ankle, before and after various plaster and surgical treatment, in children with spastic cerebral palsy.

Compensatory Posture

Equinus posture as a compensatory mechanism for leg-length inequality and hip- and knee-flexion deformities can occur. A complete musculoskeletal examination usually allows recognition of these conditions. It should be noted that there are situations where slight equinus, which induces a knee extension thrust, may be desirable as a means of obtaining stability at the knee, especially if there is weakness of the quadriceps muscle and a mild dynamic knee-flexion posture.

Structural Deformities

In addition to assessment of the possible dynamic forces leading to equinus deformity at the ankle–foot complex, evaluation should define the structural features of the deformity. This should include assessment on its severity and flexibility and the exact site of the deformity. The pathoanatomy may be divided into soft-tissue and bony abnormalities. Soft-tissue contractures are evaluated under static and dynamic conditions as well as with EMG. Osseous abnormalities are defined by appropriate standing or weight-bearing radiographs of the foot and ankle.

DIAGNOSIS

The difficulty in characterizing the pathophysiologic and pathoanatomic aspects of spastic equinus deformity in cerebral palsied children is that clinical assessment can be misleading. As described above, clinical assessment is best performed under EMG monitoring and by comparing the findings with these patients' reflexes intact as well as abolished. Because the approach to diagnosing spastic equinus deformity can be confusing, a simple diagnostic algorithm (Fig. 24-2) that incorporates the salient features of the pathophysiologic and pathoanatomic factors has been constructed. The sequence of steps taken to derive information is as follows:

1. Determine if equinus deformity is expressed during static examination or gait.
2. During static examination, with the patient awake, determine if the equinus deformity is flexible or fixed. Fixed deformity is arbitrarily defined here as the inability to dorsiflex passively the ankle to neutral position. In dorsiflexion, it is important to supinate the foot, locking the calcaneus beneath the talus as well as locking the mid-tarsal joints themselves to prevent a false appearance of dorsiflexion due to increased hindfoot valgus or a mid-foot breech. Dorsiflexion is performed with the knee flexed and extended. Limitation of dorsiflexion is also assessed with the patient standing and walking, which may bring out subtle limitation of dorsiflexion not appreciated during static

examination. If there is no significant limitation of dorsiflexion during these maneuvers, the patient probably has flexible equinus with no structural or neural abnormalities of significance. Limitation of dorsiflexion may be due to structural or neural factors or both. The following steps help to separate these possibilities.

3. Spasm is abolished by examining the patient under general anesthesia or by the method of Richet, in which a tourniquet is placed around the thigh of the involved limb and set to 200 mmHg for 20 min. At the end of this period, reflex as well as electrical activity is abolished, and the clinical examination is repeated. Local nerve blocks are not dependable. With all reflexes abolished, if there are static contractures, they will be elicited by the Silfverskiöld test. If there is limitation of dorsiflexion with the knee flexed and also extended, the soleus, or both the soleus and gastrocnemius, are contracted. If limitation exists with the knee extended but not flexed, the gastrocnemius is contracted. If with all reflexes abolished the equinus is totally correctable, i.e., flexible, then the apparent contracture with the patient tested awake was due to either local muscle spasm or to primitive extensor synergy.

4. Spasm may be distinguished from primitive extensor synergy by performing the Silfverskiöld test with EMG monitoring while the patient is awake. Quick stretch tests with the knee flexed and extended will result in differential electrical activity in the gastrocnemius, the soleus, or the whole of the triceps surae. The latter indicates activation of the primitive extensor synergy.

5. Even if it has been determined by the above steps that the equinus deformity is due to contracture and not primitive extensor synergy, the primitive reflex response, which was not expressed during the quick stretch test, may come into play during gait. A spastic muscle, when contracted, may become activated early in the gait cycle. This distortion of phase in the gastrocnemius must be differentiated from primitive extensor synergy involving triceps surae. Dynamic EMG is useful in making these distinctions.

TREATMENT

Principles

Treatment outcome is determined by four broad factors: the nature of the spastic equinus deformity, proper patient selection, the ability of the treatment

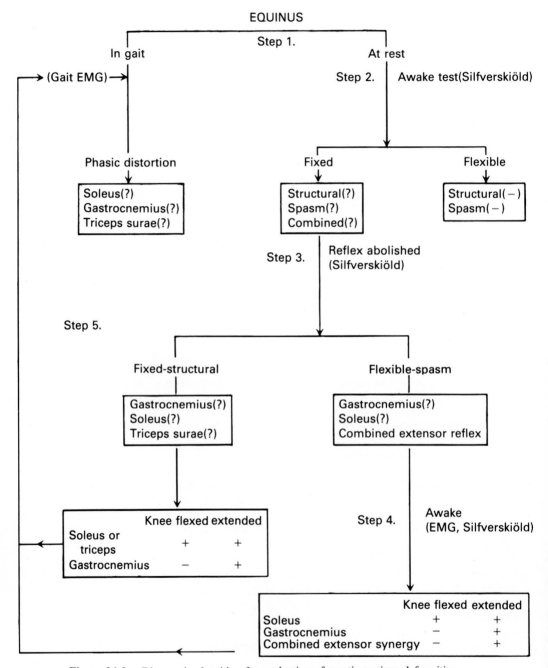

Figure 24-2. Diagnostic algorithm for evaluation of spastic equinus deformities.

team to assess, treat, and coordinate care of the many other musculoskeletal abnormalities that often accompany the spastic equinus deformity, and the availability of an effective treatment modality.

Patient Selection

Variables associated with the patient as a whole are significant determinants of successful treatment outcome. Simply because a given procedure is technically feasible does not necessarily mean it should be done. There should be realistic expectations of improved stance, ambulation, or nursing care far above the risk of surgery or recurrent deformity.

Severity of involvement. If the patient is so severely disabled with cerebral palsy that treatment of equinus deformity would not benefit overall status, treatment is not indicated. There must be a reasonable hope of success.

Intelligence. Patients must have an adequate level of intelligence to cooperate in postoperative care and rehabilitation. Truscelli and associates feel that an intelligence quotient (IQ) of at least 70 is necessary for adequate rehabilitation.[25] Where the goal is only to improve nursing care with facilitation of transfer, less intelligence is acceptable. Others feel that intelligence is not as important as motor-development level. Patients who demonstrate persistence of certain primitive reflexes, such as a tonic neck reflex, have a poor prognosis for ambulation.[3,4] Other important prognostic signs for independent ambulation include the ability to sit independently and the demonstration of reciprocal motion and balance on parallel bars. In these patients, the increased stability and decreased energy consumption after successful treatment of equinus may permit them to progress to the next level of locomotor skill—independent ambulation.[5]

Age. Age is an important indicator of success from the standpoint of recurrence. Strayer states that those operated on early, before fixation of compensatory vestibular and labyrinthine reflexes, have better results.[20] Craig and Van Vuran noted that 11 percent of patients aged 1–5 yr, 4.3 percent of those aged 6–10 yr, and none of those aged 11–15 yrs required a second operation.[6] Silver and Simon encouraged surgery as early as three years of age to decrease contractures of joint capsules and neurovascular bundles.[18] Ingram, however, feels that better results are obtained if surgery is delayed as long as possible because of the high rate of recurrence when done early.[11]

Family. A supportive family is an asset in treatment, since it provides emotional support, complies with follow-up care, and assists with postoperative care and rehabilitation.

Treatment Team

The treatment team consists of the orthopaedic surgeon, pediatrician, physical therapist, occupational therapist, social worker, and other pediatric health care providers experienced in all aspects of cerebral palsy patients and their families. Effectiveness of treatment for equinus deformity frequently depends on effective management of other associated abnormalities. The many reports on various treatment modalities stress the importance of careful postoperative management. Although not documented, Craig and Van Vuran credit their high rate of success, measured by low rate of recurrence, to the use of neurodevelopmental techniques postoperatively.[6] A well-staffed treatment center that is able to provide general support for the various needs of these patients and families probably increases compliance and follow-up care.

Methods

The reference frame for discussion of treatment of spastic equinus deformity in cerebral palsy is the circuit connecting the brain, spinal cord, peripheral motor and sensory nerves, and terminal muscle–tendon units (Fig. 24-3). It is within this organization that associated central and peripheral abnormalities interact. Operative and nonoperative treatment modalities may be applied at various levels of this organization, directed at the pathophysiology and the pathoanatomy (Table 24-1).

Pathophysiologic Factors

Treatment directed at deforming forces is to effect balance at the ankle–foot complex to prevent occurrence or recurrence of the equinus deformity.

Brain. Strayer believed that if a cerebral palsy child with spastic equinus deformity was relieved of fear of falling, the equinus-directed spasm as well as adductor spasm would be eliminated.[20] Medications of various types have been used to suppress centrally based spasm acting at the ankle–foot complex; however, the systemic effect is a disadvantage when the problem is local. One drug, dantrolene sodium, deserves further comment. There is general agreement that this drug does reduce spasticity, but there are disagreements on its ability to effect functional im-

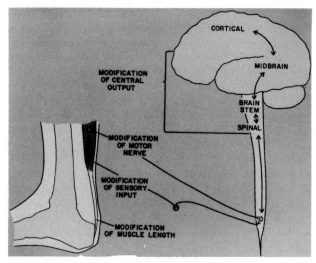

Figure 24-3. Illustration depicting the major neurologic areas for potential modification of spastic equinus deformities: brain, spinal cord, peripheral nerves (motor and sensory), and muscle–tendon unit. Table 24-1 lists the nonoperative and operative modalities of treatment of these various areas.

provement. A recent study by Joynt and Leonard concludes that dantrolene sodium is effective in reducing the force of muscle contraction in spastic cerebral palsy, but objective functional improvements were not significant.[12]

Neurodevelopmental techniques have been advocated but lack strong documentation on efficacy.[4] There is suggestion that sensory feedback may be

beneficial in treatment of dynamic equinus. Research in cerebellar stimulation also appears to have beneficial effects on spasticity in cerebral palsy.[13]

Spinal cord. Invasive and noninvasive dorsal column stimulation appear to be promising adjuncts to treatment of spasticity.[15] Posterior rhizotomy has long been used in the treatment of spasticity but has

Table 24-1

Comparison of Nonoperative and Operative Treatment Modalities According to the Level of the Neurologic Lesion

Level	Treatment	
	Nonoperative	Operative
Brain	Medications Biofeedback techniques	Electrical stimulation
Spinal cord	Electrical stimulation	Electrical stimulation Rhizotomy
Peripheral nerve	Nerve blocks	Neurectomy (partial, total; motor, sensory)
Muscle–Tendon	Manipulation Cast Brace Splints	Tendo Achilles Lengthening Translocation Gastrocnemius Recession (origin, insertion) Midbody aponeurotomy

the side-effects of ataxia and excessive hypotonia. Use of intraoperative dorsal root stimulation appears to have overcome these side-effects.[8]

Peripheral nerves. Temporary nerve blocks as a trial before partial or total neurectomies may alter muscle forces at the ankle–foot complex, but the long-term effect of neurectomy cannot be determined by this method. Complete neurectomy is generally in disfavor because it weakens the muscle and may result in reversal of the deformity and, in the case of triceps surae, poor push-off.[11] The selective neurectomy of Stoffel is advocated for severe clonus, keeping the soleus innervation intact for push-off.[19] Neurectomy, of course, does not lengthen the contracted triceps surae. Even selective neurectomy is condemned by some because it creates fibrosis and can result in a calcaneal deformity.[6,14]

Muscle–tendon unit. Lengthening of the triceps surae or lengthening and recession procedures on the gastrocnemius have dual effects of improving structural relationships as well as balancing deforming forces. This is because contractures and deforming forces are tied together by length–tension relationships. By lengthening or recessing, contracture is improved, spasticity is decreased, and the muscle is weakened.

Forward translocation of the insertion of tendo-Achilles can result in decreased equinus-directed force because the lever-arm between the insertion and axis of the ankle is decreased.[24]

In those cerebral palsy patients who lack trophic regulatory mechanisms in muscles to keep up with skeletal growth, dissociation of muscle and bone length inevitably continues. Although surgical lengthening will improve length–tension relationships in these muscles, it is only temporary, and, because of ongoing dissociation of length between muscle and bone, progression of equinus is inevitable. Manipulation and casts or orthoses usually do not alter this underlying process.[22] In those who do have intact trophic regulatory mechanism, however, equinus deformity is attributable to muscle imbalance or postural causes, and as the muscle imbalance is surgically corrected and primary causes of postural equinus treated, the equinus deformity would be expected to stay corrected. In cases of mild imbalance, serial casts, night splints, and orthoses would be expected to be of significant benefit.

The diagnostic algorithm (see Fig. 24-2) separates contractures and primitive extensor reflexes during the quick stretch test of the triceps surae and gastrocnemius spasm and primitive extensor reflex during gait. If EMG shows activity in the triceps surae, tendo-Achilles lengthening would improve length–tension relationship and decrease spasm. If the activity is localized to the gastrocnemius, then a recession of gastrocnemius would be more specific.[14]

Pathoanatomy

It is accepted that the neurologic lesion in the brain is irreversible, and one must be resigned to treating the secondary musculoskeletal abnormalities such as an equinus deformity. Limitation of dorsiflexion may be due to contractures of ligaments and capsules and to osseous changes.

Nonoperative treatment is usually ineffective once a significant equinus contracture has occurred, and when equinus cannot be corrected past neutral, when persistent toe–toe gait exists, or when secondary changes of knee recurvatum and hip flexion occur.[1] Manual stretching does not release contractures, and the heel tends to ride up inside the orthosis.[4] Serial casting is effective when the equinus deformity is mild and in those patients with an intact trophic regulatory mechanism.

The level of the surgical procedure is exemplified by the four prototypes in Figure 24-4.

Silfverskiöld procedure. The Silfverskiöld procedure converts the gastrocnemius from a two-joint to one-joint muscle like the soleus by recessing its medial and lateral heads below the level of the knee joint.[17] A partial neurectomy of the tibial motor nerves to the gastrocnemius muscle was occasionally performed to functionally weaken the muscle and decrease spasticity. Its rationale was to decrease the contracture or spasm of gastrocnemius and preserve the soleus muscle for push-off. Perry and associates have shown that isolated contracture of the gastrocnemius is not common, and this is determined under general anesthesia so that primitive extensor synergy would not imitate it.[14] Silver and Simon, before the report of Perry et al, used the Silfverskiöld procedure and partial tibial neurectomy to decrease spasm and reported 5 recurrences in 110 procedures of spastic equinus deformity.[18] This high success rate is not shared by everyone. A commonly stated contraindication to the Silfverskiöld procedure is if one anticipates simultaneous release of the hamstrings. Combined release of the gastrocnemius and hamstrings can result in genu recurvatum.

Vulpius procedure. The Vulpius procedure consists of a distal release of the gastrocnemius at its

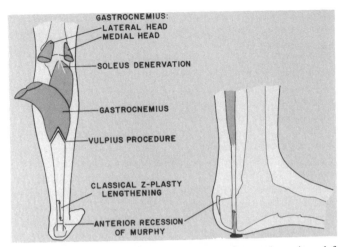

Figure 24-4. The prototypes of surgical treatment in spastic equinus deformities: gastrocnemius recession (proximal or distal), neurectomy (soleus or gastrocnemius), tendo-Achilles lengthening, and tendo-Achilles advancement.

junction with the soleus and a recession of the soleus aponeurosis.[26] This was later modified by Strayer to include resuturing the gastrocnemius tendon to the soleus.[20] The rationale was initially to decrease contracture of the gastrocnemius, but its beneficial effect was attributable to alteration of proprioceptive reflexes centrally along with modification of the stretch reflex peripherally. Its indications include children under six years of age with bilateral spastic cerebral palsy who have never walked and who show generalized extensor spasm and a positive Silfverskiöld test. It is contraindicated in athetosis and in adults with hemiplegia. Strayer reported 70 percent excellent or good results with this procedure. Postoperative care includes a toe–groin cast for four weeks followed by an ankle–groin cast. Bost, in discussing Strayer's paper, stated that he had 88 percent satisfactory results in 155 patients. Conversely, Bleck had 30 percent recurrence in 59 patients following a Strayer-type procedure, and there was 0.85 percent calcaneal deformity.[4] Sharrard and Bernstein reported 15 percent recurrence; interestingly, their postoperative regimen consisted of no orthoses or night splinting after 3–5 wk of plaster.[16]

Holt has shown with EMG that after the Strayer slide procedure, the equinus was corrected but there continued to be abnormal and excessive electrical activity in the gastrocnemius.[10] There was also evidence that the dorsiflexor anticus may have improved in neuromuscular activity. Complications in the Strayer

procedure include sural nerve damage, calcaneal deformity, and weakness of knee flexion.

Tendo-Achilles Lengthening

Multiple techniques for tendo-Achilles lengthening have been tried for various reasons. The anatomic indication is the patient's inability to dorsiflex above neutral with the knee flexed, since it implies significant contracture of the soleus or the triceps surae. Based on EMG findings during quick stretch test of triceps and distortion of gait phase, if primitive extensor reflex exists, tendo-Achilles lengthening is indicated. Contraindications to tendo-Achilles lengthening include isolated gastrocnemius contracture or spasm as determined by physical examination and EMG during static and gait analysis.

There are three ways to perform tendo-Achilles lengthening. Delpech in 1816 did it subcutaneously with early good and later poor results.[7] This was attributed by Banks to poor postoperative and follow-up care.[1] Many advocate sliding lengthening in the manner of White, since it appears to give better control of tension and the amount of lengthening, and continuity of the Achilles tendon is maintained.[2,27] Less postoperative or iatrogenic overcorrection has been reported.[2] Banks and Green had a recurrence rate of 29.9 percent at 10-yr follow-up study, however. This was thought to be due to the number of surgeons involved, and it was expressed that if one surgeon were to do the procedure, 90 percent success would be anticipated. Bleck had 90 percent success using the Hoke sliding lengthening procedure, and it has been recommended when multiple surgeons are involved because it "never results in overcorrection."[4]

Some workers advocate complete sectioning of the tendo-Achilles and suturing it back in the corrected position. Thompson and Grabe reported 87 percent success in 80 procedures at 4.5 yr follow-up study.[23] Sharrard and Bernstein performed coronal sectioning of the tendo-Achilles before reapproximation in the corrected position.[16] Twenty-three percent recurrence was reported, and it was said to be due to persistent functional weakness of the dorsiflexors not recognized preoperatively. EMG was not performed. Complications included knee-flexion weakness when hamstring release was done subsequently and also calcaneal gait.

Combined Tendo-Achilles Lengthening and Strayer Procedure

Craig and Van Vuran were dissatisfied with the results of lengthening procedures of the tendo-Achilles in the reports above.[6] Using metal markers, they confirmed their impression that the gastrocnemius could only be adequately released by a Strayer-type procedure and not by tendo-Achilles lengthening. If the Silfverskiöld test were positive, combined tendo-Achilles lengthening and Strayer procedure were performed. If the test was negative, it implied contracture of the soleus, and the treatment chosen was tendo-Achilles lengthening. There were 9 recurrences in 100 cases. Postoperatively, the forefoot was kept in 40 degrees of dorsiflexion and was in a long-leg cast for 3 wk, followed by a short-leg walking cast for 3 wk and then by a fore-foot hyperextension boot. Their success rate was said to be attributable to neurodevelopmental techniques used postoperatively. Recurrence was attributable to a strong withdrawal reflex masked before surgery by action of a posiive support reflex.

Forward Translocation of Tendo-Achilles

In forward translocation of the tendo-Achilles, the insertion of the tendo-Achilles is translocated from the dorsal tuberosity of calcaneus to the calcaneal margin of the subtalar joint—about a 2.5-cm anterior advancement.[24] Biomechanically, this results in diminution of 50 percent of equinus directed force but only 15 percent decrease of push-off. Indication for this procedure was a dynamic equinus with less than 15 degrees of fixed equinus. It was applied to predominately spastic patients, since tension athetosis

was a relative contraindication. Ninety percent satisfactory results were obtained in 79 procedures in 48 patients. Postoperative care consisted of a short-leg walking cast for six weeks followed by a short-leg brace for six months. Failures were chiefly due to technical difficulties. Objections to this procedure in this study were that it is a much more involved procedure than simple heel-cord lengthening without necessarily better results, and the follow-up period of one to four years was too short.

DETERMINANTS OF SUCCESS

Much is unknown about spastic equinus deformity in cerebral palsy. Lack of true knowledge about its essential pathophysiology and pathoanatomy breeds controversies in all its aspects. Treatment is empirical, and some procedures appear to give conflicting results of success and failure in various studies.

Perhaps it is not the specific type of treatment that is the key determinant of success, but other less-stressed considerations such as patient selection and the nature of the underlying pathophysiology. Truscelli's conclusion applies in that satisfactory results in his series were not a function of the type of procedure, but appeared to be a function of pathophysiology (absence or presence of trophic muscle regulation to bone growth). As for surgical treatment, one may expect to get 70–90 percent satisfactory results no matter what operative method is used and what postoperative care is given. Although various series are difficult to compare, any given series can expect and attain at least this range of success. This target range should be achieved with the simplest and safest method.

REFERENCES

1. Banks HH: The management of spastic deformities of the foot and ankle. Clin Orthop 122:70, 1977
2. Banks HH, Green WT: The correction of equinus deformity in cerebral palsy. J Bone Joint Surg 40A:1359, 1958
3. Beals RK: Spastic paraplegia and diplegia. An evaluation of nonsurgical and surgical factors influencing the prognosis for ambulation. J Bone Joint Surg 48A:827, 1966
4. Bleck EE: Orthopaedic Management of Cerebral Palsy. Philadelphia, Saunders, 1979
5. Campbell J, Ball J: Energetics of walking in cerebral palsy. Orthop Clin North Am 9:374, 1978

6. Craig JJ, Van Vuren J: The importance of gastrocnemius recession in the correction of equinus deformity in cerebral palsy. J Bone Joint Surg 58B:84, 1976

7. Delpech JM: Tenotomie du tendon d'Achille. Chirurgie clinique de Montepellier, ou observations et reflexions tirees de travaux de chirurgie clinique de cette ecole. Paris, Gabon, 1823

8. Fasano VA, Broggi G, Barolat-Romani G, et al: Surgical treatment of spasticity in cerebral palsy. Child's Brain 4:289, 1978

9. Gunsolos P, Welsh C, Houser C: Equilibrium reactions in the feet of children with spastic cerebral palsy and of normal children. Dev Med Child Neurol 17:580, 1975

10. Holt KS: Facts and fallacies about neuromuscular function in cerebral palsy as revealed by electromyography. Dev Med Child Neurol 8:255, 1966

11. Ingram AJ: Miscellaneous affections of the nervous system, in Crenshaw AH (ed): Campbell's Operative Orthopaedics (ed 6). St. Louis, Mosby, 1980, p 1567

12. Joynt RL, Leonard Jr JA: Dantolene sodium suspension in treatment of spastic cerebral palsy. Dev Med Child Neurol 22:755, 1980

13. Penn RD, Gottlieb GL, Agarwal GC: Cerebellar stimulation in man. Quantitative changes in spasticity. J Neurosurg 48:779, 1978

14. Perry J, Hoffer MM, Giovan G, et al: Gait analysis of the triceps surae in cerebral palsy. A preoperative and postoperative clinical and electromyographic study. J Bone Joint Surg 56A:511, 1974

15. Rekate HL: Personal communication

16. Sharrard WJW, Bernstein S: Equinus deformity in cerebral palsy. A comparison between elongation of tendo calcaneus and gastrocnemius. J Bone Joint Surg 54B:272, 1972

17. Silfverskiöld N: Reduction of the uncrossed two-joints muscles of the leg to one-joint muscles in spastic conditions. Acta Chir Scand 56:315, 1923–1924

18. Silver CH, Simon SD: Gastrocnemius-muscle recession (Silfverskiöld operation) for spastic equinus deformity in cerebral palsy. J Bone joint Surg 41A:1021, 1959

19. Stoffel A: The treatment of spastic contracture. Am J Orthop Surg 10:611, 1912–13

20. Strayer LM: Gastrocnemius recession. J Bone Joint Surg 40A:1019, 1958

21. Tardieu C, Tabary JC, Huet de la Tour E, et al: The relationship between sarcomere length in the soleus and tibialis anterior and the articulation angle of the tibia-calcaneum in cats during growth. J Anat 1241:581, 1977

22. Tardieu C, Tardieu P, Colbeau-Justin, JT, et al: Trophic muscle regulation in children with congenital cerebral lesions. J Neurol Sci 42:357, 1979

23. Thompson P, Grabe RP: Lengthening of the achilles tendon in cerebral paresis (abstr). J Bone Joint Surg 61B:255, 1979

24. Throop FB, DeRosa GP, Reech C, et al: Correction of equinus in cerebral palsy by the Murphy procedure of tendo calcaneus advancement: A preliminary communication. Dev Med Child Neurol 17:182, 1975

25. Truscelli D, Lespargot A, Tardieu G: Variations in the long-term results of elongation of the tendo Achilles in children with cerebral palsy. J Bone Joint Surg 61B:466, 1979

26. Vulpius O, Stoffel A: Orthopädische Operationslehre. Stuttgart, Enke, 1913, p 29

27. White JW: Torsion of the Achilles tendon. Arch Surg 46:784, 1943

Clyde L. Nash

25

Spinal Deformities

The spine is frequently the final common pathway for the expression of musculoskeletal deformity in children with cerebral palsy. Early in life, attention is naturally focused on the extremities, especially the lower extremities, as the child, family, and physician deal with the problems of attempted ambulation. As a practical matter, hip problems occur before spinal deformity, and, as a result, the spine is placed in the background while the more obvious deformities are managed. However, it is the head-trunk-pelvic complex that will ultimately become a major factor in how well an individual functions as a long-term member of society. The finest bracing and extremity surgery will not be of much assistance to the child who can neither sit nor stand in a reasonable "facing the world" attitude because of a severe spinal deformity. This chapter will deal with the nature of the spinal deformities seen in cerebral palsy and the variety of methods currently available to deal with them.

NATURAL HISTORY

Although the literature tends to be reasonably consistent on the incidence or prevalence of spinal deformities in the cerebral palsy population, global statements such as "deformities of the spine are fortunately rather uncommon in cerebral palsy; but all of the usual deformities do occur and can be formidably severe" are still being made.[1,2,4,5,8,12,14,17,20,22,23,26] Drennan et al. also point out that although standard techniques are being used, the problems have yet to be resolved. The reason for these apparent inconsistencies lies in the fact that there is a spectrum of spinal deformities, with the severe neurologically handicapped individuals having the more severe deformities.

Occurrence

The presence or absence of spinal deformities varies greatly in the population of cerebral palsied children being studied. Ambulatory patients have been reported to have as low an incidence as 6 percent, while severely disabled and institutionalized children may have as high an incidence as 64 percent.[4,20] As expected, the degree of deformity also parallels the degree of neurologic involvement. Monoplegics are infrequently involved or, if so, to a mild degree, while quadriplegics, particularly those with combined spasticity and athetosis, have a higher incidence of spinal deformity and curves of greater magnitude.[21,26]

Although there are some consistencies in the occurrence of spinal deformity, there are a great number of variables to consider. The cerebral palsy patient is frequently included in discussions of patients with neuromuscular disease. Although this is technically appropriate, the cerebral palsied patient is less apt to develop the long "C"-type curve patterns typical of those associated with major muscle weakness. If it does occur, it is often associated with generalized hypotonia and is manifested by hyperkyphosis. There are two basic types of curves: the rather typical right thoracic left lumbar curves (Fig. 25-1) and the thoracolumbar or lumbar curves (Fig. 25-2), frequently associated with pelvic obliquity and hip instability. In the former group, the onset of the deformity tends to be near the adolescent growth spurt, and the patients are usually ambulatory. In the latter group, the curve deformities often begin earlier and are asso-

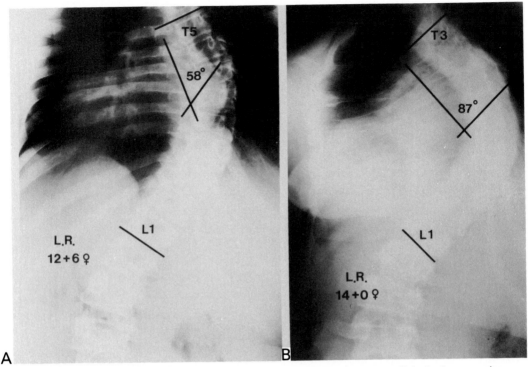

Figure 25-1. Typical right thoracic scoliosis in a young girl with spastic diplegia demonstrating progression from 58(A) to 87(B) degrees over an 18-mo period during adolescence.

ciated with nonambulation. In either case, puberty represents a threat to both groups for significant curve progression. The fact that the rate of skeletal maturation can be anywhere from normal to severely delayed requires that individuals be diagnosed early and followed well beyond the adolescent years to recognize late subtle progression of their curves. Children with associated mental retardation are more apt to have delayed growth and require continued assessment into the early adult years.

Association with Pelvic Obliquity

The question of the relationship among pelvic obliquity, scoliosis, and hip dysfunction deserves some comment. The most commonly espoused position is that progressive deformity of the spine leads to pelvic obliquity (spinopelvic deformity), which subsequently puts the hip on the high side at risk for subluxation and dislocation. Letts, however, in his recent long-term and well-documented review of 22 patients, noted that in 15 patients (68 percent), hip subluxation came first, leading to pelvic obliquity and spinal curvature (femoropelvic deformity).[13] The ad-

ductor muscles were identified as the major deforming force, with complete dislocation occurring, on the average, by seven years of age. In the patients in whom the curvature occurred first, the presence of the primitive Galant reflex was a constant finding.

Incidence

A number of factors affect the incidence and potential severity of curvatures. They can be summarized as follows:

1. Patients with spastic, athetoid, and ataxic types of cerebral palsy are all susceptible to scoliosis (15–35 percent).[17,22,24]
2. Quadriplegics have a higher incidence of scoliosis than patients with less neural damage.[25] Similarly, institutionalized patients have a higher incidence than noninstitutionalized ones.[14,15,26]
3. There is a high incidence of fixed pelvic obliquity or hip flexion contractures with scoliosis, particularly of the thoracolumbar and lumbar types.[25] These are frequently associated with hyperlumbarlordosis.

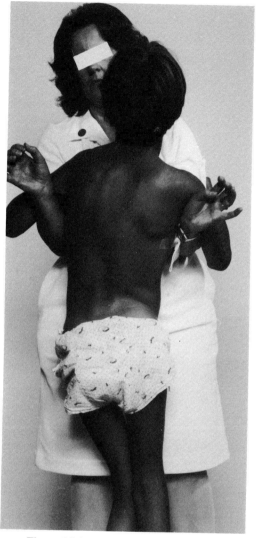

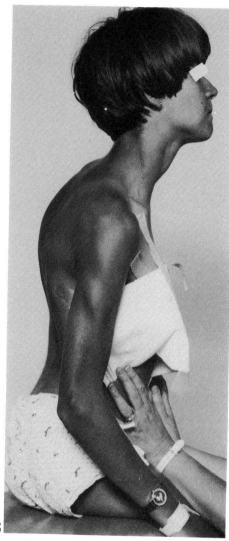

A   B

Figure 25-2. Typical sweeping left thoracolumbar curve with muscle weakness, hyperkyphosis, and potential pelvic obliquity. (A) Back view. (B) Side view.

Curve Progression

If a curvature does develop, what are the chances of its becoming severe? Riseborough and Herndon, studying a population of noninstitutionalized patients, noted that 71 percent had curves of 30 degrees or less, 19 percent had curves of 31–60 degrees, and only 10 percent had curves greater than 60 degrees (Fig. 25-3).[22] Bonnett and associates found that 42 of 294 cerebral palsy patients (14 percent) had curves greater than 30 degrees, and 33 of them (79 percent) eventually required surgery.[5] Rosenthal and associates found that only 1 of 50 mature cerebral palsy

patients screened had a curvature greater than 40 degrees, while 18 had lesser curves.[24] Lonstein, in his recent report of a series of surgical cases with cerebral palsy and significant mental retardation from a major spine center, surveyed for 31 years to collect 108 cases.[15] There was an impressive average deformity of 83 degrees, however.

It is thus important for the pediatric health care provider to be cognizant that the child with the more severe neurologic involvement has the greater chance to develop significant spinal deformity. These patients are frequently very limited in their ability to

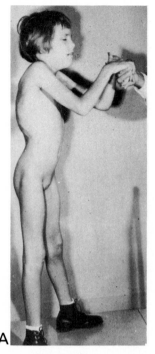
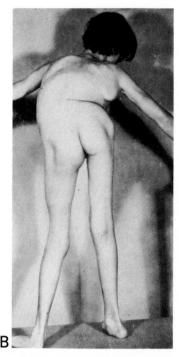
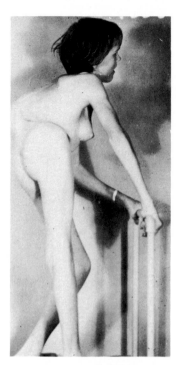

A   B

Figure 25-3. (A) This young girl has moderately severe spastic diplegia associated with moderate mental retardation. She was not followed for possible spinal deformity. (B) Ten years later she shows severe progression of her spinal deformity, affecting her balance, function, and cardiopulmonary status.

communicate and ambulate and, as a result, are apt to be ignored because of their very poor apparent rehabilitation potential. Clearly though, the presence and progression of spinal deformity with or without associated pelvic deformity reduces their level of function and social interaction. In a group where this is already limited because of mental retardation and motor dysfunction, the additional losses from spinal deformity are particularly critical.

TREATMENT

Basic Considerations

For a number of reasons, the approach to treatment of spinal deformities represents a particular challenge. Perhaps most central to any consideration is an understanding of the concepts, which, for lack of a better term, can be called *cost effectiveness*. Treatment in almost any form is expensive. Support for medical care is not unlimited, and the commitment of community resources must be balanced against the

benefits to both the patient and to society. Children with severe handicaps and mental retardation pose unique questions and evoke a wide range of moral, ethical, and very personal responses on their "worth to society."

Goals

The goals of treatment are numerous, but are all related to minimizing deformity and improving stability.

Maintenance of balance. There is an increasing recognition that the responsiveness of a mentally retarded child to the environment is affected by trunk, head, and eye posture. The inability to relate to the horizon and to the activities going on in front markedly reduces interaction with the environment. Balance, both sitting and standing, is critical not only to socialization but also to the individual's ability to be employed, albeit on a limited basis. If an individual must use the upper extremities to maintain posture, he or she cannot use them for any productive function. Conversely, in quadriplegics the upper extremities frequently cannot be used for postural support substitutes, and the ability to compensate for trunk deformity is minimal.

Pain. There are varying reports on the degree to which pain is a problem in cerebral palsy patients. Pain pathways are maintained, and, although the patient's recognition of pain may be altered, the incidence of pain increases as the deformity increases. Pelvic obliquity and hip dislocation are both sources of pain, particularly in the sitting patient. Several authors have reported incidences of back pain up to 52 percent in patients undergoing surgical correction.[5] Aside from the pelvic pain, degenerative osteoarthritis can be produced from long-standing deformity, which, in turn, causes postural deformity and eventually postural pain. Patients with athetoid involvement are particularly prone to this entity and more apt to develop degenerative osteoarthritic changes earlier, possibly because of their increased motion in the deformed position.

Hygiene. Pelvic posture, hip alignment, and hip function play an important role in the care of these patients. Since a large number of these patients will require lifetime support care, the ease with which perineal hygiene can be maintained is an important consideration. As noted above, control of trunk alignment bears directly on this matter and is an important factor in deciding on the need for treatment.

Pressure ulcers. Patients with cerebral palsy have sensory input and can perceive pain; however, there are a number of reasons why responses to the stimuli may not be normal, and areas of increased pressure can lead to ulcers. Frequently, trunk and pelvic deformity gives the patient no choice but to bear weight on an ischial tuberosity or greater trochanter unilaterally. The curvatures are rigid, and the patient's ability, first to perceive the pain input correctly and second to respond appropriately, can be markedly impaired, especially if he or she is severely mentally retarded. Upper-extremity involvement makes purposeful changes of position difficult, and spasticity and athetosis add shear components to the pressure phenomena. Although the cerebral palsy patient is not as susceptible to skin breakdown as a meningomyelocele patient, rigid deformities and inappropriate neural responses combine to make pressure sores a potential problem. This is true not only for the pelvis but also for the trunk when external spinal supports are applied.

Cardiopulmonary function. Severe deformity will adversely affect cardiopulmonary function in this group of patients, just as it will in any other patients with major spinal abnormalities. These patients will be more prone to intermittent infections and frequently will require additional institutional care to manage these episodes. These problems can eventually lead to a shortened life span.

Orthotic Management

To brace or not to brace has been a traditional discussion in the care of cerebral palsy patients.[1,3,7,12,17,18,20,22] Attempts at the effective application of orthotics share the same frustrating aspects as other care programs (Fig. 25-4). Only recently have there been reports in the literature indicating limited efficacy to this approach (Fig. 25-5).[18] The goals of bracing are the same for these patients as for those in any other group of children with spinal deformity, namely, minimization of deformity during growth either to avoid the need for surgery altogether or to permit surgery to be delayed and carried out at a more appropriate time.

The initial question is usually whether the child will tolerate the bracing process. The generally held view that bracing cannot be tolerated and is therefore ineffective has not been supported by the recent literature. Actually, reports of brace failure due to patient intolerance show that this occurs in a small percentage of total patients braced. Although there are no absolute contraindications, patients with poorly controlled hyperactivity, severe mental retardation, and pronounced hypotonicity are increased risks. Deformities greater than 50 degrees, particularly if they are rigid, will not respond to treatment any more than those would in a non-cerebral-palsy patient.

Types of Orthoses

Three basic forms of orthotics can be employed: (1) cervical–thoracic–lumbar spinal orthosis (CTLSO), or Milwaukee type, (2) thoracic–lumbar spinal orthosis (TLSO), or total-contact orthosis, and (3) the cervical–thoracic–lumbar spinal and hip orthosis (CTLSHO), or in-chair orthosis.

CTLSO. Curves in the mid- and upper thoracic area, particularly those associated with increased kyphosis, are best managed with the CTLSO. Fortunately, these comprise 15–20 percent of the deformities and are not the majority of cases.[7,18,20] The modified Boston brace with a superstructure can also be used because of its pelvic control. These patients

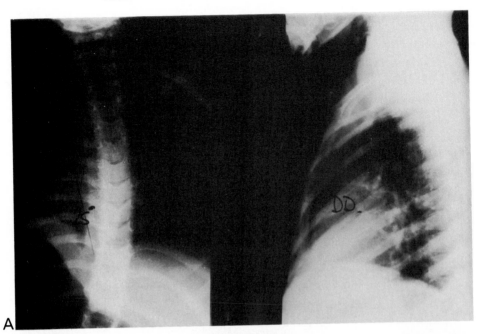

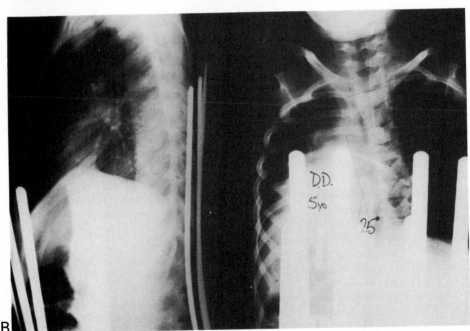

Figure 25-4. (A) Early radiographs of a child aged 5 yr showing a long, sweeping, 25-dereee right thoracic curve. (B) Attempts at bracing were made using an inadequate low total contact orthosis. (C) More appropriate bracing using a CTLSO did not prevent significant progression because of advanced deformity at 12 yr of age. (D) Progression continued with severe complications. Early appropriate bracing and surgical intervention could have prevented this severe deformity.

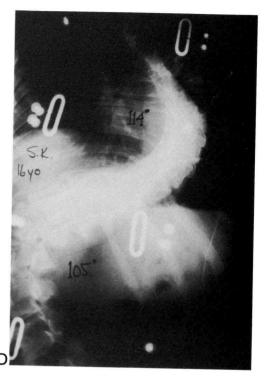

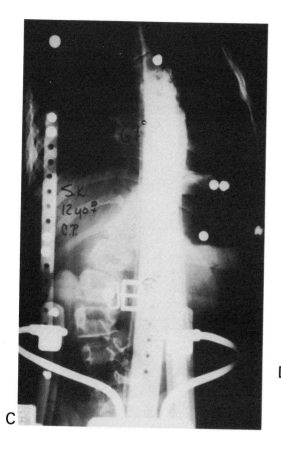

C

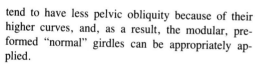

tend to have less pelvic obliquity because of their higher curves, and, as a result, the modular, preformed "normal" girdles can be appropriately applied.

TLSO. The TLSO provides the most effective approach for a number of reasons. First, the majority of curves are either thoracolumbar or lumbar with apecies below the eighth thoracic vertebrae. Second, they provide a broader area of contact with lower area pressure in each unit. The patients may require a general anesthetic in order to obtain an accurate body mold from which a custom orthosis can be fabricated (Fig. 25-6), however. This can be true for any of the orthotics used.

CTLSHO. Children with poor trunk control frequently have problems that cannot be managed with the CTLSO or TLSO. This is particularly true of those with pelvic obliquity, hip deformities, and poor head control. Maintenance of hip abduction and alignment can be a critical factor that requires positioning of the lower extremities as part of the or-

thotics. Also, this form of bracing can support the trunk to free the upper extremities for use.

A variety of seat designs and materials are being developed to not only support the child but also to help manage pressure areas due to fixed deformities. One of the more specialized forms of this orthosis is the suspension type developed at Newington Children's Hospital.[8] The trunk area is contoured to provide graduated distribution of pressure to reduce the sacral weight bearing. With proper care, it can be used for prolonged periods in patients who are unable to carry out effective weight shifts and decubitis prevention.

Results of Bracing

Despite the traditional pessimism on the efficacy of bracing, several reports in the literature indicate that modest goals can be achieved. In 1977, Bunnell and MacEwen reported that 38 of 41 patients had arrest of progression over an average 26-mo follow-up period.[7] Molded orthoplast jackets were used 23 hr a day with very few complications. The usual relative contraindications were skeletal maturity, high thoracic apex, and deformity beyond 50 degrees. McMaster and Clayton studied 20 institutionalized patients who were treated an average of 24 mo in a

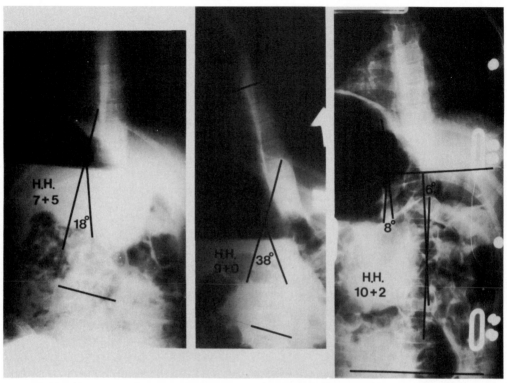

Figure 25-5. Early progression of a right lumbar curve that was flexible and controlled in a TLSO.

Boston brace with or without superstructure.[18] The traditional indications for bracing were used, but the superstructure and throat mold were avoided in patients with poor head control and in nonambulators. Initial curves averaged 42.5 degrees (30–60 degrees), with the final follow-up curves averaging 31 degrees in the brace (10–57 degrees). Problems were minor, with the most common being poor or limited application because of lack of institutional personnel cooperation. Despite this, the authors felt that the use of braces in this difficult group of patients was very worthwhile. It has been my experience that patients and family do much better if the brace training and break-in are done in the hospital, where skin care, positioning, and brace tolerance can be closely monitored by skilled personnel. If the child is from an institution, one or two key personnel should be encouraged to participate in this early training period in order to encourage dedication to long-term maintenance of the program. Without this detailed early training, successful bracing cannot reasonably be expected to occur.

Indications and Recommendations

It is apparent that there is a place for orthotics in the treatment of spinal deformity in cerebral palsy. The following summarizes my experience to date:

1. Orthotics ideally must be applied early in curves less than 30 degrees with documented progression. Early detection is therefore necessary.
2. The total contact type of bracing is particularly effective, except where excessive rotation or pelvic obliquity fixed from below (femoropelvic) exist. The Boston module can be difficult to fit in the more severe curves and may not be tolerated because of the marked anterior–posterior molding.
3. Milwaukee braces and superstructures are needed in high thoracic or hyperkyphotic curves but are best tolerated in ambulatory patients with adequate head control.
4. Orthotics can arrest progression of deformities and therefore delay or possibly prevent the need for surgery. If surgery is subsequently required, post-

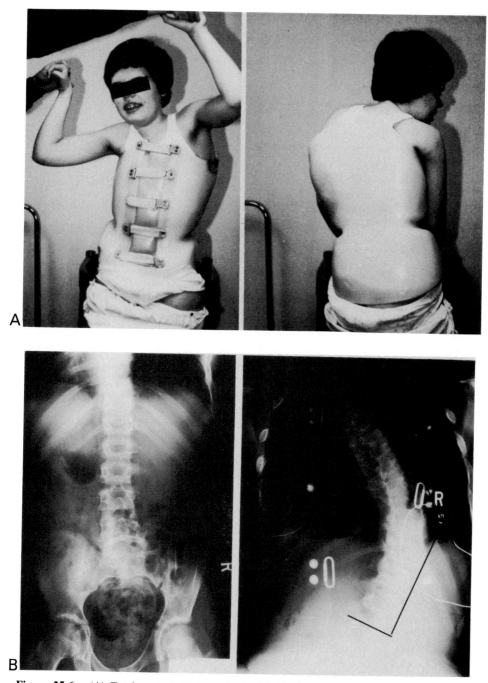

Figure 25-6. (A) Total contact plastic orthosis (TLSO) in a mentally retarded child with late progression of a right thoracolumbar scoliosis. (B) Anteroposterior radiographs demonstrating significant progression of spinal deformity.

operative immobilization will be facilitated because the patient has become accustomed to constraining devices.

5. In many cases, the individually molded orthosis is the only one that can be fitted. This includes the use of in-chair devices, which can be used to control hip adduction and pelvic obliquity as well.

6. Regardless of the type of orthosis, effective ongoing family or institutional care will be needed in order to ensure that the brace is worn for adequate periods and that potential problems are minimized. Without this support, bracing should not be undertaken. Hospital admission for initial brace adjustment and training can be very helpful and should be arranged if at all possible.

7. The early and effective application of bracing has a well-defined cost benefit in terms of the savings if surgery can be avoided or done under conditions of reduced risk of complications. Also, since most patients live for many years, minimization of deformity will require less attendant care over a long period.

Surgical Management

Indications

Under the best of circumstances, a significant number of cerebral palsy patients will need surgical spinal stabilization. A number of authors report series of spinal fusion patients with the clear recognition that this is a difficult group of patients with a high complication rate.[3,6,9,15,16,21,27] It is not always clear from these studies what the incidence is of cerebral palsy children who will need surgery, however. Bonnett and associates, as stated previously, found that 33 of 42 cerebral palsy patients (79 percent) with curves greater than 30 degrees eventually required surgery.[5] Other series report that 2–29 percent of spastic scoliosis patients need surgery.[22,27] Obviously, the distribution of the patient population and the vigor with which early detection and treatment are carried out will affect the statistics.

The indications for surgery, and consequently the cost–benefit analysis, are in many ways different from those of the idiopathic adolescent with scoliosis. Maintenance of function and the prevention of pain and pelvic deformity all play an important role in the cerebral palsy patient.

Balance. Maintenance or restoration of antigravity balance for standing or sitting is extremely important in order to maximize independent function. Loss of spinal balance can be due to lateral, anterior–posterior, or rotational deformities, pelvic obliquity, or hip soft-tissue contractures.

Pain. Back and pelvic pain have been reported in as many as 52 percent of patients undergoing surgery.[5] The sources of pain can be spine, rib–pelvis impingement, hip dysfunction, or decubitus pressure areas.

Curve progression. The progression of spinal deformity, particularly into or beyond the 30–40 degree range in a skeletally immature patient, has been increasingly cited as reason for surgery before the deformities become excessive. Deformities beyond 50 degrees are generally considered amenable only to surgical treatment.

Cardiopulmonary compromise. Cardiopulmonary compromise has been cited both as an indication and as a contraindication for surgery depending on its severity. In cases of late, severe deformity the risks of major surgery (frequently multiple surgeries) in the face of heart and lung dysfunction far outweigh any benefits to be derived. It must be remembered that spinal surgery does not reverse cardiopulmonary deficits to any great extent.[19] Therefore, preventive concepts are more important and support the need for early intervention and stabilization of spinal deformity. Also, it must be noted that measurement of cardiopulmonary function can be very difficult in this group of patients because of their poor cooperation. Early, mild changes may not be detectable, and therefore surgery is most effective in preventing future problems rather than in correcting deficits.

Freedom from bracing. Freedom from bracing can be a very desirable objective, especially in those patients requiring long-term institutionalization. Bracing is frequently a source of irritation to hospital personnel, and the brace can be a source of repeated pressure sores if inappropriately applied.

•   •   •

It should be noted that these possible indications for surgery are made independent of whether mental retardation is present. The intellectually brighter and physically more independent patients have more to lose if deformities are not controlled, but the goals are valid even for the severely handicapped child.

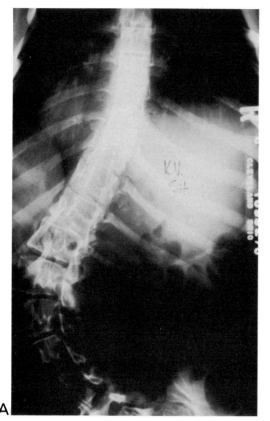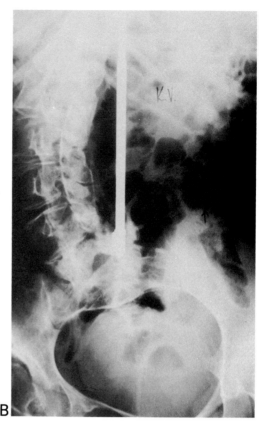

A   B

Figure 25-7. (A) Sitting anteroposterior radiograph of a severe left thoracolumbar scoliosis with pelvic obliquity. (B) Inadequate fixation with a single Harrington distraction rod. Multiple pseudoarthroses are present.

Surgical Techniques

The selection of an effective operative plan can be difficult in these patients because of the number of variables to be considered. The type of cerebral palsy (spastic, athetoid, or ataxic), severity of the deformity, presence of associated hip and pelvic deformity, mental retardation, and variety of instrumentation systems available are all important factors. Reviewing the literature, it is apparent that there are two consistent recommendations for surgical techniques:

1. Patients with single thoracic or double thoracic–lumbar curves with good compensation do well with posterior spinal fusion alone, particularly if it is done before the deformity becomes too severe (greater than 60 degrees). Corrections in the range of 40 percent, with pseudoarthrosis of 7–15 percent, can be expected.[6,15,21]

2. Patients with thoracolumbar or lumbar curves, particularly those associated with pelvic obliquity and hyperlordosis, require both anterior and posterior spinal fusions. With posterior surgery alone, pseudoarthrosis rates run 28–50 percent, while combined procedures reduce this complication to 0–18 percent.[5,6,15,21] Also, the correction obtained is increased to 50–60 percent.

Instrumentation

Systems for correcting spinal deformity continue to evolve. With this has come more flexibility of design, ease of application, and increased points of fixation. The unique biomechanical problems posed by the cerebral palsy spine all point to the need for instrumentation that is adaptable to a variety of deformities, strong, and, most of all, capable of spreading the load over a wide area of bone–instrument contacts. The more points of fixation, the more effectively the loads are distributed.

Posterior. The single Harrington distraction device will prove to be inadequate in most instances, unless it is used early in well-compensated thoracic or thoracic–lumbar curves (Fig. 25-7). Augmentation with a multisite compression system will help greatly, especially if transverse loading systems are also employed (Fig. 25-8). The recently introduced Luque system of segmental spinal instrumentation fulfills many of the criteria (Fig. 25-9).[11] The implants are quite strong, adaptable to deformity, and have multiple sites of load sharing. There are no reports as yet of such a series to document the effectiveness and complications of this approach, however.

Anterior. The Dwyer, and more recently the Zielke, forms of instrumentation are anterior systems that employ multiple sites of fixation.[10] For this reason, they add a great deal of spinal stabilization to these patients. The Dwyer system is more adaptable in spinal deformities, since its cable is flexible. The Zielke system, however, with its use of a rod rather than a cable, can be a more powerful tool for correction of deformity and is stable in more planes of motion. Both systems are not appropriate for kyphotic deformities. In these cases, anterior surgery with multiple discectomy and release of the anterior longitudinal ligament and interbody bone grafting followed by posterior instrumentation is indicated.

Bone Grafting

As in any spine stabilization procedure, long-term success directly depends on the establishment of a solid fusion mass. Unfortunately, these patients are frequently frail with reduced bone stock, not only for instrument fixation but also for bone grafting. The posterior iliac crest, including both sides, may be insufficient. These patients are frequently limited walkers or nonambulators, however, and the tibia and fibula can be used as donor sites with impunity. Supplementation with allograft bone can be quite helpful, since these patients are generally young, and incorporation of these grafts is somewhat better. This is particularly true of the anterior, interbody fusions where large cancellous surfaces are available.

Complications

Spinal surgery in cerebral palsy patients is fraught with problems even under the best of circumstances.

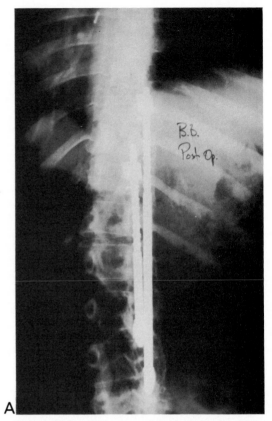

A

Figure 25-8. Three examples (A to C) of multiple posterior instrumentation including segmental wiring.

Death. Lonstein reported a 3 percent death rate in a series of severely handicapped patients.[15]

Pseudoarthrosis. Depending on the series, surgical techniques, and patient type, the rate of pseudoarthrosis can reach 52 percent. In general, rates of 15–25 percent can be anticipated. Because of the close relationship between correction and function, pseudoarthrosis will frequently need to be repaired surgically in order to achieve the original goals.

Pressure ulcerations. Pressure ulcerations may occur in up to 30 percent of patients. Even if there is no detectable decrease in pain awareness, rigidity of deformity and inappropriate muscle control and activity predispose to intolerable pressure and shear forces. Strong internal devices, removable orthosis, and well-padded and contoured casts will help minimize these risks.

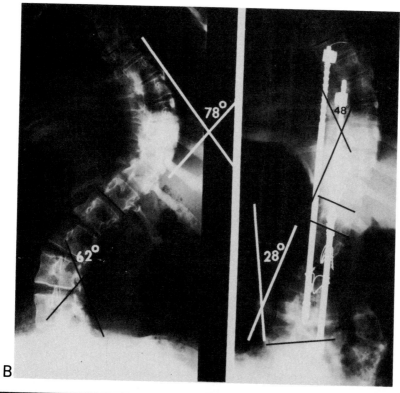

B

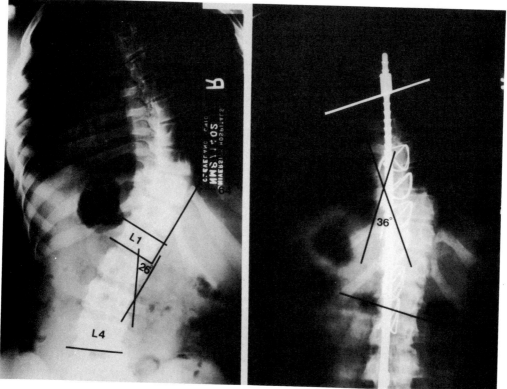

C

269

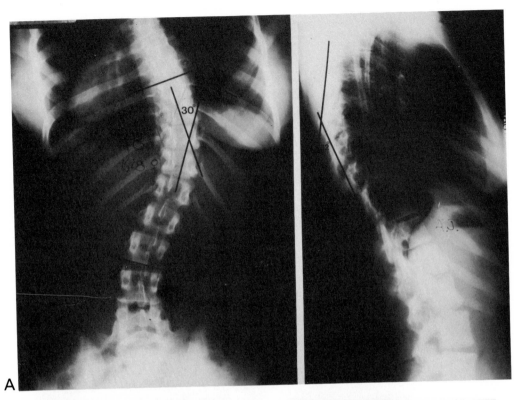

A

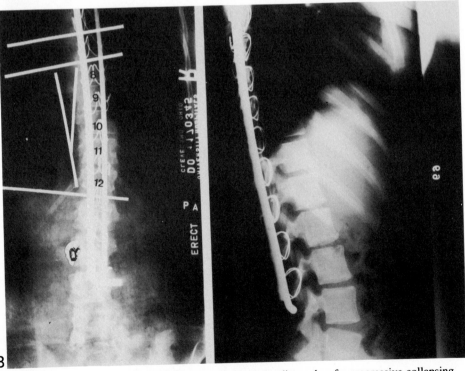

B

Figure 25-9. (A) Preoperative anteroposterior and lateral radiographs of a progressive collapsing spine in a girl aged 16 yr with cerebral palsy. (B) Postoperative radiographs of a Luque segmental spine instrumentation and posterior fusion.

Instrument failure. Asymmetric muscle forces, rigidity, cyclic loading, severe deformity, and poor bone stock all predispose these patients to instrument failure. This occurs in approximately 25 percent of patients and can occur at the bone–metal interface or in the implant itself, particularly if there is associated pseudoarthrosis.

Infection. Infection is increased modestly, in the range of .5 percent. Antibiotics and aseptic, meticulous surgical techniques are the key to keeping infection to a minimum.

Miscellaneous. A variety of other problems can be encountered, including paralysis (less than 1 percent), nontolerance of support devices, and late progression of deformity.

Contraindications

The only true contraindication to spinal surgery is severe cardiopulmonary compromise coupled with marked spinal deformity that is amenable to major reconstructive surgery (or surgeries); extensive postoperative immobilization makes the risks too high for the minimal benefits to be derived.

Self-abusive or hyperactive behavior to the extent that spinal immobilization techniques cannot be tolerated will generally jeopardize the chances for successful surgery. As noted above, the child who can tolerate a brace will tolerate postoperative support. In the child in whom there has been no preoperative bracing, a preoperative trial of cast application can be very helpful in determining ability to tolerate rigid immobilization. Even if a general anesthetic is needed to apply the cast, these patients will frequently surprise everyone with their tolerance of controlling devices. This preoperative test can be very helpful in deciding whether surgery is indicated.

REFERENCES

1. Balmer GA, MacEwen GD: The incidence and treatment of scoliosis in cerebral palsy. J Bone Joint Surg 52B:134, 1970
2. Bleck EE: Deformities of the spine and pelvis in cerebral palsy, in Samilson RL (ed): Orthopaedic Aspects of Cerebral Palsy. Philadelphia, Lippincott, 1975, p 124
3. Bradford DS, Moe JJ, Winter RB: Scoliosis, in Rothman RH, Simeone FA (eds): The Spine, vol. 1. Philadelphia, Saunders, 1975, pp 340–341
4. Bonnett C, Brown JC, Perry J, et al: The evolution of treatment of paralytic scoliosis at Rancho Los Amigos Hospital. J Bone Joint Surg 51A:206, 1975
5. Bonnett C, Brown JC, Grow T: Thoracolumbar scoliosis in cerebral palsy. J Bone Joint Surg 58A:328, 1976
6. Brown JC, Swank SM, Specht L: Combined anterior and posterior spine fusion in cerebral palsy (abstr). Presented at the Scoliosis Research Society, 16th annual meeting, 1981
7. Bunnell WP, MacEwen GD: Non-operative treatment of scoliosis in cerebral palsy: Preliminary report on the use of a plastic jacket. Dev Med Child Neurol 19:45, 1977
8. Drennan JC, Renshaw TC, Curtis BH: The thoracic suspension orthosis. Clin Orthop 139:33, 1979
9. Duckworth T: The surgical management of cerebral palsy. Prosthet Orthot 1:96, 1977
10. Dwyer AF: Experience of anterior correction of scoliosis. Clin Orthop 93:191, 1973
11. Ferguson RL, Allen BL: Segmental spinal instrumentation for routine scoliotic curve. Contemp Orthop 2:450, 1980
12. Fisk JR, Bunch WH: Scoliosis in neuromuscular disease. Orthop Clin North Am 10:863, 1979
13. Letts RM, Turenka S, Klasser O, et al: Windswept hip phenomenon and scoliosis in cerebral palsy (abstr). Presented at the Scoliosis Research Society, 15th annual meeting, 1980
14. Lonstein JE: Deformities of the spine in children with cerebral palsy. Orthop Rev 10:33, 1981
15. Lonstein JE, Akbarnia BA: Operative treatment of spine deformities in patients with cerebral palsy and mental retardation (abstr). Presented at the Scoliosis Research Society, 16th annual meeting, 1981
16. MacEwen GD: Operative treatment of scoliosis in cerebral palsy. Reconstr Surg Traumatol 13:58, 1972
17. MacEwen GD: Cerebral palsy and scoliosis, in Hardy JH (ed): Spinal Deformity in Neurological and Muscular Disorders. St. Louis, Mosby, 1974, pp 191–199
18. McMaster WC, Clayton K: Spinal bracing in the institutionalized person with scoliosis. Spine 5:459, 1980
19. Makley JT, Herndon CH, Inkley S, et al: Pulmonary function in paralytic and nonparalytic scoliosis before and after treatment. J Bone Joint Surg 50A:1379, 1968
20. Mital MA, Beklin SC, Sullivan RA: An approach to head, neck, and trunk stabilization and control in cerebral palsy by use of the Milwaukee brace. Dev Med Child Neurol 18:198, 1976
21. Molloy MK, Kuhlmann RF: Severe mental retardation, scoliosis, and spinal fusion (abstr). Presented at the Scoliosis Research Society, 16th annual meeting, 1981
22. Riseborough EJ, Herndon JH: Scoliosis associated with neuromuscular diseases, in EJ Riseborough and JH Herndon (eds): Scoliosis and Other Deformities of the Axial Skeleton. Boston, Little, Brown, and Co., 1975, pp 222–223

23. Robson P: The prevalence of scoliosis in adolescents and young adults with cerebral palsy. Dev Med Child Neurol 10:447, 1968

24. Rosenthal RK, Levine DB, McCarver CL: The occurrence of scoliosis in cerebral palsy. Dev Med Child Neurol 16:664, 1974

25. Samilson RL: Orthopaedic surgery of the hips and spine in retarded cerebral palsy patients. Orthop Clin North Am 12:183, 1981

26. Samilson RL, Richard R: Scoliosis in cerebral palsy: Incidence, distribution of curve patterns, natural history, and thoughts on etiology. Curr Pract Orthop Surg 5:183, 1973

27. Stanitski CL, Micheli LJ, Hall JE, et al: Surgery for spinal deformity in cerebral palsy (abstr). Presented at the Scoliosis Research Society, 15th annual meeting, 1980

Harold Rekate

26

Neurosurgical Aspects

The role of the neurosurgeon in the comprehensive management of children with cerebral palsy has been limited in the past but now, with the advent of neurostimulation and other neurosurgical procedures to modify spasticity, there has been renewed participation. Neurosurgical consultation should therefore be considered for disabled children, especially those with spastic diplegia and a moderate or higher level of intellectual function, since they will receive the greatest benefits in prevention of musculoskeletal deformities, maximization of ambulatory ability, and enhancement of mental development.

ANATOMY AND PHYSIOLOGY

Voluntary movement, such as the grasping of an object or walking, is the result of a complex interaction of fasciatory and inhibitory stimuli acting on the anterior horn cells in the anterior gray matter of the spinal cord. This is the "final common pathway" of the motor system (Fig. 26-1). The efferent neurons from the anterior horn cells stimulate contraction of skeletal muscle. The movement thus effected is superimposed on the resting tone of the muscle innervated. The resting tone of the muscle is likewise under central nervous system (CNS) control through gamma efferent fibers.[14] *Cerebral palsy* is a general term for perinatal injury to areas of the motor system, interfering with the fine performance of voluntary coordinated movements.[1]

The pathology and pathophysiology of cerebral palsy are diffuse. Various descriptive terms such as *ulegyria* or *focal narrowing of the cortical gyri* and *status marmoratus*, a marbled appearance of the basal ganglia, are used to describe the gross pathology.[4,16] The major areas of involvement of the brain leading to the motor abnormalities that are regarded as cerebral palsy occur in the basal ganglia, thalamus, and cerebellum, although the cerebral hemispheres and brain stem are not necessarily spared.

Disorders of motor function that are included in the general complex referred to as cerebral palsy can be divided into two distinct categories. In the first, the major disability lies in the abnormality of resting tone and includes spasticity and rigidity. Spasticity is an extremely complex abnormality involving markedly increased resting muscular tone with a marked increase in deep tendon reflex activity and alternating facilitation of antagonistic muscle groups, leading to clonus.[24] Spasticity is usually associated with lesions of the corticospinal tract and may occur anywhere in this tract from the precentral gyrus to the lateral and anterior columns of the spinal cord. Spasticity tends to involve some muscle groups more than others. In the upper extremities the flexor groups are more affected, and in the lower extremities the extensors and adductors are more severely affected, with the exception of the hip, where flexor involvement predominates over the extensors. In rigidity, as in spasticity, the resting tone of muscles is increased but, in contrast, the reflexes are diminished or absent and there is no clonus. Rigidity is often associated with lesions of the basal ganglia and occurs with other extrapyramidal movement disorders. Flaccidity, which is lack of normal resting tone, will not be discussed here because it is not a symptom of CNS disease.

The second category of motor disturbance in cerebral palsy is movement disorder with normal resting tone. This form of movement disorder may be as

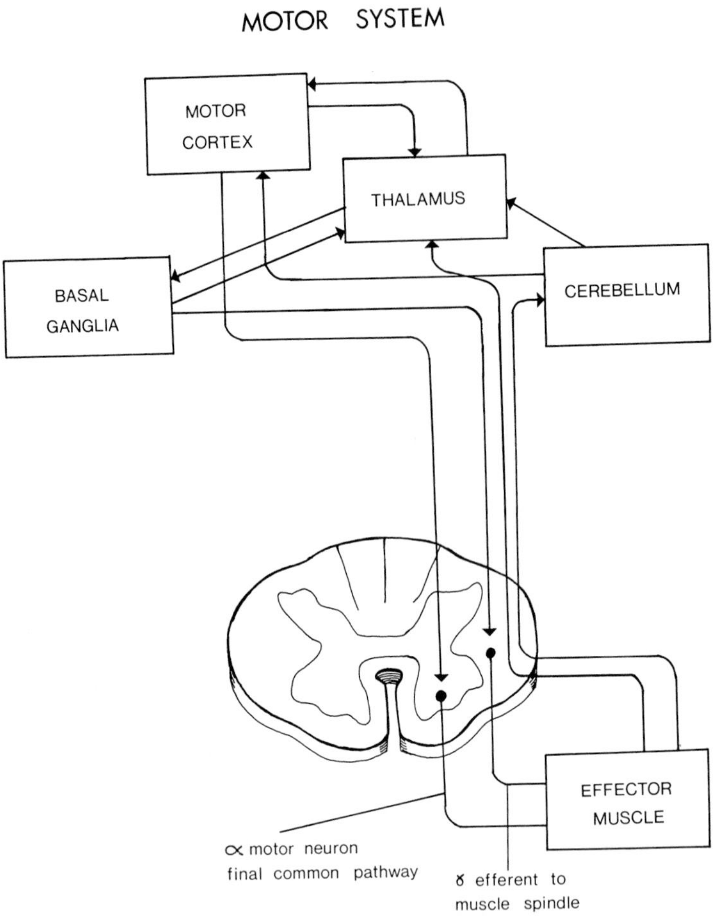

MOTOR SYSTEM

Figure 26-1.   Diagram of the neuroanatomy of the motor system demonstrating the complex interactions of facilitory and inhibitory mechanisms that lead to smooth coordinated movements.

devastating to the patient's functional level as spasticity or rigidity but tends to disappear in sleep. Generally, it is secondary to lesions in the basal ganglia (striatum or pallidum) but can be due to lesions in the subthalamic nucleus (hemiballismus), substantia nigra, red nucleus, or cerebellum and its central connections. Included in this category are chorea—wild jerky forcible rapid movements, athetosis—uncontrolled slow sinuous motor activity, dystonia—maintenance over time of an athetoid position in its extreme, and incoordination—due to damage to the cerebellum.[19]

This catagorization of abnormalities of movement into abnormalities of resting tone and active movement is extremely important in deciding among the multiple neurosurgical modalities available to treat

these problems. Although occasionally these conditions exist in the same child with cerebral palsy, it is usually evident which of the problems has led to the most serious disability. Although some neurosurgical procedures are purported to help both the spasticity and the extrapyramidal movement disorders, most neurosurgical intervention in the functioning of the motor system affects either resting tone or movement disorders.

**NEUROSURGICAL PROCEDURES
IN CEREBRAL PALSY**

The various neurosurgical procedures in cerebral palsy can be divided into two parts: ablative surgery

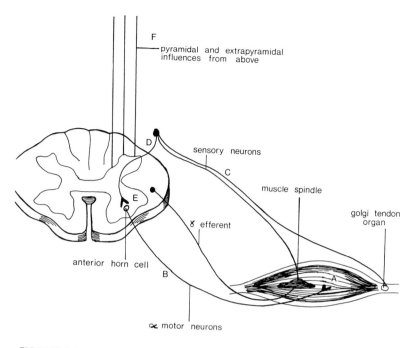

TARGETS FOR ABLATION TO RELIEVE SPASTICITY

A. MUSCLE OR TENDON

B. MOTOR NEURON EITHER AT ROOT LEVEL
     OR PERIPHERAL NERVE

C. SENSORY NERVE

D. POSTERIOR ROOT

E. DISCONNECTION WITHIN CORD

F. MODIFICATION OF SUPRASEGMENTAL INFLUENCES

Figure 26-2. Targets for ablation to relieve spasticity. These are based on the concept that spasticity is related to increased resting tone of the deep tendon reflex.

and neural stimulation as it relates to the motor system. The history, rationale, and, as much as possible, the results of these procedures should be familiar to physicians caring for disabled children.

Ablative Procedures

The precise nature and cause of spasticity is unclear, but its sine qua non clinically is the abnormally active monosynaptic deep tendon reflex. Landau has postulated the lowering of the threshold for firing of motor neurons to asynchronous low-level excitation of spindle receptors due to lesions of the upper motor neurons as the physiologic basis of spasticity.[24] In both experimental animals and humans it has been shown that spasticity can be ablated by the

disruption of the monosynaptic circuit in the deep tendon reflex. It is this disruption of the monosynaptic deep tendon reflex that forms the basis of most ablative procedures for the relief of spasticity, and it can be accomplished at any point in the reflex arc (Fig. 26-2).[10–13,17,18,23,28–30,46] The most peripheral forms of this concept, sectioning of peripheral nerves and lysis of effector organs (skeletal muscles), fit into the schema but are not considered in this discussion.

Clearly, spasticity can be relieved by sectioning of the anterior roots of the spinal cord or of the motor nerves.[30] The effects of such procedures are unsatisfactory in patients with cerebral palsy even when there is no motor power in the involved muscles. The resulting flaccidity leads to marked reduction in muscle mass and predisposes to ankylosis of joints and

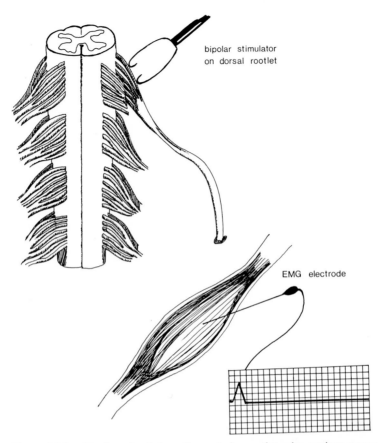

bipolar stimulator
on dorsal rootlet

EMG electrode

Figure 26-3.   Bipolar stimulation of a posterior rootlet using various parameters of stimulation allows differentiation of two populations of rootlets for
selective section.

decubiti. If motor function is retained in a spastic
extremity even though functionless secondary to the
spasticity, all hope for usefulness of the extremity is
lost. In 1908, Forster demonstrated relief of spasticity
without total muscular flaccidity by sectioning the
dorsal or sensory roots.[12] Forster's procedure did,
however, have its disadvantages as well because of
the lack of sensation and particularly because of the
loss of position sense, which prevented the functional
use of the extremity. Several modifications of posterior rootlet section have been advanced. Gros has
recommended the salvage of only one or two rootlets
in each root, and Guidetti and Fraioli feel that it is
better to hemisection all the nerve roots in an attempt
to preserve sensation.[17,18] In each case, results have
been encouraging and the degree of sensory loss surprisingly little.

   Fasano et al. reported on a technique that they
call functional posterior rhizotomy; it represents an
attempt to demonstrate abnormal interconnections
scientifically and, conversely, to spare these interconnections, which are not participating in the spasticity.[10,11] The operative technique involves the exposure of the posterior nerve rootlets from T11 to S1.
With continuous electromyographic (EMG) recording of involved musculature, each nerve rootlet is
separated and stimulated with bipolar stimulation 1
cm apart (Fig. 26-3). The rootlets are sectioned using
multiple parameters of frequency and strength, but
the rootlets that fail to suppress stimulation at high
frequency (50 Hz) are felt to be involved in the process leading to spasticity and are therefore sectioned.
Side-effects of the procedure are minimal, yielding
little or no objective sensory loss and good relief of
spasticity in a large percentage of patients. Fasano
has recommended continuous ketamine anesthesia
because of the effect of other anesthetic agents on
the EMG. Limited experience with this technique at

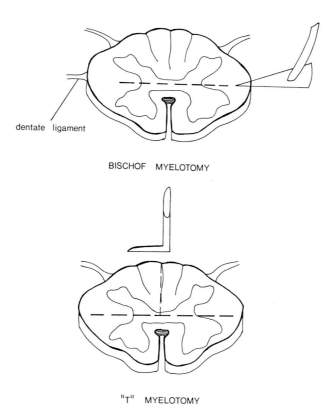

dentate ligament

BISCHOF MYELOTOMY

"T" MYELOTOMY

Figure 26-4. Spinal cord myelotomy for spasticity was first performed by Bischof and required a lateral approach and retraction of the spinal cord. The procedure was later modified to the T myelotomy, which can be performed for the midline dorsum of the spinal cord.

Rainbow Babies and Children's Hospital in Cleveland, Ohio, tends to confirm their conclusions. The patients awaken with a subjective feeling of numbness in the lower extremities but with little objective loss of pinprick sensation, voluntary motor activity is fascilitated secondary to the decreased spasticity, and pain is relieved. The subjective numbness clears with time. My experience with children with spastic diplegia clearly confirms that there are two distinctly definable populations of posterior roots separable by the effect that their stimulation had on the involved musculature by EMG recording.

The reflex arc for the deep tendon reflex may be interrupted within the substance of the spinal cord. Theoretically, such a procedure could affect resting tone without also affecting the independent functioning of either the motor or sensory system. The original description of the technique was by Bischof in 1952, and the first series was reported by Tonnis and Bischof in 1962 (Fig. 26-4).[3,42] Their technique involved the identification of the dentate ligaments laterally

and the horizontal sectioning of the cord at this level from L1 to S1 and unilaterally to S5 if spastic neurogenic bladder was a prominent part of the symptom complex. A variation of this procedure, the so-called T myelotomy, has been recommended more recently because rotation of the cord is unnecessary, and therefore this procedure is, to some extent, more likely to retain preserved motor function (see Fig. 26-4). The technique involves midline dorsal myelotomy with extensions laterally to disconnect the anterior and posterior gray matter of the spinal cord. Myelotomy has been shown to preserve motor function in the majority of the patients in whom it has been used, but at present the prime indication for the procedure is traumatic paraplegia with flexor spasms, and the procedure has limited usefulness in children with cerebral palsy.[7,23,29,46]

Ablative procedures have been recommended for spasticity whose effect is not on the reflex arc itself but on the suprasegmental influences on the reflex arc. Several authors have recommended cervical posterior rhizotomies at the C1–C3 level for the relief of spasticity in the upper extremities. Theoretically, the effect here is in the abolishing of the tonic neck reflexes. This has also been reported to benefit patients with athetosis.[2,20,22] Manipulation of suprasegmental influences can potentially modify both abnormalities of tone and motion. The posterior rhizotomy C1–C3 or its extended variant has been recommended for choreoathetosis of severe degree, and some successes have been reported. Guidetti has reported postoperative respiratory difficulty in some patients.[18]

Lesions of the deep cerebellar nuclei have been shown to lead to hypotonia as well as tremor and dysmetria. Neurosurgeons have attempted to use this information to modify movement disorders and spasticity in patients with cerebral palsy. Nashold was able to produce ipsilateral hypotonia and reduce intention tremor in five patients using a medial dentate nucleus target.[32] Guidetti reported an extensive experience using stereotaxic dentatolysis with good results in choreoathetosis and little, if any, effect on spasticity.[18] At present, too little is known about the effects of deep cerebellar nuclear ablations to determine its place in the neurosurgical armamentarium in the treatment of cerebral palsy.[40,47] Schneider has reported his experiences in the surgical removal of large areas of the cerebellum for the relief of various movement disorders, with some amelioration being obtained in some patients.[38]

The most rostral target for neurosurgical ablative surgery is the thalamus. Various targets have been proposed, including the ventralis lateralis (VL) nucleus, pulvinar, and various areas of the fields of Forel.[16,18,21,31] Substantial reductions in uncontrolled movement disorders have been obtained. Pulvinolysis has been abandoned by those with experiences with the lesion.[16,18] VL thalamotomy should be reserved for patients who are totally disabled by their constant writhing movements.[21,31] In patients with preexisting disease in the area of the thalamus and basal ganglia, there is an increase in the risk of side-effects of the procedure, including language impairment.

Neurostimulation Procedure

Chronic electrical stimulation of various areas of the CNS is, at present, the area of primary interest to neurosurgeons involved in the management of children with cerebral palsy. A substantial volume of literature, much of it contradictory, is growing about the effects of stimulation of dorsal surface of the cerebellum and the dorsal columns of the spinal cord on the motor system, and other targets for stereotaxic placement of stimulating electrodes are being evaluated. A detailed analysis of the potential physiologic mechanisms, electronics and engineering considerations, and critical review of the various studies showing or not showing efficacy is complex and will not be discussed.[26,36,37] Suffice it to say that several physiologic parameters can be modified by chronic stimulation of various areas within the CNS. The mechanisms for these modifications remain to be elucidated, but two primary theories are currently popular. The first is that direct stimulation of heavily myelinated tracts electrically modify neural pathways directly. In cerebellar stimulation this would result in an increase in the inhibitory outflow from the cerebellum to the remainder of the motor system. In the spinal cord, stimulation would result in a fascilitation of the fast proprioceptive fibers to cerebellum or thalamus. An alternative theory postulates the release of various peptide neurotransmitter substances acting on the motor system. There is some evidence for each of these theories, and each may have some element of truth.[9]

Care must be taken in the interpretation of clinical data from studies of CNS stimulation. Patients and their families desperately desire improvement in motor function, and subjective improvement without objective improvement in measurable function will not result in improvement in the patient's quality of life. Even objective change in physiologic parameters are not necessarily convincing that the procedure is effective and worthwhile. The above disclaimer notwithstanding, some patients with cerebral palsy have been benefitted to the point of a modicum of improvement in functional status by neurostimulation. The problem remains which patients with which motor abnormalities will respond to which form of neurostimulation and using which parameters of stimulation.

Chronic cerebellar stimulation, first introduced by Cooper, has been advocated for movement disorder as well as for spasticity. An array of platinum electrodes is placed by craniectomy on the medial dorsal surface of each cerebellar hemisphere, and stimulation is produced through a radiofrequency-coupled receiver in the clavicular region (Fig. 26-5). The procedure is usually performed with the patient sitting so that the cerebellar hemispheres fall away from the tentorium, facilitating the placement of the electrodes. Multiple studies of large numbers of patients have shown the effectiveness of the procedure.[6,8,25,33,34] Other careful studies have shown little or no effect.[35,45] Penn and co-workers have shown definitive ameliorating effects on rigidity but little or no effect on speech function.[34,35] Cerebellar stimulation at present is controversial and expensive, and there is little ability to select in advance patients who will respond to stimulation.[33–35]

Chronic stimulation of the dorsal columns of the spinal cord was first proposed by Shealy for relief of chronic pain based on the "gate theory" of Melzack and Wall.[27,39] Somewhat through serendipity, it was found that patients with multiple sclerosis who also had pain were relieved of some aspects of their motor disturbances.[5] This finding has also led to the study of spinal cord stimulation in numerous pathologic processes involving the motor system, including cerebral palsy. These studies have been greatly facilitated by the availability of percutaneously implantable epidural stimulating electrodes (Fig. 26-6). The procedure can be performed under local anesthesia and permits the patient to undergo a period of trial stimulation before the implantation of the expensive receiver. If there is no improvement in the condition during the period of trial stimulation, the electrodes are removed.[15,41,43,44]

Chronic dorsal column stimulation has been advocated for all motor abnormalities associated with cerebral palsy. The evidence for the effectiveness of this procedure in spasticity, especially the spasticity of spastic diplegia, is compelling. Results of this procedure in patients with choreoathetosis have been less successful using the currently available percutaneously implantable electrodes. Initial reports of experiences with stimulation at high cervical levels

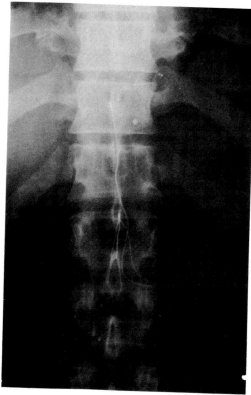

Figure 26-5. Radiograph of the lower thoracic spine showing position of epidurally placed leads for spinal cord stimulation.

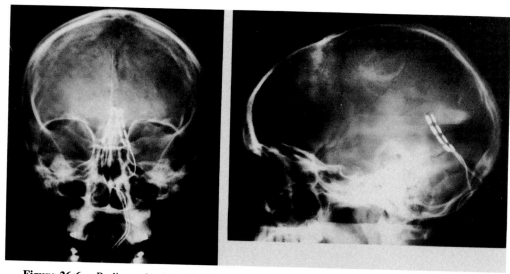

Figure 26-6. Radiograph of the skull demonstrating placement of platinum electrode array over the medial dorsal surface of the cerebellum for chronic cerebellar stimulation.

have been encouraging in patients with abnormalities of active movement.

REFERENCES

1. Adams RD, Victor M: Principles of Neurology. New York, McGraw-Hill, 1977, pp 872–876
2. Benedetti A, Carbonin C, Colombo F: Extended posterior cervical rhizotomy for severe spastic syndromes and dyskinesias. Appl Neurophysiol 40:41, 1977
3. Bischof W: Die Longitudinale Myelotomie Erstmaligzervikal durchgefuhrt. Zentralbl Neurochir 12:205, 1952
4. Blackwood W, Corsellis JAN: Greenfield's Neuropathology. Chicago, Year Book Medical Publishers, 1976, pp 423–442.
5. Cook AW, Weinstein SP: Chronic dorsal column stimulation in multiple sclerosis. NY State J Med 73:2868, 1973
6. Cooper IS, Upton ARM: Effects of cerebellar stimulation on epilepsy, the EEG and cereral palsy in man, in Cobb WA, Van Duijn H (eds): Contemporary Clinical Neurophysiology (EEG suppl 34). Amsterdam, Elsevier, 1978, pp 349–354
7. Cusick JF, Larson SJ, Sances A: The effect of T-myelotomy on spasticity. Surg Neurol 6:289, 1976
8. Davis RM, Cullen RF, Flitter MA, et al: Control of spasticity and involuntary movements. Neurosurgery 1:205, 1977
9. Dimitrijevic MR, Sherwood AM, Faganel J: Mechanisms of motor control augmentation using continuous epidural spinal cord stimulation, in International Symposium on External Control of Human Extremities, Dubrovnik, 1978. Advances in External Control of Human Extremities. Belgrade, Yugoslavia, Committee for Electronics and Automation, 1978, pp 657–663
10. Fasano VA, Urciuoli R, Broggi G, et al: New aspects in the surgical treatment of cerebral palsy. Acta Neurochir (suppl). 24:53, 1977
11. Fasano VA, Broggi G, Barolat-Romana G, et al: Surgical treatment of spasticity in cerebral palsy. Child's Brain 4:289, 1978
12. Förster O: Ueber eine neu operative Methode der Behandlung spasticher Lähmungen mittels Resektion hinterer Ruckenmarkswurzeln. Z Orthop Chir 22:203, 1908
13. Fraioli B, Guidetti B: Posterior partial rootlet section in the treatment of spasticity. J Neurosurg 46:618, 1977
14. Friede RL: Developmental Neuropathology. New York, Springer-Verlag, 1975, pp 57–93
15. Gildenberg PL: Treatment of spasmodic torticollis by dorsal column stimulation. Appl Neurophysiol 41:113, 1978
16. Gillingham FJ, Walsh EG, Zegada LF: Steriotactic lesions of the pulvinar for hypertonus and dyskinesias. Acta Neurochir (suppl) 24:15, 1977
17. Gros C, Oyaknine G, Vlahavitch B, et al: La radicotomie selective posterieure dans le traitement neurochirugical de l'hypertonie pyramidale. Neurochiurgie 13:505, 1967
18. Guidetti B, Fraioli B: Neurosurgical treatment of spasticity and dyskinesias. Acta Neurochir (suppl) 24:27, 1977
19. Haymaker W: Bing's Local Diagnosis in Neurological Diseases. St. Louis, Mosby, 1969, pp 404–418
20. Heimburger RF, Slominski A, Griswold P: Cervical posterior rhizotomy for reducing spasticity in cerebral palsy. J Neurosurg 39:30, 1973
21. Hitchcock ER: Stereotaxic surgery for cerebral palsy. Nurs Times 74:2064, 1978
22. Kottke FJ: Modification of athetosis by denervation of the tonic neck reflexes (abstr). Dev Med Child Neurol 12:236, 1970
23. Laitenen L, Singounas E: Longitudinal myelotomy in the treatment of spasticity of the legs. J Neurosurg 35:536, 1971
24. Landau WM: Spasticity and rigidity, in Plum F (ed): Recent Advances in Neurology. Philadelphia, Davis, 1969, pp 1–32
25. Manrique M, Oya S, Vaquero J, et al: Chronic paleocerebellar stimulation for the treatment of neuromuscular disorders. Appl Neurophysiol 41:237, 1978
26. McLellan DL, Selwyn M, Cooper IS: Time course of clinical and Physiological effects of stimulation of the cerebellar surface in patients with spasticity. J Neurol Neurosurg Psychiatry 41:150, 1978
27. Melzack R, Wall PD: Pain mechanisms: A new theory. Science 150:971, 1965
28. Milner-Brown HS, Penn R: Pathophysiologic mechanisms in cerebral palsy. J Neurol Neurosurg Psychiatry 42:606, 1979
29. Moyes PD: Longitudinal myelotomy for spasticity. J Neurosurg 31:615, 1969
30. Munro D: The rehabilitation of patients totally paralysed below the waist: Anterior rhizotomy for spastic paraplegia. N Engl J Med 233:453, 1945
31. Narabayashi H: Experiences of stereotoxic surgery on cerebral palsy patients. Acta Neurochir (suppl) 24:3, 1977
32. Nashold BS, Slaughter DG: Effects of stimulating or destroying the deep cerebellar regions in man. J Neurosurg 31:172, 1969
33. Penn RD: The Neurosurgical treatment of cerebral palsy. Pediatr Ann 8:72, 1979
34. Penn RD, Gottlieb GL, Agarwal GC: Cerebellar stimulation in man: Quantitative changes in spasticity. J Neurosurg 48:779, 1978
35. Ratusnik DL, Wolfe VI, Penn RD, et al: Effects on speech of chronic cerebellar stimulation in cerebral palsy. J Neurosurg 48:876, 1978
36. Richardson RR, Nunez C, Siquera EB: Histological reaction to percutaneous epidural neurostimulator. Med Prog Technol 6:179, 1979
37. Sances A, Larson S, Myklebast J, et al: Studies of electrode configuration. Neurosurgery 1:207, 1977

38. Schneider RC, Crosby EC: The interplay between cerebral hemispheres and cerebellum in relation to tonus and movements. J Neurosurg 20:188, 1963

39. Shealy CN, Mortimer JT, Hagfors NR: Dorsal column electroanalgesia. J Neurosurg 32:560, 1970

40. Siegfried J, Verdie JC: Long-term assessment of stereotactic dentatotomy for spasticity and other disorders. Acta Neurochir (suppl) 24:41, 1977

41. Siegfried J, Krainiek JU, Haas H, et al: Electrical spinal cord stimulation for spastic movement disorders. Appl Neurophysiol 41:134, 1978

42. Tonnis W, Bischof W: Ergebnisse der Lumbalen Myelotomie Nach Beschof. Zentralbl Neurochir 23:120, 1962

43. Waltz JM, Pani KC: Spinal cord stimulation in disorders of the motor system, in International Symposium on External Control of Human Extremities, Dubrovnik, 1978. Advances in External Control of Human Extremities. Belgrade. Yugoslav Committee for Electronics and Automation, 1978, pp 545–556

44. Waltz JM: Spinal cord stimulation for palsies? Patient Care 13:188, 1979

45. Whittaker CK: Cerebellar stimulation for cerebral palsy. J Neurosurg 52:648, 1980

46. Yamada S, Perot PL, Ducker TB, et al: Myelotomy for control of mass spasms in paraplegia. J Neurosurg 45:683, 1976

47. Zervas NT: Long term review of dentatectomy in dystonia musculorum deformans and cerebral palsy. Acta Neurochir (suppl) 24:49, 1977

James R. Gage

27

Surgical Complications

This chapter will discuss problems specific to cerebral palsy surgery. Complications such as infection, loss of fixation, or nonunion will not be included, since they are common to orthopaedics in general. The major pitfalls, problems, and principles relevant to each type of cerebral palsy are discussed separately.

Cerebral palsy is one of the more difficult treatment problems in orthopaedics, since the primary problem cannot be attacked directly. The orthopaedist is limited to correcting the peripheral manifestations of the central nervous system (CNS) lesion.

Clinical evaluation, although useful, is not sufficient by itself for presurgical decision making. Two patients may have a similar clinical problem; the same surgical approach may be used, yet the functional results may be dramatically different. In retrospect, it is apparent that, although the clinical appearance of the two patients was similar, they had different underlying muscular problems. More sophisticated methods of analysis thus are needed to distinguish these neuromuscular lesions, or nonpredictability becomes the cardinal feature of surgery in the cerebral palsied child (Fig. 27-1). Even when the objectives of surgery are met, the results may fall far below the expectations of the patient, the parents, and even the surgeon.

Reasons for this include (1) inability to correct the primary CNS lesion, (2) inadequate or incorrect preoperative assessment, (3) unrealistic goal setting or expectations on the part of the physician, the patient, or the parents, (4) failure to assess the effect of surgery on other joints, (5) inability to understand the effect of surgery on the primitive reflexes, and (6) absence of proven solutions.

Cary lists five principles that can be applied to cerebral palsy surgery:[4]

1. The surgeon will redefine his end product, not in terms of the result of a single treatment episode, but in terms of his long-range treatment objectives.
2. He will identify with precision his patient's problems, not only immediate, but future, and do so in terms of interference with function.
3. He will analyze the effects of growth, not only on the problems identified, but also on the treatment procedures considered.
4. He will make valid alternatives in order to make an intelligent choice of optimum treatment plan.
5. He will recognize that the whole child, not just his motor-skeletal parts, must function in society, and will avail himself of the experience and help that can be provided by other professionals working as members of the rehabilitation team.

Diligent application of these principles will enable the orthopaedist to avoid most common complications.

SPASTIC CEREBRAL PALSY: HEMIPLEGIA

Results from surgery in patients with hemiplegia are more predictable than in other types of cerebral palsy.

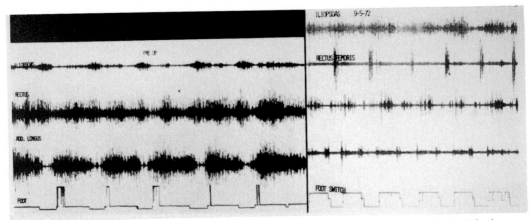

Figure 27-1. Dynamic EMG of two patients with clinically similar gait patterns. On the left, the rectus femoris and adductors are spastic throughout the gait cycle and the iliopsoas is operating phasically, whereas on the right the converse is true. It is apparent that if identical surgical procedures, e.g., iliopsoas recessions, were carried out on both patients, the outcome would not be the same.

Lower Extremity

Surgery is most frequently indicated in the lower extremity for equinovarus deformity and generally produces favorable results. Overlengthening of the hemiplegic heel cord will result in triceps weakness and a suboptimal gait pattern but will not produce the crouch gait that would occur after overlengthening of the tendo-Achillis in spastic diplegia. The most common error is a recurrent deformity because the tendo-Achillis was lengthened insufficiently, at too early an age, or the surgical result was not protected from the effects of growth by night splinting. A minor limb length inequality is common but usually not great enough to warrant correction.

Upper Extremity

Unrealistic expectations are the most common reason for dissatisfaction after upper-extremity surgery. Motor disability is combined with loss of proprioception on the affected side. Both elements prevent normal use of the hand. Benefits of surgery will be largely cosmetic and not functional, although the ability to use the affected hand as an assist may be improved.

Hoffer has noted that wrist flexion deformity may develop because of spasticity of the wrist flexors or weakness of the extensor digitorum relative to the long finger flexors.[7] When the classic Green transfer of flexor carpi ulnaris to wrist extensors is performed in the former case, function of the hand will be im-

proved; if done in the latter, the patient may be unable to open the hand for grasp, since the wrist can no longer be flexed sufficiently. To open the hand before surgery, the patient had used wrist flexion to increase the excursion and power of the extensor digitorum relative to the finger flexors. Hoffer recommends dynamic electromyographic (EMG) studies of the upper extremity to differentiate between these two conditions—another situation that demonstrates the need to analyze problems precisely in terms of interference with function.

SPASTIC CEREBRAL PALSY: DIPLEGIA

Spastic diplegia is the type of cerebral palsy most amenable to surgical correction. Although there are relatively few major gait patterns, many subpatterns exist, with subtle differences between them. Since clinical examination is not sufficient to elucidate these differences, preoperative high-speed gait photography and dynamic EMG often are necessary to assess gait patterns. Without such analysis, treatment errors are likely to occur.

Lower Extremities

One of the most frequent postoperative complications in spastic diplegia is crouch gait after overlengthening of the heel cords. In reality, the etiology is more likely a failure to recognize and correct co-

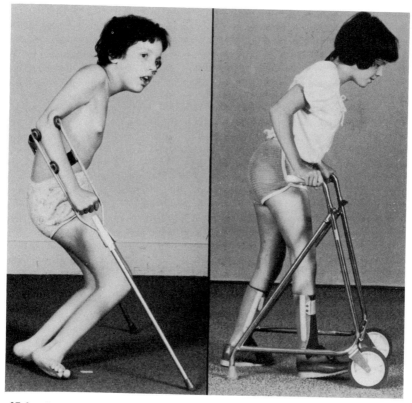

Figure 27-2. Preoperative and postoperative photographs of a child with spastic diplegia. Hindfoot stability was restored with bilateral subtalar arthrodesis followed two weeks later by bilateral lengthenings of the medial hamstrings and iliopsoas recessions. The triceps surae was not lengthened in this patient since the physician wished to preserve the knee-extension moment it generates.

existing fixed or dynamic contractures at the hips and knees. Before surgery, the equinus contracture of the ankle produces an extension moment at the knee that partially offsets the static or dynamic hamstring contracture. When this moment of extension is removed by surgical lengthening of the triceps surae, the knees are carried into further flexion by the spastic hamstrings. Similarly, if the hamstrings alone are lengthened in hopes of correcting a crouch gait, the postoperative result may, paradoxically, be a deeper crouch. In this situation, release of the hamstrings, which are flexors of the knee and extensors of the hip, allows the antagonistic spastic hip flexors to carry the hips into even more flexion. Since the patient must keep a center of gravity over the feet to maintain balance, increased knee flexion is required—hence the paradoxic effect.

Surgical lengthening of the triceps surae tendon may convert the predominant tone pattern in the lower extremities from extension to primarily one of flexion through modification of the afferent impulses to the tone centers in the brain stem and midbrain. These impulses emanate from the stretch receptors in the triceps or the intrinsic muscles of the foot. The problem can generally be avoided by carrying out a measured tendo-Achillis lengthening that permits the triceps to come under tension at 5 degrees of equinus. The Newington experience suggests that the triceps surae should be slightly overlengthened in a hemiplegic and slightly undercorrected in a diplegic.

Simultaneous lengthening or recession of spastic overactive muscles at the hip, knee, and ankle as advocated by Bleck and Rang probably lessens the chance of a crouch gait postoperatively (Fig. 27-2).[1,10] The possibility of other untoward effects is greater because of the greater degree of intervention, however. Careful, objective, preoperative assessment is even more critical when this approach is taken.

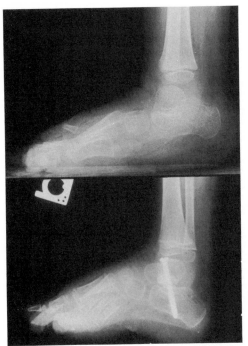

Figure 27-3. Roentgenograms of the foot of a child with an iatrogenic vertical talus produced by attempting to cast the foot out of equinus. A tendo-Achillis lengthening was performed along with subtalar arthrodesis using the technique of Dennyson and Fulford. Note the amount of bone in the sinus tarsi at the time of the four-week cast change. The subtalar arthrodesis was clinically and roentgenographically solid eight weeks postoperatively.

The Feet

Simplification of foot and ankle motion is a valid principle. The method of subtalar arthrodesis advocated by Dennyson and Fulford is effective in correcting hindfoot valgus, provided that fixed bony deformity is not present in the midfoot (Fig. 27-3).[5] When midfoot deformity is present, triple arthrodesis usually will be necessary. These procedures may be accompanied by appropriate tendon lengthenings, but tendon transfer should be avoided, since the results of transfers are unpredictable in cerebral palsy. Similarly, the McKeever arthrodesis of the first metatarsophalangeal joint has been an effective procedure, whereas the McBride procedure, which obtains correction partially through tendon transfer, has produced unpredictable results and has been abandoned at Newington.[11]

Torsional Deformities

Inconsistent results are also the hallmark of attempts to correct torsional deformities in spastic diplegic gait. Undercorrection or overcorrection seems to be much more common than ideal correction in these children. Even when correction is obtained, recurrence of deformity with growth is common, since the muscle imbalance that produced the deformity is frequently allowed to persist. There is a great deal of controversy over the precise cause of femoral anteversion in spastic diplegia. The anterior gluteal muscles and medial hamstrings are known internal rotators of the hip, whereas the role of the adductors and the iliopsoas is subject to some debate.[1,8] Bleck feels that the iliopsoas contributes to femoral anteversion through maintenance of a hip-flexion contracture. He also has noted that an increase in this contracture almost invariably follows femoral osteotomy for correction of anteversion unless it is accompanied by an iliopsoas recession. Bleck therefore, advocates iliopsoas recession routinely when using derotation osteotomy of the femur to correct anteversion in spastic diplegia.

Gait Analysis

In the future, the inconsistent results that are now so prevalent in cerebral palsy surgery may be decreased by pattern recognition. There are now three major patterns of spastic diplegic gait that can be differentiated clinically.[2] Each of these is heterogeneous, however, since Sutherland has been able to elucidate 10 patterns of spastic diplegic gait using computer-analyzed force plate, dynamic EMG, and video data.[13] It should soon be possible to divide spastic diplegia into homogeneous subtypes and develop treatment protocols for each type. Consistent surgical results in this complex surgical disorder will be possible only when this has been achieved.

SPASTIC CEREBRAL PALSY: TOTAL BODY INVOLVEMENT

The major pitfall in spastic quadriplegia is unrealistic goal setting. Many children who are marginal ambulators are subjected to futile surgical procedures in an effort to maintain ambulation (Fig. 27-4). Root in 1977 pointed out that 78 percent of patients with total body involvement are confined to a wheelchair.[12] For the majority of these patients, wheelchair mobility with independent or assisted transfer is thus a much more realistic goal than ambulation. For most

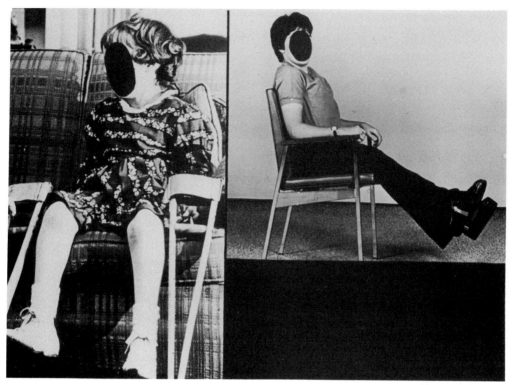

Figure 27-4. A spastic diplegic patient shown at ages 6 and 18 yr. In the intervening years she had several surgical procedures "to improve ambulation," with the result that she lost all motion of her knees. Despite the fact that she has good use of her upper extremities and normal intelligence, she is unable to transfer independently without knee flexion. In an attempt to gain the unrealistic goal of ambulation, the more realistic goal of independence in activities of daily living was lost.

of these children, the major orthopaedic goals are to preserve a straight spine and a level pelvis, prevent hip dislocation, minimize knee-flexion contracture to allow assisted or independent transfer, and maintain plantigrade, shoeable feet. Attainment of these goals will maximize the child's potential for independence in activities of daily living or wheelchair mobility.

The majority of unsatisfactory surgical results occur because fixed deformities were allowed to develop before corrective measures were attempted. For example, early hip subluxation may respond to measures as simple as adductor tenotomy and abduction splinting, whereas a painful hip dislocation with concurrent fixed pelvic obliquity may be a nearly insoluble problem.

Lower Extremities

The ability to make independent or assisted transfers as an adult may determine whether a patient can remain at home or whether institutional care is required. Since plantigrade feet are required for transfer, maintaining the feet in this position should be a high priority. Subtalar or triple arthrodesis may be needed to control varus or valgus deformity. Judicious heel cord lengthening will control equinus, but overlengthening may result in loss of the extensor thrust necessary for even assisted transfers. Hallux valgus also may become severe enough to produce pain or limit shoe wear. We have found that since precise muscle balance is difficult to obtain and maintain, deformity frequently recurs after soft tissue releases have been performed to correct hallux valgus. Surgical arthrodesis of the first metatarsophalangeal joint, the McKeever procedure (Fig. 27-5), has been more successful in the Newington experience.[11]

The Spine

Scoliosis in cerebral palsy differs from idiopathic scoliosis in that the curvature continues to progress beyond maturity. This occurs because the

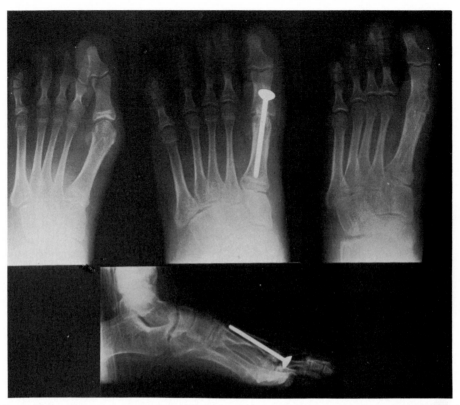

Figure 27-5.   Roentgenograms of an adult with spastic quadriplegia. A McKeever arthrodesis of the first metatarsophalangeal joint was used to treat the hallux valgus. Note the solid arthrodesis attained after screw removal.

muscle imbalance producing the spine deformity continues throughout life. Most of the severe scoliosis seen in adult patients could have been prevented had effective orthotic management been employed until the spine was mature enough for surgical fusion (Fig. 27-6).

Failure to fuse a sufficient number of vertebrae to prevent progression is the most frequent surgical error. In general, lumbar curves should be fused to the sacrum. Failure to fuse the spine to the pelvis in patients with neuromuscular scoliosis will almost invariably lead to decompensation. The pelvis must be level to ensure a stable sitting platform with good weight distribution. Pelvic obliquity must therefore be corrected before fusion. This frequently requires release of tight hip musculature, particularly the adductors and the iliopsoas, or preoperative traction.[3]

In the past, scoliosis surgery in cerebral palsy was often complicated by loss of fixation, nonunion, or pressure sores. The incidence of these complica-

tions was higher than in idiopathic scoliosis because of hypertonicity or athetoid movements. More recently, segmental spinal stabilization (Fig. 27-7) has been able to avoid many of these complications.[6] Two L-shaped rods are wired to the lamina at each vertebral level. The excellent correction and secure internal fixation obviate the need for postoperative plaster. This avoids potential skin problems associated with casting.

ATHETOID CEREBRAL PALSY

Complete unpredictability characterizes operative treatment of athetoid cerebral palsy. In general, fixed extremity contractures are less common than in spastic cerebral palsy. When tenotomies or tendon lengthenings are performed for athetoid patients, there

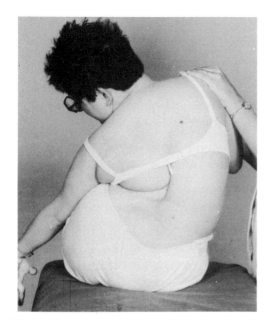

Figure 27-6. Loss of sitting balance secondary to severe scoliosis in a young adult with spastic quadriplegia. A deformity of this magnitude is easier to prevent than to correct.

is a propensity for antagonists that had been silent preoperatively to become dominant postoperatively. For example, a child dominated by hip adductor tone preoperatively may develop fixed hip abduction after adductor releases. For this reason, a minimal adductor release without anterior branch neurectomy is recommended in children who have developed hip subluxation despite prophylactic night splinting. If it is determined under anesthesia that each hip can be abducted to 45 degrees or more, isolated tenotomy of the adductor longus and gracilis combined with postoperative abduction night splinting during the remainder of growth will usually be sufficient. Should the child's hips assume a postoperative abduction posture, night splinting should be discontinued and the child's thighs swaddled in a diaper splint to prevent the development of a fixed abducted position.

Surgery directed toward improving athetoid ambulation should be avoided, since it is invariably unsuccessful. Surgery should be confined to problems of fixed bony deformity, e.g., impending hip dislocation and structural scoliosis. Even in these cases, surgery should be undertaken only after thoughtful analysis, and parents should be forewarned of the unpredictability of the result.

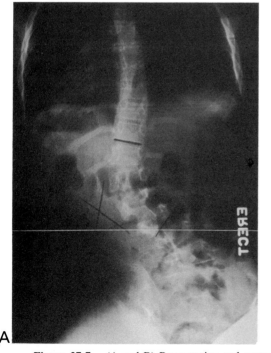

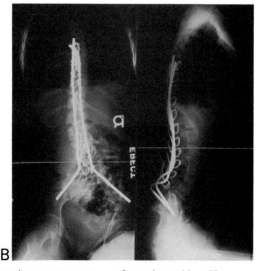

A   B

Figure 27-7. (A and B) Preoperative and postoperative roentgenograms of a patient with a 65-degree lumbar scoliosis treated with segmental spinal stabilization. (C) Eight days after surgery. Sitting balance has been restored.

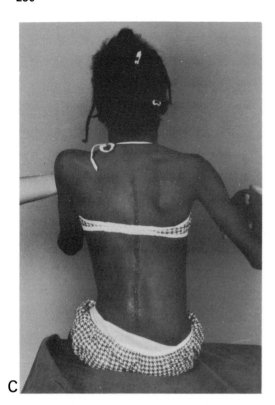

C

MIXED CEREBRAL PALSY

The surgeon may be confused by the child with mixed cerebral palsy in whom the clinical presentation is primarily one of spasticity. Despite the predominance of spasticity, the athetoid component renders the result unpredictable. Perry and Hoffer have found that variability in dynamic EMGs preoperatively is an indication of athetosis and that the more variable the EMG recording preoperatively, the more likely an unpredictable postoperative result.[9]

They suggest the following guidelines for surgery in patients with athetoid or mixed cerebral palsy:

1. Reserve surgery for problems of fixed bony deformity and do not attempt surgery for the purpose of improving functional ambulation.
2. Avoid tendon transfers and neurectomies. In general, use judicious lengthenings rather than tenotomies.
3. Where practical, obtain correction and maintain it with arthrodesis. This is particularly true in the foot; e.g., marked equinovalgus deformity interfering with independent transfer in the young child might well be controlled by subtalar arthrodesis, or a severe hallux valgus interfering with shoe

wear would be controlled by a McKeever arthrodesis of the first metatarsophalangeal joint in a skeletally mature patient.

•   •   •

Most of the poor or inconsistent results following attempts at surgical correction in cerebral palsy are not "acts of God;" they are iatrogenic. Many of these unsatisfactory results could be avoided if realistic goal setting, accurate, objective preoperative analysis, and careful, thoughtful problem analysis in conjunction with known surgical principles were routinely carried out. In fairness to those physicians who are involved in cerebral palsy surgery, however, it should be noted that the technically accurate, objective assessment methods that have been so long needed are only now becoming available at a clinical level, and many problems in the clinical treatment of cerebral palsy remain unsolved.

REFERENCES

1. Bleck EE: Orthopaedic Management of Cerebral Palsy. Philadelphia, Saunders, 1979, pp 134–207
2. Bleck EE: Postural and gait abnormalities caused by hip-flexion deformity in spastic cerebral palsy. Treatment by iliopsoas recession. J Bone Joint Surg 53A:1468, 1971
3. Bonnett C, Brown JC, Grow T: Thoracolumbar scoliosis in cerebral palsy. Results of surgical treatment. J Bone Joint Surg 58A:328, 1976
4. Cary JM: Personal communication, 1980
5. Dennyson WG, Fulford GE: Subtalar arthrodesis by cancellous grafts and metallic internal fixation. J Bone Joint Surg 58B:507, 1976
6. Ferguson RL, Allen BL: Segmental spinal instrumentation for routine scoliotic curve. Contemp Orthop 2:450, 1980
7. Hoffer MM: Personal communication, 1980
8. McKibbin B: The action of the iliopsoas muscle in the newborn. J Bone Joint Surg 50B:161, 1968
9. Perry J, Hoffer MM: Preoperative and postoperative dynamic electromyography as an aid in planning tendon transfers in children with cerebral palsy. J Bone Joint Surg 59A:531, 1977
10. Rang M: Strategy of treatment in children with cerebral palsy. Presented at the 15th annual Orthopaedic Clinical Meeting, Newington Children's Hospital, Newington, Conn., 1977
11. Renshaw TS, Sirkin RB, Drennan JC: The management of hallux valgus in cerebral palsy. Dev Med Child Neurol 21:202, 1979
12. Root L: The totally involved cerebral palsy patient. Instructional Course Lectures, 44th annual meeting, The American Academy of Orthopaedic Surgeons, Las Vegas, 1977
13. Sutherland DH: Personal communication, 1981

PART V

Social, Educational, and Maturational Considerations

Nancy Neuer
Gerald A. Strom

28

Guidance and Support for Parents

Parents with a child handicapped by cerebral palsy encounter a multitude of problems, not normally experienced with raising a nonhandicapped child, that can have a profound effect on themselves, their family unit, and other siblings as well as on the involved child. The role of the social worker who deals with these parents is to have a thorough understanding of these various problems and to attempt to minimize or prevent their sequelae by appropriate education and counseling.

PSYCHOSOCIAL FACTORS AFFECTING THE CHILD AND FAMILY

The birth of a child precipitates a period of developmental adjustment for every family. During pregnancy, each parent engages in a process of psychologic preparation that focuses on the imagery associated with the expected child. Fantasies involving the infant's sex, appearance, personality, and potential achievements enable parents to form beginning emotional bonds to their child. When a normal, healthy baby is born, parents must adjust their expectations and fantasies to comply with the reality of the actual infant born. In part, they relinquish the imagery of the idealized child and gradually incorporate the reality of the actual baby.[10]

Problems Following Birth of a Handicapped Child

The birth of a handicapped child can intensify the reality process to the extent of creating a family crisis. Many parents initially view the baby as frightening and as somewhat of a threat, yet societal values dictate that an immediate investment be made in the child as a love object.[17] The altered images comprising the reality of a handicapped child often constitute a narcissistic insult to parents. Children are viewed most definitely as an extension of self—a blending of a family's legacy for the future. When a child is born with a known defect, parents often feel personal failure and shame.[5,10]

The spectrum of feelings parents experience in response to a handicapped child include anger, denial, repulsion, disappointment, guilt, and depression. These reactions may occur singly or in combination. Many parents engage in an introspective process to explain reasons for causality and to assign responsibility for this event. Differential responses to the impact of a defective infant reflect societal values as well as professional practices. Mothers tend to use the mechanism of guilt to cope initially with the crisis. In part, this may be viewed as an internalization of society's communication of responsibility to a mother for the physical and emotional well-being of her child.[10] Hospital personnel who prefer to share information initially with the father serve to reinforce the mother's sense of implicit guilt. This practice tends to ally the father with the attending health care professionals, further isolating the mother and delineating the dyad of mother and child. Professionals often act precipitously to dispel parental guilt without recognizing that guilt serves as a beginning step in mastering a potentially overwhelming situation or may be a synonymous statement of beginning control and reorganization during a critical period.

Alterations in Maternal–Infant Bonding

Bonding is a difficult process that parents confront with conflicting emotions. Attachments formed during pregnancy must be adjusted to encompass the reality of the disabled child. There are potential interferences in the bonding process specific to families of cerebral palsied infants, involving difficulties related to muscle tone, positioning, and feeding.

Cuddling the baby may prove difficult because of muscular rigidity or floppiness. The resulting lack of gratification of tactile nurturance leaves parents with residual feelings of rejection coupled with a sense of inadequacy. Feedings may also be extremely labored and tedious if the oral musculature is so affected. This process impedes parents' basic need to nurture their infant, again reinforcing feelings of rejection and failure. The cerebral palsied child who experiences an organic failure to thrive further complicates parents' feelings of loss because of the visible absence of very basic nurturing interactions parents provide. A substantial number of infants and toddlers with spasticity appear extremely irritable and are reported to cry for long intervals during the day and night. Many infants reverse their days and nights, which adds an additional burden to the parent–child attachment process.

Mourning

Parents move from initial critical responses involved in bonding with their handicapped infant to the process of mourning the loss of the expected, perfect child. Olshansky defines this process of adaptation to a handicapped child as a state of "chronic sorrow."[14] Unlike more transient life crises, where readjustments occur and closure is achieved within six months after the event, the ongoing nature of parenting a handicapped child negates this principle.[15] The very presence of the child, whether within or outside of the context of the family, serves as a constant reminder of grief and loss. Olshansky defines his conceptualization of chronic sorrow as encompassing the life span of the parents. Feelings of grief, anger, loss, guilt, and depression reach periods of quiescence yet are exacerbated by the child's developmental milestones. Feelings of grief and loss are felt when milestones are not achieved by specifically accepted chronologic dates and if these achievements differ markedly from those of nonhandicapped peers. Some of the most potent stages of developmental mastery for parents include achievement of ambulation, functional speech, school entry, adolescence, and adulthood. The expectations parents anticipate from each maturational stage must be potentially adjusted or relinquished as the child reaches each level. Parents may thus again face feelings of disappointment and sorrow as they experience and anticipate their child's growth.

The concept of mourning is not specific to parents of handicapped children. Many children with disabilities confront issues and experience the emotions that parallel the early responses of their parents. Adolescence characterizes a time of emotional turbulence that may become intensified for the disabled.[1,11] The handicapped teenager may feel the permanence of the disability; fantasies of "outgrowing" physical limitations will not be actualized. There is a period of introspective searching for causality, which naturally leads to anger at parents, who have historically been the most powerful people in adolescents' lives. Anger at parents may trigger an exacerbation of dormant feelings in the parents. Ultimately, the handicapped adolescent is faced with mourning the loss of the fantasized self and accepting the reality of the limitations the specific disability imposes.

WORKING WITH PARENTS OF CEREBRAL PALSIED CHILDREN

Eventual attempts at accepting the handicapping condition are not smooth; rather, parents move both forward and backward as they deal either consciously or unconsciously with their ambivalent feelings. It is essential to remember that acceptance is not a stable condition but fluctuates through different life crisis, developmental stages, and the prognosis and diagnosis of the disability.[9,12,13]

It is important to allow parents to adjust to their feelings of having a handicapped child at their own pace. Each family comes with its own history and coping mechanisms, and it is the responsibility of the professional working with them to identify and assess the family's ability to use help. The important point is to demonstrate basic concern and interest and to be available to give the parents the arena to ventilate their feelings. It is necessary to share complete information with the family and then allow members to express their feelings, both positive and negative, and in return offer them acceptance, trust, and interest.[18]

A fundamental belief is that people are uncomfortable with circumstances and events over which they have no control. When one looks at the difference between acute and chronic illnesses, this is highlighted. Although an acute illness may be a transient, anxiety-producing episode, a chronic illness carries with it the threat of a lifelong commitment, both emotional and financial, that can immobilize a parent or family unit.[2]

Problems in Dealing with Parents

Social workers must be aware of a number of problems in working with parents of children with cerebral palsy. Parents may have (1) difficulty understanding the diagnosis, (2) trouble accepting the diagnosis, (3) differing degrees of guilt about causation, (4) anger that this has happened to them, which can at times lead to the projection of blame outside themselves, and (5) a tendency to look for magical solutions.[2,7,19]

Whatever the reason, having a handicapped child does produce change, not only within the family but in their functioning outside the home. Sometimes crisis serves as a positive motivation and sometimes as a very disruptive element within a family. The professional will try to aid the family to look at the total situation and not just at the handicap. This can help a family move from a helpless state to a more active role in the treatment process, which, in turn, can help maximize the child's potential for development.[4]

This leads to the question of how much, when, and how to tell the family of the diagnosis of cerebral palsy. When the diagnosis is clear and the prognosis is favorable, the discussion is easy. When there are multiple problems with an uncertain outlook, the discussion will inevitably produce anxiety. Professionals must thus be constantly aware of the family's psychologic needs.[6]

The National Association for Retarded Children conducted a study indicating that approximately 40 percent of the parents surveyed stressed the importance of the professional's attitude when sharing the diagnosis with the family. One parent wrote, "We shall always be greatful to our young doctor for his skillful sympathetic handling of our case—he took as much interest in us as he did in our child, and spared us what may have been a dreadful shock." The parents studied felt that the thoroughness of the diagnostic assessment that preceded the medical interpretation, and the clarity and directness with which it was presented, helped in their receiving of the diagnosis. Parents also felt that the professionals should not only stress the limitations, but also the assets, of their child. Another key factor was to discuss the diagnosis in terms of parental expectations for their child on a day-to-day basis, if at all possible.[19]

Professionals must be sensitive to feelings of ambivalence, since family members are attempting to bond with the child, they are seeing a lack of developmental progress, are given information on a lifelong problem, and are learning of the uncertainty that accompanies the diagnosis. One must also be alerted to the guilt that this may evoke, which can result in overprotective and overindulgent attitudes toward the child. Feelings of depression can also be anticipated. Disappointment in the child and concern for his or her future are appropriate reactions to accompany feelings of unhappiness.[8]

It is the general consensus of professionals in the field that satisfactory emotional development of the handicapped child and adolescent depends more on the manner in which parents and family relate to the child than to the extent of the handicap itself. Of utmost importance is the degree to which the parents and other significant family members confront and integrate their feelings about the handicapped child. At this point, it is necessary to add that an important variable to address is the child's age at the time of diagnosis. Research has revealed that the cases where the diagnosis was made at the time of birth, parents were better able to nurture their children emotionally than were parents who learned of the diagnosis later on. This again illustrates the mourning process parents must confront when faced with the birth of a defective child. Parents informed of the diagnosis soon after birth were able to begin the mourning process when the child was an infant. Beginning mastery of this mourning allowed them to use emotional energy to nurture the child when the child required this investment. For parents who learn of a child's handicap later on, the mourning begins at the point of diagnosis. Many times this may occur when the child is old enough to be cognizant of the "upheaval" facing the family. The child might not be aware of all the parameters involved in the parents' reactions but definitely feel the upset and know that he or she is the focus or "cause" of the emotional crisis.[2]

Counseling Parents

In counseling parents of cerebral palsied children, professionals must keep in mind some basic points. First, and most basic, is treating the family with respect and acceptance. (Initially, it is not only important what is said, but how it is said.) Second, professionals must be willing to work together with the family as a team. Third, they must create an atmosphere in which the family feels comfortable in expressing themselves and their feelings. Fourth, they must help family members develop the self-determination they need to make appropriate decisions. Families are put into very helpless situations for they cannot undo the condition; however, they can gain some control by making decisions in areas that they can control. Finally, honesty is a very basic premise to all counseling situations and should be implicit in all professionals actions.[6,16]

PRACTICAL CONSIDERATION

The theoretic framework discussed above provides an intellectual base for understanding the emotional impact sustained by families of handicapped children. In order to gain a more complete perspective of this experience for the family system, however, it is necessary to address the practical and concrete obstacles imposed by the presence of a handicapped child.

Financial concerns may be paramount for families whose children require intensive medical and rehabilitative treatment. Each state administers a program governing monetary services available to families of handicapped children. Eligibility requirements preclude many families from participation in these programs, however. Of equal concern is the difficulty of locating appropriate medical, rehabilitative, counseling, educational, and other community resources to serve the child and family.

Numerous services available for the child's treatment directly and extensively use a parent as therapist, teacher, and transporter. With the majority of appointments scheduled during "working hours," the working parent may naturally be excluded from participation in the child's care and feel isolated by the resulting expertise demonstrated by the spouse.[3]

Siblings may receive a disproportionate amount of their parents' time, energy, and attention because of the handicapped child's needs. This may result in a strained parental and sibling relationship. In addition, a cyclic pattern may emerge where parents experience an inability to reduce any input to the handicapped child for fear that it will further damage him or her. Inevitably, parents are left with little opportunity to fulfill their own needs.

In short, each member of the family is directly affected by the presence of the handicapped child as well as by the treatment prescription. Professionals must be sensitive to the needs of each family member and consider restructuring the service delivery system to preserve the family's equilibrium.[3]

REFERENCES

1. Carson AS: Technical alterations in the psychotherapy with an adolescent cerebral palsy patient, in Turner FJ (ed): Differential Diagnosis and Treatment in Social Work. New York, Free Press, 1968, pp 369–378
2. Davis RE: Family of the disabled child. NY State J Med 75:1039, 1975
3. Doernberg NL: Some negative effects on family integration of health and educational services for young handicapped children. Rehabil Lit 39:107, 1978
4. Drayer C, Schlesinger EG: The informing interview, in Noland RL (ed): Counseling Parents of the Mentally Retarded. Springfield, Ill. Charles C Thomas, 1970, pp 99–109
5. Drotar D, Baskiewicz A, Irvin N, et al: The adaptation of parents to the birth of an infant with a congenital malformation: A hypothetical model. Pediatrics 56:710, 1975
6. Gardner RA: Psychogenic problems of brain injured children and their parents. J Am Acad Child Psychiatry 7:479, 1968
7. Gardner RA: Guilt reaction of parents of children with severe physical disease. Am J Psychiatry 126:636, 1969
8. Giannini M, Goodman L: Counseling families during the crisis reaction to mongolism, in Noland RL (ed): Counseling Parents of the Mentally Retarded. Springfield, Ill., Charles C Thomas, 1970, pp 110–121
9. Hewett S, Newson E: The Family and the Handicapped Child. Chicago, Aldine, 1970
10. Klaus M, Kennell J: Maternal–Infant Bonding. St. Louis, Mosby, 1976
11. Mende KK: Coping styles of 34 adolescents with cerebral palsy. Am J Psychiatry 135:1344, 1978
12. Miller LG: Toward a greater understanding of the parents of the mentally retarded child. J Pediatr 73:699, 1968
13. McMichael JK: Handicap: A study of physically handicapped children and their families. Pittsburgh, University of Pittsburgh Press, 1971
14. Olshansky S: Chronic sorrow: A response to having a mentally defective child, in Younghusband E (ed): Casework With Families and Children. Chicago, University of Chicago Press, 1965, p 100

15. Poznanski EO: Emotional issues in raising handicapped children. Rehabil Lit 34:322, 1973

16. Roos P: Psychological counseling with parents of mentally retarded, in Noland RL (ed): Counseling Parents of the Mentally Retarded. Springfield, Ill., Charles C Thomas, 1970, pp 133–142

17. Solnit AJ, Stark MH: Mourning and the birth of a defective child. Psychoanal Study Child 16:523, 1961

18. Zissermann L: Sex of a parent and knowledge about cerebral palsy. Am J Occup Ther 32:500, 1978

19. Zwerling I: Initial counseling of parents with mentally retarded children, in Noland RL (ed): Counseling Parents of the Mentally Retarded. Springfield, Ill., Charles C Thomas, 1970, pp 83–98

Naomi Breslau

29

Family Care: Effects on Siblings and Mothers

DISABLED CHILDREN: A RISING PROPORTION

Recent U.S. statistics indicate that the proportion of children with disability due to chronic illness, including cerebral palsy, has increased markedly. The percentage (and number) of children with activity limitation due to chronic conditions in the noninstitutionalized population has risen from 2.1 percent (1,418,000) in 1967 to 3.9 percent (2,309,000) in 1978.[31,32] This rise is due in part to improvements in medical therapies that increased the survival rate and prolonged the life of children born with severe physical disabilities. The shift from institutional care to care in the home is undoubtedly reflected in these statistics as well. The burden on families may have become not only more common but also more intense, since in addition to providing custodial care, families are expected to obtain a widening range of professional services on behalf of disabled children as well as administer therapeutic procedures directly. Although these trends have important implications for families, the questions of how families nurse and support disabled children and at what cost to their members have not yet been adequately addressed.

This chapter will examine the effects of childhood physical disability on family members and how the conditions of life with a disabled child in the home might contribute to personal distress and maladjustment in siblings and mothers. Previous studies have

reported that severe disability in children has adverse effects on their families.[5,9,10,18,19,22,26,30] The daily care of the child often depletes parents' energy, causes withdrawal from social relationships, and restricts activities. There is evidence that marital tensions increase, although several reports suggest that in some families, parents are drawn closer together. Two studies found that mothers of disabled children scored higher than control mothers for emotional distress and depression.[11,29] Although maladjustment in siblings has been reported in several studies, the evidence is mixed for who is at risk—boys or girls, younger or older—and what types of pathologic conditions they are at risk for.[3,7,8,13,27,29]

It should be noted that although reports on disabled children and their families are abundant in the literature, few are based on rigorously designed studies in which control groups are used. Furthermore, previous research, as a rule, has not been based on explicit conceptual frameworks designed to explain why and how a disabled child in the home might contribute to adverse outcomes in family members.

This chapter examines the proposition that the presence of a disabled child in the home alters the conditions of family life thereby increasing the likelihood of psychological impairment in siblings and mothers. If indeed families of disabled children reduce their extra-domestic activities, if home life becomes duller and more monotonous, if marital solidarity is undermined and conflict is heightened, could not then these changes themselves explain the reported maladjustment in siblings and mothers? The hypotheses to be tested, the variables and their operational definitions will be introduced in the course of data presentation.

*This study was supported by grants from the Cleveland Foundation, the Charles S. Mott Foundation and the Easter Seal Research Foundation.

CLEVELAND STUDY

In the Cleveland study, data were collected in a comprehensive study conducted in 1978–1979 to assess the impact of childhood disability on families and on the adjustment of the disabled children themselves. Families of children with cystic fibrosis, cerebral palsy, myelodysplasia, and multiple physical handicaps were selected from four pediatric specialty clinics of two teaching hospitals in Cleveland, whose caseloads are representative of area children in these diagnostic categories. All families of patients 3–18 yr of age who resided in the Cleveland area were asked to participate in the study. From 460 eligible families, 369 (80 percent) complete interviews were obtained. For a comparison (control) group, a 3-stage probability sample was designed to represent all Cleveland area families with 1 or more children 3–18 yr of age. From 530 eligible control families, 456 (86 percent) complete interviews were obtained.

In all 825 study families, data were gathered from mothers in home interviews using a structured questionnaire that includes several self-administered instruments. Trained female interviewers, matched according to respondents' race, conducted the interviews. A wide range of variables was covered, including the health status of several individuals in the family, sociodemograpbic cbaracteristics, and aspects of the family's social environment.

In control families a randomly selected child aged 3–18 yr served as the index child and was the object of a detailed inquiry, analogous to that of the disabled child. In study families in which there were siblings aged 6–18 yr, data were obtained on the psychologic functioning of a randomly selected sibling in this age group. Data were gathered on 237 siblings of disabled children and 248 control siblings. The effect that the disabled child had on other siblings and their mothers was studied and contrasted for important variables.

Effect on Siblings

Hypothesis

An hypothesis about the impact on siblings was stimulated by an intriguing theme in previous research that siblings' birth order in relation to the disabled child influences their psychologic adjustment.[3,17] Specifically, younger siblings are said to be at greater risk than older siblings because they might be displaced in the family as their ill sibling assumes a more dependent role.[17] Displacement, such as an

unexpected change in the status of the sibling within the family, might explain psychopathology in siblings when the disability is acquired, not congenital.

An alternative concept was tested in this study (in which all the disabled children had congenital conditions). Since congenitally disabled children are born with their disabilities, their age relationship to siblings indexes a pertinent factor in the early family environment of the siblings: older siblings of disabled children have lived their earliest years in a normal family, whereas younger siblings were born into families with a disabled child. Reports about the impact on parents of the birth of a child with a congenital abnormality characterize the event as a crisis and the parents' response as an emotional turmoil.[6,12,13] This would suggest that a normal sibling born into a family with a disabled child might experience, in the early years of life, an environment incapable of providing adequate care, maternal love, and stimulation. Robertson has suggested that there might be important developmental consequences of even temporary but intense maternal preoccupations that interfere with the mother's attentiveness to the infant in the first year of life.[24] Since parents' initial response to the birth of a disabled child is likely to change with time, the early biography of a younger sibling should be further differentiated by the age spacing between the sibling and the disabled child. It was therefore hypothesized that (1) younger siblings of disabled children would be more psychologically impaired than older siblings and that (2) among younger siblings, those in close age-spacing relationship to the disabled child would be worse off than those who were not.

In terms of the general formulation outlined above, which asserts that the presence of a disabled child may deprive the family's environment of those conditions that enhance psychologic functioning, the siblings hypothesis focuses on a particularly strategic period in their lives, i.e., their early life experience. It should be kept in mind, however, that in this study there are no direct measures of the early family environment of the siblings. Instead, the early environment of siblings is inferentially measured by relative birth order and age spacing. The interpretation of the results is necessarily tentative.

Psychologic functioning. Psychologic functioning of siblings was measured by the screening inventory developed by Langner et al.[16] The inventory is based on mothers' answers to 35 dichotomously coded items and comprises 7 subscales, each measuring a different area of child behavior. The sum

Table 29-1

Aggressive Behavior of Siblings by Disability, Sex, and Relative Birth Order
(n = 485)*

	Disabled				Controls			
	Male	(No.)	Female	(No.)	Male	(No.)	Female	(No.)
Younger	2.294	(34)	0.852	(54)	1.339	(62)	0.736	(52)
Older	1.536	(69)	1.650	(80)	1.315	(75)	0.712	(59)

*A three-way interaction effect (sample, sex, birth order) is statistically significant (p < 0.05).

of the 35 items provides a composite measure of psychologic impairment, and a cut-off point of 6 distinguishes those severely impaired (scoring 6 and over) from those moderately impaired or well. This study employed two broad indexes based on this inventory: (1) an index of aggressive behavior, which combined 15 items in 3 subscales, and (2) an index of depression–anxiety, which combined 15 items in 3 other subscales. Internal consistency reliability of each index was approximately 0.80.

Before discussing the pertinent results, some general findings are of interest. The overall comparison of 237 siblings of disabled children with the 248 control siblings revealed that the proportions of siblings classified as psychologically severely impaired were approximately the same in the two samples: 16 percent of siblings of disabled children and 13 percent of control siblings were so classified. (The difference is likely to be due to chance.) On aggressive behavior, however, siblings of disabled children score significantly higher than control siblings: 1.51 and 1.07, respectively (p < 0.02).

Birth Order and Age Spacing

In the analysis of the effects of relative birth order and age spacing, siblings' sex was controlled on the grounds that children's response to environmental influences may vary by sex.

To test the hypothesis that younger siblings of disabled children are more psychologically impaired than older siblings and that this difference is not simply a birth-order effect observable in all families, an ordinary least-squares linear model was used on the combined sample of 485. Siblings' psychologic scores were regressed first on three dichotomous variables: sample (disabled versus control), sex (male versus female), and relative birth order (younger versus older). These were followed by the addition of the two- and three-way interactions of these three variables. The results indicated a statistically significant three-way

interaction: among siblings of disabled children, the effect of birth order was significantly different for males and for females, whereas among control siblings birth order had no effect. This was the case for both aggressive behavior and depression–anxiety.

To describe these interactions more clearly, Table 29-1 presents the means of aggressive behavior by sample, sex, and relative birth order, as calculated from the regression results. As can be seen, among male siblings of disabled children, those younger than the disabled child scored higher than those older, whereas among female siblings of disabled children those younger scored lower than those older. Among control siblings, relative birth order had neither a uniform nor a sex-specific relationship with psychologic functioning. The means for depression–anxiety, which appear in Table 29-2, showed the same interaction pattern as in aggressive behavior.

The effects of *age spacing* on the psychologic functioning of younger siblings were examined by a series of sex-specific comparisons between those less than two years and those two or more years younger than the disabled child. For younger *male siblings* of disabled children, the mean score of aggressive behavior was markedly higher for those in the close age-spacing category than for those in the wide one: 4.6 and 1.0, respectively (p < 0.005). Age spacing, however, was unrelated to depression–anxiety in this group; the difference between the means of those in the close and wide age-spacing categories, 1.7 and 1.1, respectively, was not statistically significant.

For *younger female siblings* of disabled children, mean scores of aggressive behavior were actually in the reverse order to that hypothesized; the difference between the two age-spacing categories was not statistically significant. On depression–anxiety, however, female siblings in the close age-spacing category scored higher than those in the wide age-spacing category, 1.2 and 0.7, respectively, a difference nearly reaching statistical significance (p < 0.10).

Table 29-2

Depression–Anxiety of Siblings by Disability, Sex, and Relative Birth Order
(n = 485)*

	Disabled				Controls			
	Male	(No.)	Female	(No.)	Male	(No.)	Female	(No.)
Younger	1.295	(34)	0.833	(54)	0.903	(62)	0.924	(52)
Older	0.740	(69)	1.300	(80)	0.699	(75)	0.729	(59)

*A three-way interaction effect (sample, sex, birth order) is statistically significant (p < 0.05).

Among younger siblings in the control group, age spacing had no effect on the psychologic functioning of either males or females.

Clinical relevance. These findings taken together indicate that a normal male sibling born into a family with a disabled infant less than 2 years of age is at risk for later psychologic impairment. It is unclear why a similar influence is not evident for female siblings. It should be pointed out, moreover, that the sex difference observed here is consistent with previous findings on children's responses to adverse life experiences.[2] In a review of research findings on this point, Rutter concluded that although many studies found no sex differences, where there has been a sex difference, both in young subhuman primates and in children, the male has usually been found to be the more vulnerable.[25] He suggests that "young males may be more susceptible than females to psychological stress, as certainly they are to biological stress." A detailed analysis of the effects of child disability on siblings is presented elsewhere.[3,4]

Effects on Mothers

Hypothesis

The analysis of the impact of child disability on mothers employed a more elaborate study model and a more direct measurement of its key variables. It was hypothesized that a disabled child in the home exerts a negative influence on (1) family cohesion and support and (2) the richness and variety of family stimuli. These changes, together with other experiences associated with caring for a disabled child, impair a mother's internal resources for dealing effectively with life problems and increase the probability that she will experience distress. It was also hypothesized that the effects vary between blacks and whites, on the grounds that the impact of child disability on family economic resources might vary by race.

Family environment. The rationale for focusing on the family environment as a key variable in this context can be summarized as follows. The care of a disabled child tends to preempt a mother's employment, curtail her opportunities for other extradomestic activities, and confine her to the home. When child disability is severe, these restrictions might be experienced by mothers as particularly compelling for two interrelated reasons: (1) the anticipation of prolonged child care responsibilities, inasmuch as severely disabled children are not expected to outgrow their dependence, and (2) the lack of psychic rewards that parents ordinarily receive in the form of children's achievements in mastering developmental tasks. Unrewarding child care efforts tend to undermine pedagogic goals and reduce the meaning of child care to a custodial chore, making the associated sacrifices seem worthless.

Family cohesion and activities. The proposition that family cohesion exerts an influence on the emotional well-being of mothers requires little explanation, since the literature on social supports and mental health has demonstrated this relationship repeatedly. The connection between the variety of family activities and maternal well-being might require an explanation, however. Recent empiric and theoretic developments in the area of social structure and personality have suggested that people's competencies for dealing with cognitively complex phenomena are formed in environmental settings.[28] The central characteristic of a given setting is the variety and complexity of the stimuli that it offers. In this general framework, the family setting figures primarily in the development of intellectual abilities and motivations in childhood, whereas occupational settings are viewed as the arena in which competencies continue to be shaped during adult life.[14,15] If the substantive complexity of men's work influences their internal resources, as previous research has revealed, could not, then, the family setting affect mothers' internal resources, especially when it consitutes their principal or sole environmental setting?

Internal resources. Two classes of internal resources for dealing with stress or with complexity have been delineated in the literature: intellectual flexibility and orientations toward self and social reality.[33] Although intellectual flexibility can be viewed as general competency, orientations toward self and social reality (the extent to which one perceives one's action as effective in mastering the environment) are relevant to coping in that they influence the degree of effort people exert in dealing with problematic situations. Those with a firm sense of mastery over their lives are more likely to approach problems with persistent effort than those with fatalistic perspectives. Although analytically distinct, these two dimensions of people's internal resources (intellectual flexibility and orientation toward self and the social environment) are correlated empirically. Their association may reflect their common social antecedents or the dependance of self-directed orientations on intellectual flexibility.[14] In this study, a mother's internal resources were defined as her orientation toward self and the social environment, i.e., her sense of mastery.

Mastery and distress. Mastery was viewed in this study as a factor affecting maternal distress. Implicit in this formulation is a distinction between the two concepts, the first defined as a cognitive dimension, the second as an affective dimension. That is to say, mastery describes a generalized belief about the social environment, whereas distress refers to negative affective experiences such as worry, anxiety, and sadness. This distinction, and the notion that the two variables are linked together in a causal sequence, are embedded in current theories of the genesis of psychologic disorder.[23,33]

Maternal distress was measured by a 7 item scale developed by Pearlin and Schooler.[21] It describes "the unpleasant feelings of which people are aware" and is specific to a woman's experience as a mother. Answers to each item range from 1 to 4, and possible scores are from 7 (low distress) to 28 (high distress). Mastery is measured by a 7 item scale also developed by Pearlin and Schooler.[21] Answers to each item range

from 1 to 4, and possible scores are from 7 (low mastery) to 28 (high mastery). Family repertoire of activities is measured by combining two scales, each with nine items, from Moos' Family Environment Scale (FES), namely, intellectual–cultural and active–recreational.[20] Family cohesion is measured by combining two other scales from the Moos FES, also with nine items each, namely, cohesion and conflict. Internal consistency reliability of each of these measures exceeds 0.80. Disability status is defined as a dichotomous variable with a value of 1 for a family with a disabled child and 0 for a control family.

Study Model

Figure 29-1 is a diagramatic representation of the study model. Since stressful demands on mothers have other sources apart from a disabled child, the model includes five indicators of social class and of family composition as covariates. To simplify the presentation, the path diagram does not depict these variables. All path coefficients were, however, computed in a model that includes these variables. The presence of a disabled child in the home and five covariates—race, family income, maternal education, number of children, and age of youngest child—were taken to be *exogenous* or *predetermined variables*; i.e., the model says nothing about how values of these variables are themselves determined. It was supposed that two sets of family variables—family repertoire of activities and family cohesion—depended on the six predetermined variables as well as on other factors that are not specified in the model. It was further felt that a mother's internal resources (her sense of mastery) depended on the two family factors as well as on the six predetermined variables and unspecified residual factors. Finally, maternal distress was seen as a function of a mother's sense of mastery, the two sets of family factors, and the six predetermined factors as well as unspecified residual factors. The model thus considered four successive outcomes of child disability.

It should be noted that this cross-sectional study has limitations in the causal inferences that can be drawn from it. Some variables in the model may be reciprocally related, whereas the model focuses only on influences that move in a single direction. For example, maternal distress may affect family cohesion, although interest was focused only on the influence that goes from family cohesion to maternal

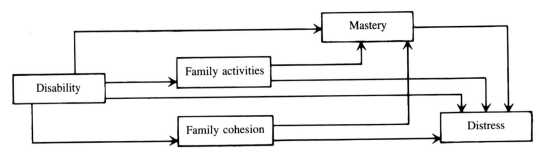

Figure 29-1. Path Diagram Representing a Model of the Impact of Child Disability on Maternal Distress.

distress. The statistical approach—path analysis—like statistics in general, cannot solve issues entangled with causality. These must be answered by study design. It should be noted, however, that there is no ambiguity in the direction of the relationship between child disability and each of the dependent variables in the model. Clearly, an association between child disability and maternal distress, for example, must be interpreted as an indication that the presence of a disabled child in the home affects maternal distress. As to the relationships between family factors and mastery or maternal distress, longitudinal data may provide more definitive answers about directionality. Figure 29-2 presents the estimates of the model using data on the 639 two-parent families in the study.

Maternal Distress

The results show that certain factors initially conceived to be causes of later outcomes are not sufficiently important empirically as direct influences (Fig. 29-2). Mastery and family cohesion thus had direct paths to maternal distress, while child disability, the key variable, as well as family repertoire of

activities did not. What was revealed by the path model that would not be revealed in a conventional regression model, however, is that factors not directly influential may nevertheless have indirect influences. Child disability thus, influences maternal distress indirectly through family repertoire and mastery. The model explains 40 percent of the variance in maternal distress.

These results provided general confirmation of the hypothesis: the presence of a disabled child in the home, uninfluenced by its interrelatedness with other aspects of the environment, has a significant negative effect on family repertoire of activities, which in turn affects a mother's sense of mastery, a factor that looms large among the determinants of maternal distress.

Effects of Race

Separate analyses were performed for black and white two-parent families. Results from these analyses are presented in Figures 29-3 and 29-4. The first result to emphasize is that the overall picture was rather different in black and white families. The causal

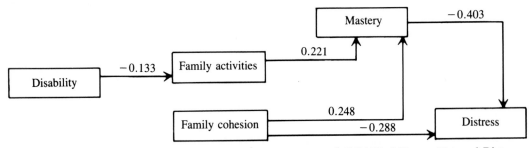

Figure 29-2. Path Diagram Representing a Model of the Impact of Child Disability on Maternal Distress: Estimates for Two-Parent Families (n = 639). A *straight line* with an *arrowhead* at one end represents a direct relationship; the variable at the head of the arrow depends directly on the variable at the tail. The degree of dependence is estimated by a path coefficient, which is a standardized partial regression coefficient. In this diagram, paths whose coefficients are less than 0.100 are omitted as empirically unimportant.

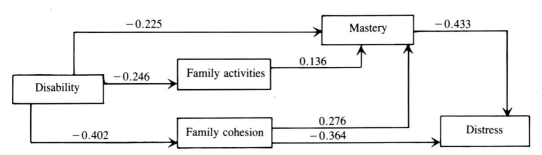

Figure 29-3. Path Diagram Representing a Model of the Impact of Child Disability on Maternal Distress: Estimates for Blacks (n = 105).

chain that connects the presence of a disabled child in the home to maternal distress is substantially stronger for blacks than for whites. Although in white families child disability affects mothers through a single string of connecting paths, in black families its effect spreads in several directions and its consequences for maternal distress are amplified by multiple connections. In black families, child disability has direct negative effects on family cohesion, family repertoire, and mothers' sense of mastery. Among these, the effect on family cohesion is first in order of magnitude. In white families, child disability has a direct negative effect only on family repertoire. In statistical terminology, key variables in the model "interact" with race.

Path coefficients are standardized so that there is meaning in the comparison between different variables in a single population. To compare effects between the two samples and to ascertain concretely the degree of dependence, however, unstandardized regressions are presented in Table 29-3.

As can be seen in Table 29-3, the dependence of maternal distress on mastery and on family dimensions and the dependence of mastery on family dimensions were similar in sign and size for blacks

and whites. For example, the regression coefficient of maternal distress on mastery was −0.633 in blacks and −0.592 in whites; the regressions of maternal distress on family cohesion were also similar in blacks and whites, −0.536 and, −0.422, respectively. Although the internal mechanisms within the family are similar for blacks and whites, the effects of child disability on these mechanisms showed marked differences. Among blacks, the presence of a disabled child in the home reduced family cohesion by 2.685 units. This change is translated to an increase of 1.44 in maternal distress (−2.685 × −0.536). In addition, the adverse effect of a disabled child on family cohesion reduced mastery by 0.746 (−2.685 × 0.278), which, in turn, is translated to an additional increase in maternal distress of 0.472 (−0.746 × −0.633). Child disability also affects family repertoire of activities and, through it, mastery and ultimately maternal distress. This indirect effect increased maternal distress by 0.120. In addition, child disability affected maternal distress in a fourth way, through its effect on mastery. This indirect effect is by 0.954 (−1.508 × −0.633). The total effect of the presence of a disabled child in the home on distress in black mothers was 2.985. For whites, the

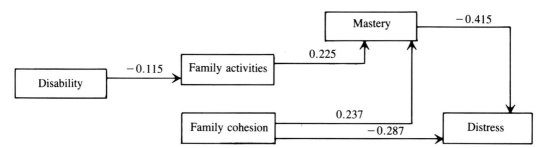

Figure 29-4. Path Diagram Representing a Model of the Impact of Child Disability on Maternal Distress: Estimates for Whites (n = 534).

Table 29-3
Partial Regression Coefficients in Successive Multiple Regressions
of Maternal Distress (Two-Parent Families)

Independent Variable	Family Activities	Family Cohesion	Mastery	Distress
	Blacks (n = 105)			
Income	0.039	−0.020	−0.022	−0.110*
Education	0.723*	−0.065	0.448*	0.388
Number of children	0.546*	−0.135	0.024	0.329
Youngest	0.150*	−0.054	0.101	0.003
Disability	−1.885*	−2.685*	−1.508*	−0.234
Family activities			0.119	0.059
Family cohesion			0.278*	−0.536*
Mastery				−0.633*
Constant	−0.296	9.181	13.422	10.369
R²†	0.217	0.185	0.289	0.461
	Whites (n = 533)			
Income	0.038*	0.022*	0.016	0.003
Education	0.406*	0.017	0.074	0.031
Number of children	0.202	−0.566*	−0.107	−0.203
Youngest	0.017	0.029	−0.118	−0.026
Disability	−0.836*	−0.062	−0.369*	0.723*
Family activities			0.189*	−0.056
Family cohesion			0.245*	−0.422*
Mastery				−0.592*
Constant	5.417	5.316	17.432	6.308
R²	0.138	0.068	0.196	0.353

*Coefficient exceeds twice its standard error.
†R² is the proportion of variable in the dependent variable explained by the model.

indirect effect of child disability on maternal distress is only through family repertoire and is calculated to change this score by 0.096. The total effect on maternal distress in whites was 0.82.

This comparison indicates that child disability has a far greater impact on black than on white mothers. Among blacks, child disability weakens those family processes that constitute important social conditions that enhance the psychologic well-being of all mothers, as well as erodes mothers' sense of mastery directly. In contrast, among whites a cohesive family climate and a mother's firm sense of mastery over her fate continue to shield her from experiencing distress. Neither of these important factors is weakened by child disability.

Effects of Family Income

Analysis of the effects of child disability on maternal distress in low- and high-income families revealed analogous results: the effect was almost twice as large in families with income of less than $10,000 as in families with income greater than $10,000. The difference, however, does not reach statistical significance (p < 0.12).

Some explanations for these differential vulnerabilities of black and white families (and perhaps also of low- and high-income families) might be found in results from an analysis of the impact of child disability on maternal employment.

Maternal Employment

Using the data on 639 two-parent families from this Cleveland study, the following question was addressed: Does child disability have a greater negative effect on maternal employment in low-income and in black families?

Black and low-income mothers are more likely to hold blue-collar, low-skilled jobs and thus be more affected by the presence of a disabled child in the home. First, conflicts between child-care demands and demands of the workplace would be greater for them, since the types of jobs they have access to do not accommodate easily to flexible or part-time schedules or frequent absences. Second, the net monetary benefits of hourly wage, low-paid work (part time or full time), considering the high cost of non-family care for disabled children, may be too low to constitute an effective incentive for market work. Third, since the primary motivation for maternal employment in these families is more likely to be financial need, their decision to work for pay would more likely be governed by these monetary considerations.

To examine this question, an ordinary least-squares linear model was used. Factors identified in previous research as having an influence on mothers' employment were controlled in this analysis. Differential effects of child disability were tested as interactions between child disability and husband's income and between child disability and race.

Controlling for mothers' age and education, number of children, age of youngest child, mothers' health, race, husbands' income, and the presence of a disabled child, partial regression coefficients for the two interaction terms are statistically significant ($p < 0.01$). The negative impact of child disability on maternal employment was greatest for families with the lowest level of income and decreased as family income rose. For example, the probability that a mother of a disabled child with husband's income of $5,000 (in 1977 dollars) is employed is, on the average, 10 percent lower than that of a mother of children free of disabilities but with the same income. When family income is $10,000, the deficit is by 6 percent. For families with income of $19,000, the effect of a disabled child on maternal employment was near zero.

As to the interaction of child disability with race, the results indicated that the negative effect of a disabled child on the probability that a mother is employed is almost three times as strong among blacks as among whites. For whites, the presence of a disabled child in the home reduces the probability of maternal employment by 13 percent, whereas for blacks the reduction is by 36 percent.

In order to assess the significance of these findings fully, it is necessary to take into account the economic conditions that induce black married women and wives of low-income husbands into the labor market in higher numbers. Low-income families are more likely to depend on wives' paid work for income needed for the purchase of nondiscretionary market goods. There is, in addition, an excess in the employment rate of black as compared to white wives,

an excess that persists even when husbands' income and other compositional differences are controlled. This may be due in part to the fact that a husband's income does not measure long-term earnings or the expected stability of his employment. The difficulty of maintaining a modest standard of living in unsettled economic times and in insecure jobs is probably greater for black than for white families. Such uncertainties may motivate black wives to remain in the labor market when white wives withdraw in response to increases in husband's income.

Since low-income and black families depend more closely on wives' earnings for their standard of living, child-care responsibilities that deter wives' employment are economically far more damaging for them than for other families. Although in high-income families the withdrawal of the wife from market work reduces income, the loss of this increment does not threaten a family's capacity to meet its basic needs. In low-income and black families, on the other hand, such losses often threaten the foundation of subsistence.

Conclusions

This chapter represents a statistical analysis of the effects of child disability on the psychologic adjustment of siblings and mothers. The results suggests that the presence of a disabled child in the home increases the likelihood of psychologic problems in siblings and mothers through its negative effects on family life.

With respect to *siblings,* birth order and age spacing are employed as indexes of the early life environment of siblings. Two interrelated hypotheses were tested: (1) younger siblings, specifically those born into a family with a disabled child, would be worse off than older siblings, whose early years were lived in a normal family, and (2) Among younger siblings, those in close age-spacing relationship to the disabled child would be worse off than those who were not. The results partially support these hypotheses. A *male* sibling born into a family with a disabled infant less than two years of age is at risk for psychologic impairment later on. For *female* siblings, a similar effect is not in evidence.

With respect to *mothers,* it was hypothesized that a disabled child in the home increases maternal distress through its negative effects on family cohesion and the range of family activities. The results supported this formulation. Analysis also revealed that the negative impact of child disability is far greater for blacks than for whites. A similar trend emerged for family income: the inpact of child disability on maternal distress is greater among low-income than high-income families. Data on the impact of child disability on maternal employment (and hence on family economic resources) indicate analogous race and income differences.

The finding that the economic impact of child disability varies across income levels and between blacks and whites suggests a link between social class, family vulnerability, and the economic consequences of child disability. The differential economic impact of child disability between blacks and whites parallels the differential impact of child disability on family functioning. In black families, where economic losses associated with child disability are more probable and far more severe, we find that child disability is associated also with substantial losses in family cohesion and in mothers' internal resources. In contrast, among whites, where the economic consequences of child disability are milder, the family appears to be a stable environment. The finding that family stability in the face of one type of stressful life problem is race related and the possibility that the association might be linked to socioeconomic factors have implications that go beyond the specific question addressed in this chapter. The complex picture that emerges from this analysis challenges the dominant view of the family in social and behavioral science.

In the current behavioral science discourse on sickness, the family is viewed primarily as therapeutic. This perspective is a logical extension of the concept of "therapeutic milieu," which dissolved the boundaries between specialized agents of therapy and the context of therapy. This extension, however, has gone further than underscoring the relevance of the family for the health of individuals. Instead, it constitutes a bias toward viewing the family as a shelter from harsh environments and a protective mediator of stressful stimuli. The label *social support* connotes this bias. What it tacitly emphasizes is the stability of the family and its autonomy. The family is said to be, in the words of one representative writer, "a remarkably effective buffer" between the individual and society at large.[1]

Yet despite its prominence, this model of the family has little theoretic and empiric support. Moreover, research on socialization and on status achievement strongly suggests that factors in the larger social environment exert a powerful influence on the conditions of family life. It emphasizes the predictable ways in which parents transmit to children conceptions of reality and general competencies, determined primarily by their experiences in the larger social environment. It suggests that the family, as a system intervening between the individual and society, is less often a powerful buffer than it is a transmitter of behaviors and orientations shaped in other settings.

These observations, as well as the findings presented here, which emphasize socioeconomic disparities in the capacities of families to withstand extraordinary burdens strongly suggest that in defining the family as social support, professionals have unwisely prejudged what should be assessed empirically. It is now time to devote more effort to the empiric examination of the conditions that foster or impair the capacity of families to shield individuals from the adverse consequences of illness and other life problems.

REFERENCES

1. Beiser M: Etiology of mental disorder: Sociocultural aspects, in Wolman BB (ed): Manual of Child Psychopathology. New York, McGraw-Hill, 1972
2. Bentzen F: Sex ratios in learning and behavior disorders. Am J Orthopsychiatry 33:92, 1963
3. Breslau N, Weitzman M, Messenger K: Psychological functioning of siblings of disabled children. Pediatrics 67:344, 1981
4. Breslau N: Siblings of disabled children: Birth order and age-spacing effects. J Abnorm Child Psychol 10(1):85–96, 1982
5. Burton L: The Family Life of Sick Children: A Study of Families Coping with Chronic Childhood Diseases. London, Routledge and Kegan Paul, 1975
6. Drotar D, Baskiewicz A, Irvin N, et al: The adaptation of parents to the birth of an infant with a congenital malformation: A hypothetical model. Pediatrics 56:710, 1975
7. Farber B: Effects of a severely mentally retarded child on family integration. Soc Res Child Dev 24:2, 1959
8. Farber B: Family organization and crisis: Maintenance of integration in families with a severely mentally retarded child. Soc Res Child Dev 25:1960
9. Friedrich W: Ameliorating the psychological impact of chronic physical disease on the child and family. J Pediatr Psych 2:26, 1977
10. Gath A: The school-age siblings of mongol children. Br J Psychiatry 123:161, 1973
11. Gayton WF, Friedman SB, Tavormina JF, et al: Children with cystic fibrosis. I. Psychological test findings of patients, siblings and parents. Pediatrics 58:888, 1977
12. Hare EH, Laurence KM, Paynes H, et al: Spina bifida cystica and family stress. Br Med J 2:757, 1966
13. Johns N: Family reactions to the birth of a child with a congenital abnormality. Med J Aust 7:277, 1971

14. Kohn ML, Schooler C: Occupational experience and psychological functioning: An assessment of reciprocal effects. Am Sociol Rev 38:97, 1973

15. Kohn ML, Schooler C: The reciprocal effects of substantive complexity of work and intellectual flexibility: A longitudinal assessment. Am J Sociol 84:24, 1978

16. Langner TS, Gersten JC, McCarthy ED, et al: A screening inventory for assessing psychiatric impairment in children 6 to 18. J Consult Clin Psychol 44:286, 1976

17. Lavigne JV, Ryan M: Psychological adjustment of siblings of children with chronic illness. Pediatrics 63:616, 1979

18. McMichael JK: Handicap: A Study of Physically Handicapped Children and their Families. London, Staples Press, 1971

19. Meyerowitz JH, Kaplan HB: Familial responses to stress: The case of cystic fibrosis. Soc Sci Med 1:249, 1967

20. Moos RH: The Family Environment Scale Preliminary Manual. Social Ecology Laboratory, Department of Psychiatry, Stanford University, Palo Alto, 1974

21. Pearlin LI, Schooler C: The structure of coping. J Health Soc Behav 19:2, 1978

22. Pless IB, Pinkerton P: Chronic Childhood Disorder: Promoting Patterns of Adjustment. Chicago. Year Book Medical Publishers, 1975

23. Radloff LS, Rae DS: Components of the sex difference in depression, in Simmons RG (ed): Research in Community and Mental Health, vol. 2. Greenwich, Conn., Jai Press, 1981, pp 111–138

24. Robertson J: Mother-infant interaction from birth to twelve months: Two case studies, in Foss BM (ed): Determinants of infant behavior. London: Methuen and Co., 1965

25. Rutter M: The Qualities of Mothering: Maternal Deprivation Reassessed. NeW York, Jason Aronson, 1974, p 31

26. Satterwhite BB: Impact of chronic illness on child and family: An overview based on five surveys with implications for management. Int J Rehabil Res 1:7, 1978

27. Shere MO: Socio-emotional factors in the family of twins with cerebral palsy. Except Child 22:197, 206, 1956

28. Spaeth JL: Characteristics of the work setting and the job as determinants on income, in Sewell WH, Hauser RM, Featherman DL (eds): Schooling and Achievement in American Society. New York, Academic Press, 1976, pp 161–176

29. Tew BJ, Laurence KM: Mothers, brothers and sisters of patients with spina bifida. Dev Med Child Neurol (Suppl 29) 15:69, 1973

30. Turk J: Impact of cystic fibrosis on family functioning. Pediatrics 34:67, 1964

31. U.S. National Center for Health Statistics: Current Estimates From the Health Interview Survey: United States—1967. DHEW pub no. 1000, Series 10, No. 52. Washington, D.C., U.S. Government Printing Office, 1969

32. U.S. National Center for Health Statistics: Current Estimates From the Health Interview Survey: United States—1978. DHEW pub no. (PHS) 80-1551. Washington, D.C., U.S. Government Printing Office, 1979

33. Wheaton B: The sociogenesis of psychological disorder: An attributional theory. J Health Soc Behav 21:100, 1980

Bernard H. Shulman

30

Legal Aspects of Education for the Handicapped

The enormous and complex problems of educating handicapped children are succintly stated in Sec. 601 of the Act, Education for All Handicapped (20 (USC 1401), where Congress found the following:

1. There are more than 8 million handicapped children in the United States today.
2. The special education needs of such children are not being fully met.
3. More than half the handicapped children in the United States do not receive appropriate educational services that would enable them to have full equality of opportunity.
4. One million of the handicapped children are excluded entirely from the public school system and will not go through the educational process with their peers.
5. There are many handicapped children throughout the United States participating in regular school programs whose handicaps prevent them from having a successful educational experience because their handicaps are undetected.
6. Because of the lack of adequate services within the public school system, families are often forced to find services outside the public school system, often at great distance from their residence and at their own expenses.
7. Developments in training teachers and in diagnostic and instructional procedures and methods have advanced to the point that, given appropriate funding, state and local educational agencies can and will provide effective special education and related services to meet the needs of handicapped children.

8. State and local educational agencies have a responsibility to provide education for all handicapped children.
9. It is in the national interest that the federal government assist state and local efforts to provide programs to meet the educational needs of handicapped children in order to ensure equal protection of the laws.

ATTITUDES

The laws that grant protection and rights to the handicapped student reflect both attitudinal changes and public acceptance of children who are different. This acceptance evolved over a period of recent years as a result of greater understandings that have been reached by communities of people. National and local attention has focused on the rights and struggles of children with handicaps, and the courts and legislatures have responded to this attention.

In 1919, the parents of a sixth grader aged 13 yr were not allowed to enroll their child in a Wisconsin school. When the lower court ordered the school board to enroll the child, the school board appealed. The appellate court described the child as follows:

He has been a crippled and defective child since his birth. . . . He is slow and hesitating in speech and has a peculiarly high, rasping and disturbing tone of voice, accompanied with uncontrollable facial contortions, making it difficult for him to make himself understood. He also has an uncontrollable flow of saliva which drools from his mouth on his clothing and books, causing him to present an unclean

311

appearance. . . . He is normal mentally. . . . It is claimed on the part of the School Board that his physical condition and ailment produces a nauseating effect upon the teachers and school children; that by reason of his physical condition he takes up an undue portion of the teacher's time and attention, distracts the attention of other pupils, and interferes greatly with the discipline and progress of the school.

The court, after reviewing the facts, ruled that the attendance of this child would be harmful to the best interests of the school. The balance between this child's rights and the general welfare resulted in the court's refusal to reinstate the child. This was the state of the law in 1919.[1]

In testimony before Congress before 1975, statistical evidence was given that more than 4 million handicapped children in the United States were not receiving appropriate educational services, and that 1 million handicapped children were excluded entirely from the public school system.[2] In 1975, Congress enacted Public Law 94–142, which provides requirements and money for the educational needs of such children. Some states, e.g., Massachusetts, had a similar law already. It is evident now that the "education for the handicapped" law has resulted in educators' directing attention to the need to identify these children, evaluate their needs, and design and implement appropriate programs.

IMPORTANT DEFINITIONS

Under 94–142 regulations, a child is not handicapped unless he or she needs special education. Pertinent sections of 94–142 regulations concerning definitions are described below.

The regulations of 94–142 require that each state shall ensure that full appropriate public education is made available to all handicapped children age 3–21 yr. In addition, a child search requirement must be 0–21 yr of age to enable the states to plan for children's full educational opportunity. There are no specific provisions of 94–142 regulations concerning class size or student–teacher ratios. There is only the requirement (Sec. 121a.551) that each public agency shall ensure that a continuum of alternate placements is available to meet the needs of handicapped children for special education and related services.

Handicapped. As used in Sec. 121a.5(a), the term *handicapped* means those children evaluated in accordance with Sec. 121a.520–121a.534 as being mentally retarded, hard of hearing, deaf, speech impaired, visually handicapped, seriously emotionally

disturbed, orthopaedically impaired, other health impaired, deaf-blind, multiply handicapped, or having specific learning disabilities, who, because of these impairments, need special education and related services. The definition gives further details on each handicap type.

Special education. Special education is defined in Sec. 121a.14(a) as specially designed instruction at no cost to the parent to meet the unique needs of each child, including classroom instruction, instruction in physical education, home instruction, and instruction in hospitals and institutions. The term includes speech pathology or any other related service, including vocational education if it consists of specially designed instruction.

Related services. Related services is defined in Sec. 121a.13 as transportation and such developmental, corrective, and other supportive services as are required to assist a handicapped child to benefit from special education and include speech pathology and audiology, psychologic services, physical and occupational therapy, recreation, early identification and assessment of disabilities, counseling services, and medical services for diagnostic or evaluation purposes. The term also includes school health services, social work services in school, and parent counseling and training.

SEC. 504 REGULATIONS

There also exist important relationships among 94–142, Sec. 504 of the Rehabilitation Act, and local laws (e.g., Ch. 766 in Massachusetts). The regulations under Sec. 504 of the Rehabilitation Act of 1973* deal with nondiscrimination on the basis of handicap and basically require that recipients of federal funds provide equal opportunities to handicapped persons; i.e., that they meet the needs of handicapped persons to the same extent that the needs of nonhandicapped persons are met. Subpart D of Sec. 504 contains requirements very similar to those in Part B of the Education of the Handicapped Act.

It is also important to note that both parts require that the education be provided free and that handicapped students be educated with nonhandicapped students to the extent appropriate. Evaluation pro-

---

*45CFR, Part 84, published as 42 FR 22675, May 4, 1977.

cedures must be adopted to ensure appropriate classification and procedural safeguards must be established. In several respects, however, the Sec. 504 regulations are broader in coverage than Part B. For example, the definitions of *handicapped person* and *qualified handicapped person* under Sec. 504 cover a broader population than the definition of *handicapped children* under Part B. Under the Part B definition, a handicapped child is a child who has one of the impairments listed in the act, who because of that impairment requires a special education and related services. Under Sec. 504, a *handicapped person* is a person who has a physical or mental impairment that substantially limits one of more major life activities, has a record of that type of impairment, or is regarded as having that impairment (Sec. 84.3 [j]).

The regulations for Sec. 504 also deal with a number of subjects not covered by the Part B regulations, e.g., barrier-free facilities and program accessibility, employment, postsecondary education and health, welfare and social services. Sec. 84 33 (b) (2) refers to the proper drafting of an individualized educational plan as a primary means of meeting the requirements dealing with appropriate education.

INDEPENDENT EVALUATION

Under 94–142, the parent has a right to an independent evaluation. This right, however, is limited by the school system's right to initiate a hearing to determine if its evaluation was appropriate. If so, the independent evaluation does not have to be paid for by the system (Sec. 121a.503).

If the parent initiates an independent evaluation, the results of the evaluation must be considered by the public agency (school) in any decision made with respect to the provision of a free appropriate public education to the child and may be presented as evidence at a hearing under 121a.502.

Cost sharing. An important fiscal issue for states involves cost sharing between education and human services. In Sec. 121a.301 and Sec. 121a.302 of the 94–142 regulations, mention is made that "each state may use whatever state, local, federal, and private sources of support are available in the state to meet the requirements of this part." For example, when it is necessary to place a handicapped child in a residential facility, a state could use joint agreements between the agencies involved for cost sharing the placement.

Individualized education plan. Public Law 94–142 and the adopted regulations were developed with considerable public participation. The essential element in the services rendered is the individualized education plan (IEP). The term *IEP* means a written statement (program) for each handicapped child that includes the following:

1. A statement of present levels of educational performance
2. A statement of annual goals, including short-term instructional objectives
3. A statement of specific educational services to be provided
4. A statement on the extent to which child will be able to participate in regular programs
5. A projected date for initiation and anticipated duration of such services
6. Appropriate objective criteria and evaluation procedures to see if instructional goals are met (annually)

The IEP is developed in a planning conference, which the local education agency is responsible for initiating. For a handicapped child who is currently receiving special education, a planning conference must develop an IEP for the following year. If a child is handicapped and is not receiving special education, however, an individualized planning conference must be held within 30 days of a formal determination that the child is handicapped.

As a minimum, the planning conference must include a representative of the local education agency (other than the child's teacher) who is in the field of school administration, the child's teacher or teachers, one or both of the child's parents, and, where appropriate, the child. Planning conferences may be held without parents if a parent furnishes a written waiver of both parents' right to participate or if the local agency is unable to convince the parents that they should attend. If a local school department or agency places a child in a private school setting, then that agency is responsible for the development of the IEP. The financial responsibility for the child's education remains with the state or local education agency.

PROCEDURAL SAFEGUARDS

A number of specific procedures are written into the law and expanded in the regulations. To protect the rights of children and parents, these safeguards include due process, nondiscriminatory testing, least restrictive alternative, native language, confidentiality, and the right to representation. Written notice must be given to the parents of a handicapped child before the education agency proposes to initiate or change the identification, evaluation, or educational placement of the child or the provision of a free appropriate public education. Consent must be obtained before a formal evaluation begins.

The formal evaluation must be conducted before any action is taken on placement or denial of a handicapped child in a special education program. Any change in a child's plan should be made with the knowledge and input of the parents. The basis for the plan or change of plan should be existing evaluation information that is not more than two years old.

RECENT COURT CASES

In 1972, a federal district court ruled that the equal protection clause of the U.S. Constitution is violated when handicapped children are denied a specialized education in public schools in *Mills v. Board of Education of District of Columbia,* 348 F. Supp. 866 (D.D.C. 1971). In *Panitch v. State of Wisconsin,* 371 F. Supp. 955 (E.D. Wis. 1974), the federal district court held that the handicapped child is entitled, at public expense, to an appropriate education that meets his or her needs and that is generally equivalent to the education provided to nonhandicapped children.

In a recent interesting case, *Southeastern Community College v. Daws,* 442 U.S. 397 (1979), the U.S. Supreme Court agreed with a district court decision that held that the "otherwise qualified" requirement of Sec. 504 did not require that a nursing school accept a candidate with a hearing disability. The application was denied.

In *Mattie v. Holladay,* 3EHLR 551:109 (N.D. Miss. 1978), the plaintiffs entered into a consent decree that granted some relief for their claim that Mississippi used racially biased testing that resulted in the classification of a disproportionate number of black children as mentally retarded. The question of test validity was raised and will continue to be an issue of litigation in the future.

A court in California, in *Larry P. v. Wilson Riles,* 3EHLR 551:295 (N.D. Cal. 1979), also found that standardized intelligence quotient (IQ) tests were racially and culturally biased and enjoined their use in California for the placement of children in classes for the educable mentally retarded. On a similar issue in *Parents in Action of Special Education v. Joseph P. Hannon,* 3EHLR 552:108 (N.D. Ill. 1980), however, the Illinois court disagreed with the California decision and, after a careful review of each test item on the Stanford–Binet and WISC–R tests, ruled that the tests were not unfair and indicated that the California court did not, in fact, examine the items on the test to determine whether bias did or did not exist. As for tests in general, the courts may in future litigation analyze the data for disparate impact, as did California, or elect to follow the Illinois court in judging the validity of items in a particular test.

In a recent and surprising decision, the Supreme Court of New Jersey ruled on the issue whether all mentally impaired children were protected under 94–142, no matter what degree of brain damage. In *Levine v. State of New Jersey,* the parents sought to compel the full public payment of the costs of institutional care of their children. The parents argued that the state was responsible for providing such care as part of a "free education" under both the state constitution and the federal law. State law in New Jersey provided that parents who had the ability to pay could be required to contribute to the costs of institutional maintenance. The state contended that the parents should pay because the care was custodial rather than educational. The children were both severely mentally retarded and were judged to be incapable of learning as much as a child aged five years.

The New Jersey court recognized that a great number of mentally handicapped children can benefit from education toward the achievement of valid goals (competitor in the labor market) and would, therefore, be entitled to the full educational benefits afforded by the state constitution. The court, however, concluded:

> Nevertheless, the sad fact endures that there is a category of mentally disabled children so severely impaired as to be unable to absorb or benefit from education. It is neither realistic nor meaningful to equate the type of care and habilitation which such children require for their health and survival with 'education' in the sense that that term is used in the Constitution. . . . The Constitutional mandate for a free public education simply does not apply to these unfortunate children.

It is important to note that uncertainty will prevail for some years as courts review the language of the law and regulations that are designed to protect the handicapped. A court-ordered training program has helped New York school officials understand federal handicapped education law and recognize the legal rights of parents. The year-long staff development program brought a greater awareness of responsibilities that schools have in providing a free and appropriate education to all students. Improved special education services require school systems to address problems such as time required between referral and evaluation (waiting lists), sufficient personnel for evaluation and service delivery, class size, budget cuts, need for support, and reluctance of some parents to cooperate or consent to evaluations. Staff development practices and the school's relationship with parents must be reviewed regularly for proper implementation of 94–142. The July 1979 ruling in *Lora v. Board of Education of New York* reinforces this need.

Another issue recently brought before the courts involves "related services." Causes of action in behalf of the handicapped child now allege violations of 94–142, the 1973 Rehabilitation Act, and, indeed, the Fifth and Fourteenth Amendments to the U.S. Constitution. Suits have asked the court to order the state to provide the handicapped children with appropriate diagnosis, evaluation, therapy, counseling, and emergency inpatient and long- or short-term community-based residential mental health services in an environment "least restrictive" of personal liberty. Suits have urged the courts to mandate the state to develop procedures, policies, and contracts necessary to provide handicapped education services, and, where the state has placed some handicapped children in institutions or facilities far from home, the parents have alleged that such restricts the contact of the child with his family and friends. One such suit was filed in Idaho in August 1980.

CURRENT ISSUES

A federal court in Pennsylvania recently ruled that some emotionally disturbed and profoundly retarded students are entitled to public education beyond the normal 180-day school year. Courts will inquire whether regression during the summer could be demonstrated to occur to such an extent that the child could not make effective progress toward an otherwise attainable goal of self-sufficiency *(Armstrong v. Kline)*.

In *Hoffman v. Board of Education,* a New York trial court awarded a judgment of $750,000 against the New York City school board for mistakenly placing a child of normal intelligence into a class for the mentally retarded. The child attended this class for his first 11 yr of schooling. The child suffered from a speech defect and, at age five, scored one point less on a verbal IQ test than was needed for placement in a regular class. The school psychologist diagnosed the child as retarded but recommended reevaluation within two years. The psychologist's recommendation was ignored, and the plaintiff student left school with less than a second-grade level of reading and computational skills. On appeal, however, the court reversed its decision and held for the school department as a matter of public interest. The courts thus far have been reluctant to establish an educational malpractice cause of action.

The California courts have also indicated that the dictates of public policy and the difficulty of assessing wrongs, as well as a lack of clear definition of educational malpractices, generally disfavor ruling against school systems in such suits.

The issue of "related services" will continually surface and be subject to court analysis and review. Is psychotherapy a related service? Is it educationally related or is it a medical problem? The line of demarcation cannot be simplified, and the determination as to whether a refused related service is in violation of the Rehabilitation Act of 1973 can be subject to argument (see below).

In Texas, a girl aged three years was presented to the school district for educational assessment and placement, with, among other physical problems, a neurogenic bladder secondary to myelodysplasia. Myelodysplasia often results in hydrocephalus and spina bifida with or without associated myelomeningocele. The urologists had developed the technique of clean intermittent catheterization (CIC) of the bladder. This is accomplished by catheterization of the urinary bladder by an adult on a set time sequence. This, with associated antibiotic therapy to prevent infection, is clearly the treatment used most extensively by most major medical centers today. The school department's evaluation noted the child's condition as orthopaedic handicap with some speech impairment but did not include the provisions for furnishing CIC in the plan. This request for catheterization was made by the child's parents.

On appeal, the parents claimed that the child could not avail herself of educational programs without the availability of CIC. The office of civil rights later affirmed a state board of education order and concluded that the refusal of the school district to provide the requested service was an effective denial of access to the school programs in violation of Sec. 504, specifically, 45 C.F.R. 84.37. The parents brought an action in the federal district court asserting a course of action under the Fourteenth Amendment, Sec. 1983 of the 1971 Civil Rights Act, Sec. 1415 of the Education of All Handicapped Children Act, and Sec. 504 of the 1973 Rehabilitation Act.

The Court found that "to be related in the statutory sense, the service requirement must arise from an effort to educate. There is a difference between maintenance of life-systems and enhancing a handicapped person's ability to learn." It is uncertain as to how Congress will react to a differentiation between a life system and learning skills. The court of appeals held that catheterization was needed as an entitlement to education and found such failure of service a violation of 504. Courts may yet define related services broadly, but the financial burden of such may cause Congress to act and set forth a narrower definition.

The case described above gives rise to the issue of medical- versus education-related services. Is psychotherapy a medical service or a psychologic one? If the medical service is diagnostic or evaluative, then it will be regarded as related. If it is medical per se, however, it need not be provided. In such cases, the Bureau of the Handicapped will look to state law for assistance. If state law permits the service to be supplied by a psychologist, then it can be argued that it must be supplied by the school. In a 1979 Montana case, psychotherapy was not defined in the federal regulations. The state courts went to the police dictionary and found a definition of "by psychological means." The court said the service must be provided by the schools. Litigation will continue, but it still must be asked whether Congress intended schools to accept the responsibility for psychiatric services.

As financial burdens are imposed on school districts, more and more school boards can be expected to plead lack of funds in response to mandated special education services. Several decisions have made it clear that the courts will reject a plea of lack of funds as a defense. In a recent New York City case, a federal district court ruled that the city's fiscal crisis provided no excuse for violating the statutory and constitutional rights of emotionally disturbed children. Lack of money was no reason for placing children in largely segregated special day schools. The court acknowledged in *Lora v. Board of Education* "the inescapable fact that to spend substantially more on this pupil population may well necessitate a sacrifice in services now afforded children in the rest of the system."

Proper management of cerebral palsy may involve both short and long-range goals and objectives. The main objective of Sec. 504 of 93–112 was to bring handicapped people into the mainstream of American life. The mandate applies to any program or activity receiving federal financial assistance in excess of $2500. Failure to comply with Sec. 504 can result in a cut-off of federal funds.

As to long-range plans, the physician will want to know if employment is possible in particular situations and cases. The degree of handicap will be viewed with inquiry as to self-sustaining probability

and possibility. It is wise to know that Sec. 504 mandates specific requirements for three major areas: employment of the handicapped, removal of architectural barriers, and education. Sec. 504 prohibits *employers* from discriminating against any otherwise qualified job applicant on the basis of handicap. Also, a qualified handicapped person cannot be denied a job because the employer's facilities are not accessible to him. The employer must make the necessary refinements and possible reconstructions to accommodate the qualified handicapped person.

An inventory of aptitudes, interests, and functional abilities must therefore be clearly set forth for the palsied child, with the expectation that the physician can help establish those functions that make a child otherwise qualified for the world of work. Career orientation and counseling, where indicated, will enable the child and the parents to better prepare for those opportunities that can be supported for the individual by an "otherwise qualified" status. In addition, handicapped employees must be allowed to work with nonhandicapped employees to the maximum extent possible. Sec. 504 is a civil rights law and pertains to many areas that do not directly involve a school.

CARNEGIE STUDY

Of all American children, those who are handicapped are the least identifiable as a distinctive social group. They share no common physical, psychological, or cultural characteristics; the blind child, the child with cerebral palsy, and the child with minimal brain damage are generally less like each other than each is like his or her able-bodied mates. What distinguishes handicapped children is above all a social fact: they differ from the able-bodied norm, and for this reason they are assigned a stigmatized and deviant social role.[3]

The above report, from the foreword by Kenneth Keniston, chairman of the Carnegie Council on Children, notes that "far from having to be exiled by their defective biology . . . there is every reason for handicapped children to enter the social mainstream as adults . . . to hold jobs and make careers for themselves."

The courts in the future may take judicial notice of studies and recommendations of the Carnegie Council on Children. This commission was established in 1972 by the Carnegie Corporation of New York to investigate the current status of children in American society and to develop policy recommendations for ways in which the future needs of children could be met.*

DISCIPLINE

Although special-needs students are subject to a school's disciplinary code, they are also entitled to the due process procedural safeguards other students are; however, their discipline creates unique problems.

In *Stuart v. Happi,* 443 F. Supp. 1235 (Conn. 1978), the plaintiff, a student with severe learning and emotional disabilities, was involved in a disruptive incident at school. A written request for a review of the plaintiff's special education was lodged with the defendant before the scheduled disciplinary hearing which would determine whether to expel the plaintiff. The court granted a preliminary injunction to prevent the expulsion hearing from taking place and held that 94–142 entitles school authorities to take swift disciplinary measures against disruptive handicapped children, such as suspension. The child's placement, however, can only be changed through a review of the child's special education program and a determination of whether the child's present placement is appropriate.

The court indicated that handicapped children could indeed be suspended or their placements may be changed. The clear implication of the court's decision is that handicapped children may not be expelled, however.

In *S-1 v. Turlington,* 3EHLR 551:353 (S.D. Fla. 1979), the court held that there had not been an adequate determination of the relationship between the students' handicaps and their behavior problems. The court held that the evaluation team must determine whether the disruptive behavior was the primary result of the handicap. Any change in program, plans, or placement must be recommended by an evaluating team rather than be a school board decision.

In Iowa, a court held in *Southeast Warren Com-* *munity School District v. Department of Public Instruction,* 285 N.W. 2d 137, 3EHLR 551:378 (Iowa, 1979), that school districts can expel a handicapped child if there is no reasonable alternative placement available. A recommendation must first come from the team on any possible alternative placement or expulsion, however.

In Indiana, the court held that schools may not expel students whose handicaps cause them to be disruptive. Again, it would seem that the school must first determine if the handicap is the cause of the child's misbehavior.

Although many school districts have not adopted formal guidelines for disciplining special needs students, the following guidelines should be noted:

1. When devising an IEP, the team should consider what types of disciplinary measures would be appropriate for a child.
2. The procedural safeguards applicable to all students must be followed. A series of continuous suspensions may be regarded as a change in placement.

THE FUTURE

It is important to recognize that there will be a future acceleration of litigation under 42 U.S.C. 1983. The law is yet to be clarified in the areas enumerated in this chapter, but the issues are present for changing legislation or a clearer definition by case holdings. Denial of an appropriate education to a handicapped child is a violation of the U.S. Constitution. Attorneys' fees based on *Maine v. Thibontot,* 100 S. Ct. 2502 (1980), will be assessed even for purely statutory violations of federal law.

In the management of cerebral palsy, one must be aware of the appropriate legislation as interpreted by court decisions. This will enable the physician and family to include in their diagnosis, evaluation, and educational planning such rights provided by law.

---

*The council's previous publications are (1) Keniston K: All Our Children: The American Family Under Pressure, 1977, (2) Clarke–Stewart A: Child Care in the Family: A Review of Research and Some Propositions for Policy, 1977, (3) Ogbu J: Minority Education and Caste: The American System in Cross Cultural Perspective, 1978, and (4) deLone RH: Small Futures: Children, Inequallty, and the Limits of Liberal Reform, 1979.

REFERENCES

1. *Beattier v. Board of Education,* 169 Wis. 231, 172 N.W. 153 (1919).
2. 20 USC—Sections 1401–1461.
3. Gliedman J, Roth W: The Unexpected Minority: Handicapped Children in America. New York, Harcourt Brace Jovanovich, 1979.

PARENT–PHYSICIAN RESOURCES

1. Albert RE, Emmons ML: Your Perfect Right. San Luis Obispo, Cal, Impact, 1970
2. Koppelman M, Adkerman P: Between Parent and School. New York, The Dial Press, 1977
3. NICSEM Master Index to Special Education Materials: University of Southern California, Dept. C., University Park, Los Angeles, CA 90007, 1980
4. Seligman M: Strategies for Helping Parents of Exceptional Children. New York, The Free Press, 1979

SUGGESTED RESOURCES

1. American Association on Mental Deficiency
   5201 Connecticut Avenue, N. W.
   Washington, D. C. 20015
2. American Public Health Association
   1015 18th Street N. W.
   Washington, D. C. 20036
3. American Speech and Hearing Association
   9030 Old Georgetown Road
   Washington, D. C. 20014
4. Association for Children with Learning Disabilities
   5225 Grace Street
   Pittsburgh, Pennsylvania 15236
5. Children's Defense Fund (Legal Rights)
   1520 New Hampshire Avenue N. W.
   Washington, D. C. 20036
6. Council for Exceptional Children (Legal Division)
   1920 Association Drive
   Reston, Virginia 22091
7. National Association for Mental Health, Inc.
   1800 North Kent Street
   Arlington, Virginia 22209
8. National Association for Retarded Citizens
   2709 Avenue E East, P. O. Box 6109
   Arlington, Texas 76011
9. National Society for Autistic Children
   169 Tampa Avenue
   Albany, NY 12208
10. United Cerebral Palsy Associations, Inc.
    66 East 34th Street
    New York, NY 10016

Jean M. Zadig

31

The Education of the Child with Cerebral Palsy

The 1975 Education for All Handicapped Children Act (Public Law 94-142) requires that every child with a handicapping condition receive a thorough evaluation to determine the nature of the problems, need for special education services, type of program that can best meet the need for special education services, and type of program that can best meet the child's needs. The law then guarantees an appropriate education to the child, whatever the nature and degree of the handicap. Although implementation is far from complete and the quality of available services remains uneven, there has never been a time when so many handicapped children were so well served.

The pediatrician and other medical specialists who provide continuing supervision for children with cerebral palsy are often asked to give advice and advocacy in educational matters. It is essential that they be aware of student and parental rights under federal and state laws (see Chap. 30) and knowledgeable about the child's educational needs. It is also helpful if they know local school personnel and resources.

When a disabled child is studied for educational planning, medical diagnosis will seldom be the determining factor in the choice of a school placement. Instead, level of intellectual functioning, expressive and receptive language skills, and the presence or absence of sensory, perceptual, and motor handicaps will be considered.[17] The law requires that a pupil be placed in the least restrictive placement consistent with his or her needs; for the student with normal intelligence, this will often be a regular class. The law further requires that placement decisions be made on the basis of multidimensional and nonbiased as-

sessment; however, the degree to which this is possible with students who have cerebral palsy is open to question. Intelligence is less easily assessed, and, in a sense, all tests are biased against them. Motor and perceptual deficits reduce performance scores, while communication handicaps and restricted social experience reduce verbal scores. Time constraints unfairly penalize, and even when noncognitive measures are employed, children with cerebral palsy tend to have lower scores because of their secondary handicaps. Regular class teachers who are prepared to accept a student with mild cognitive impairment may balk at accepting a handicapped child, insisting that he or she will require too much individual attention. The resource room teacher, responsible for providing academic support, may offer similar objections, and the student becomes relegated to the least desirable placement, often with pupils who are more limited in academic potential. In such classes, where academic achievement is a low priority, the student may fail to acquire reading skills, which would be enormously satisfying and useful for adult adjustment and leisure.

Socioemotional maturity must, of course, be considered in educational planning. Limited social experiences, parental overprotection and even small size may cause the child to behave and be perceived as a much younger child. If placed with normal children far below chronologic age, the child's own immature behaviors will be reinforced by the inappropriate models provided. In most cases, therefore, it is preferable to limit the age discrepancy to only one or two years. Types of placement available to these pupils are shown in Table 31-1.

Table 31-1

Placements for Pupils with Cerebral Palsy

Placement (from Least to Most Restrictive)	Pupils for Whom Appropriate
Regular class with adaptations and consultation	Pupils with fully normal intelligence and no major specific learning disability or communication or sensory handicap (degree of motor involvement less important)
As above, but with tutorial or resource room support for academics	Pupils with normal or near normal intelligence who have mild, specific learning disability or mild to moderate communication, hearing, or visual handicap
Self-contained special class with some mainstreaming where appropriate	Pupils with normal or near-normal IQ who have moderate-severe learning disabilities *or* severe communication or sensory handicap (also mildly retarded)
Self-contained class within public school, minimal interaction with normal peers	Pupils of all cognitive levels who have serious sensory or emotional handicap, unintelligible speech, poorly controlled seizure disorder (two or more)
Regional or collaborative class or private day school program	Pupils whose needs cannot be met in local district because district is small or pupil needs many specialized services (also preschoolers and adolescents)
Combination of foster, group, or pediatric nursing home and day school in community	Pupils of all degrees of handicap who cannot be at home, older pupils whose local school districts cannot meet their specialized needs
Private residential school, state institution, or pediatric home with stimulation program	Severely multihandicapped children who need nursing care, older pupils with severe problems who have exhausted all other resources, short-term alternative for others
Home or hospital tutoring	Not appropriate for any pupil except on interim basis

HISTORICAL CONTEXT

In the 19th century a few private and state schools provided education and habilitation for homogeneous groups of handicapped students, but it was not until the early decades of the 20th century that public schools began making serious efforts to serve children with handicaps. The first classes were for "slow-learning" pupils who were considered educable but were unable to progress at the rate of their normal peers. By modern standards, these children would be classified as "borderline," learning disabled, and disadvantaged; a few might be considered mildly mentally retarded. In urban areas, immigrant children were also placed in segregated classes. Children with cerebral palsy or other congenital or developmental disabilities were not accepted, and there were none of the special services that such children require. The emphasis was on the acquisition of basic academic skills, moral values, and manual skills, the last having presumed vocational relevance. The likelihood that students would eventually be integrated into the adult working community was enhanced by excluding more challenging pupils.

State residential schools had in the meantime, failed to demonstrate that institutions could habilitate most retarded persons for return to the community and now opened their doors to infants and children with severe mental retardation, cerebral palsy, and other multihandicapping conditions, where the prognosis was thought to be poor. The term *school* was a misnomer, since only the more capable residents were offered any educational program. Teachers selected pupils on the basis of their perceived educability, leaving the rest to languish in the notorious "day rooms" depicted so movingly in Blatt's and Kaplan's *Christmas in Purgatory*.[2] In contrast, private schools for physically handicapped students catered to children with poliomyelitis or other physically disabling conditions. Their strict entrance criteria virtually ensured that only the brightest children with cerebral palsy were accepted.

By the middle of this century, parent and professional advocacy had begun to effect significant change.

Public school classes for the "trainable" mentally retarded began serving large numbers of moderately retarded children of elementary-school age. Children with cerebral palsy who were ambulatory were welcome if they did not have seizures, toileting problems, drooling, or significant handicaps in hearing, vision, or communication! Some school districts also provided a class for pupils with physical handicaps, usually children aged 7–13 yr. Although such classes served a very heterogeneous population, they usually required that the children have normal or near-normal intelligence and the ability to use the toilet and move about independently.

Some communities had privately funded or state-supported day care programs for children who were low-functioning and multihandicapped, who could not qualify for public school programs. Often these classes were held in church or community halls supervised by teachers with very limited training. In some cases they provided little more than a change of scene and respite for the mother. As the number of polio victims declined sharply, some programs began to redefine their entrance criteria, and more opportunities became available for children with cerebral palsy. After 1950, there was increasing school and community awareness of this population, with its enormous heterogeneity and complex needs. Unfortunately, many children still remained at home, with, at best, four hours of home tutoring weekly.

The rationale for early education is accepted today by most professionals and certainly by most parents of children with developmental delay, but preschool programs for children with handicaps are largely a product of the last two decades. By 1960, state departments of mental health and public health had opened programs for children with mental retardation and multiple handicaps. United Cerebral Palsy established classes that were tailored to these children's needs. The Association for Retarded Children and other advocacy groups also began programs that included children with cerebral palsy. All these efforts offered a challenge to the public school to make appropriate plans for preschool "graduates."

The civil rights activities and consumer advocacy movement of the 1960s paved the way for comprehensive state legislation in the early 1970s, establishing the right of every child to a free, appropriate education based on interdisciplinary study of his or her needs. Parental rights were also safeguarded by provisions that parents must be involved in evaluation and planning for their child and could appeal decisions about placement, services, or educational objectives.

Public Law 94–142 established minimum guidelines for all the states. No longer could regular class teachers dispose of their more troublesome and challenging pupils (usually boys) by arranging for them to enter the class for educable mentally retarded (EMR) students. In fact, EMR classes have been profoundly changed by that law. Vast numbers of EMR students were returned to regular classes and received academic support in resource rooms, which offered individual or small group instruction.

A study by MacMillan and Borthwick suggests that children currently classified as EMR differ significantly from the "educables" of the 1960s.[6] They cite the example of California, where EMR enrollment was decreased by 50 percent simply by lowering the intelligence quotient (IQ) cut-off and applying more appropriate evaluation criteria to minority children. The remaining EMR pupils thus constitute a lower functioning subset of the original population. Mild mental retardation has become a lower-incidence handicap, and pupils are now more apt to have identifiable organic handicaps, such as cerebral palsy and Down's syndrome. The participation of this new EMR population in mainstreamed activities, particularly after the primary school years, is often a token gesture, valued chiefly in terms of peer socialization. Limited academic skills, and reduced ability to participate in nonacademic activities, often preclude more extensive peer contacts. In contrast to the parents of the EMR students under the old terminology, who fought the segregation of their children in special classes, the parents of EMR pupils today may prefer the more restrictive placement on the basis that the quality of educational services is superior. They often regard efforts to increase time spent in the regular class as cost-cutting measure on the school's part; they may also recognize a lack of flexibility on the part of school staff in arranging for appropriate mainstreaming (see the following case study).

Tom is 11 yr of age and has spastic hemiplegia and mild mental retardation. He is assigned to an EMR class. His speech is intelligible, but academic skills are very deficient, being appropriate for a child of seven to eight. Written work is laborious for him. Tom's parents rejected the suggestion that he be mainstreamed with grade 2 for lunch, art, and music, arguing that Tom considers second graders babies, and that, furthermore, he has no particular artistic interests. They requested that Tom instead be allowed to participate in a grade 4 social studies project involving oral and audiovisual presentations and group discussion. They pointed out that minimal reading was involved and that Tom already knew several of the students from the Cub Scouts. The school refused this request on the basis that Tom could not complete the written homework and would require a disproportionate amount of teacher time.

When school resources are limited or personnel are inflexible, parents may be able to locate outside activities. Courses for children of different ages are sponsored by museums, community and religious organizations, and public and private educational institutions. Usually entrance criteria and achievement expectations are flexible enough to allow participation by mildly handicapped children. If Tom had participated in extracurricular social studies programs, local museum programs, or societies, his parents might have used this as "justification" when requesting that he be allowed to participate in similar activities at school.

CATEGORIES OF STUDENTS

The Preschool Child with Cerebral Palsy

A motor handicap has a number of obvious implications for early development and education. An infant who lacks the ability to support his or her head may be deprived of the visual stimulation that the normal infant gets. Exploration of the world may also be severely restricted by poor ability to reach for and grasp objects or to move the body toward a goal. If, in addition to motor impairment, the child has sensory and perceptual deficits such that information obtained through the senses is limited or distorted, understanding of spatial concepts, even with relation to the body, will be delayed. By the time this child reaches the age of school entrance (three years), it will be apparent that experiences in almost all areas have inadequately prepared him or her for the developmental tasks presented to normal children of the same age. Critical sequences in sensorimotor development have been missed, and continuing limitations may further prevent the child from manipulating toys and materials, which could aid the development of concepts (see the following case studies).

Tony was four years of age when first seen. His parents had moved to the city from a state that had no early education program for a multihandicapped child. Although he had been evaluated by an interdisciplinary team at age three, no program recommendations had been made. The child spent his days lying supine on the floor, propped up only at meals. His working class family loved him, and they provided him with social stimulation, but they had not developed any system for communicating with him. He had no toys and no adapted equipment for manipulating his environment.

When enrolled in a preschool, Tony showed initial rapid gains, but family problems resulted in frequent school absence and missed therapy appointments. There was no carryover between the school program and the home, and progress slowed.

Jeremy, a boy of 5 years with spastic quadriplegia, was the only child of upper-middle-class parents who were devoted to his care. They demonstrated his ability to follow conversations and to communicate with his eyes, facial expressions, and very limited pointing. Jeremy had been enrolled in a cerebral palsy nursery program since age three, where he was the most physically limited pupil. Electronic communication devices were being adapted for his use at home and at school, and consultants provided his parents with suggestions for new technologic aids and ideas. Although Jeremy was an alert child who effectively used his limited physical resources, he required virtually one-to-one teaching in order to learn.

The individual education program (IEP) for each child (see Chap. 30) presupposes that the dimensions of the handicap and its implications for education are understood, but evaluations of the preschool child with cerebral palsy can be very difficult, particularly if there is a suspicion that home experiences have been limited. The evaluation team must seek to provide as much information as possible about the child's cognitive abilities, communication skills, sensory functioning, and other skills or weaknesses. Statements that the child is too young or too handicapped for testing are not as helpful as impressions, however tentative, which will guide in the initial placement decisions. The experienced clinician will usually have some idea of a child's abilities, and, if time permits, might visit two or three alternatives and suggest which should be tried first. He should also be ready to assist parents in gaining a realistic picture of their child at this stage in development (see the case studies below).

Mark, 4 years, with spastic quadriplegia would clearly indicate the proper sequencing of picture cards depicting various concepts by looking at the next card to be placed. When the interviewer deliberately misread his signals, he at first "protested" with subtle facial changes and then, recognizing the joke, smiled his appreciation. His parents rightly considered a placement for multihandicapped retarded children inappropriate for Mark, and the school provided a tutor instead until transportation to another district could be arranged.

Aaron, 5 years, was severely disabled. He seemed to have only random eye movements when asked to indicate yes or no, but his mother would continue to state questions, giving obvious cues on which response was correct. She had convinced herself that this preschool child could read and answer questions on the subject matter, and she spent many hours on educational instruction that appeared misguided. Since the public school program was unacceptable to her, she continued to teach Aaron at home.

Mary, also aged 5 years, could neither speak nor manipulate objects. A pediatrician had implied to the parents that she was retarded "to the level of a newborn infant." However, they kept a record of instances when Mary's grasp of a situation or of conversations in her presence suggested understanding. Her teacher quickly learned that Mary delighted in being teased; her relatively good intelligence could be inferred by her comprehension of the literal message conveyed by a statement and the intended meaning, which might be diametrically opposed. She seemed appropriate for her class, which had children with mental ages of 18–30 mo.

The Student with Mild Cerebral Palsy and Minimal Cognitive Impairment

The use of cognitive and linguistic variables for educational classification allows the child to be placed, as nearly as possible, with children who are equally bright. The child whose impairment is primarily motor should be placed in a regular classroom even if this involves accommodation to orthopaedic appliances and modification of the way he or she completes assignments (Chap. 18, 19). Some adjustments will be needed, including removal of architectural barriers, flexibility in the use of space, adaptation of equipment, and possible exemption from physical education activities. Increased teacher and peer sensitivity are critical, particularly at the secondary level, for ensuring optimal integration of the student with peers. It is also important that consultants be available to teachers to suggest alternative strategies when there are educational problems. A guidance counselor can be very helpful in assisting the adolescent to deal with feeling about the handicap and its effects.

During the elementary years the focus is on the acquisition of academic skills; usually this continues into the middle school or junior high school years, but with some increase in nonacademic course work. In the past, the inappropriate suggestion was often made that the handicapped student should begin his vocational education in early adolescence, as though he had a precocious need to enter the world of work. It is true that some bright students with cerebral palsy will have made limited academic progress, because of their specific learning disabilities, but it remains important for them to continue academic instruction, albeit with orientation toward what is practical for their adult needs. Gradually there may be a shift in emphasis, favoring nonacademic learning, with the areas of concentration tailored, insofar as possible,

to the abilities and interests of each student (see the following case studies).

Bill, aged 13 yr, is a sixth-grade pupil with spastic cerebral palsy and speech that is 75 percent intelligible in context. He has average intelligence, with a mild attentional deficit. His normal peers like him but tend to treat him as a somewhat younger child, although he is, in fact, a year older than they. He spends one 90-min period a day in the resource room, where he receives reading and math instruction at the fourth-grade level. He receives speech therapy twice a week, adaptive physical education once a week, and typing instruction (modified keyboard) once a week. He is excused from many assignments requiring writing or copying of figures, but other assignments are typed or dictated. Bill, his parents, and teachers are comfortable with the current plan but are concerned about the coming year, when he will be assigned to a large junior high school.

Michael is a personable youth aged 16 yr with spastic quadriparesis; his intelligence falls in the low average range, but with considerable scatter. He can move his own wheelchair, given enough time, and can make himself understood verbally. His parents have sought to encourage independence in their son, but have chosen to place him in a private day school for physically handicapped students. (Because of the school's endowment, funding was not an issue.) The parents believe that the educational advantages with extracurricular activities at their own expense ensured peer contacts with both normal and handicapped boys. Psychologic evaluation found him somewhat depressed and anxious about his future.

Jeff, aged 15 yr, was ambulatory but had an IQ that fell at the bottom of the low average range. His speech was moderately intelligible, and his reading was at a late third-grade level. His upper-middle-class family had provided him with rich social learning experiences, however. He related well to peers and adults, enjoyed classical music and the care of tropical fish, and was an accomplished cook. His educational plan called for three hours daily of academic instruction with emphasis on functional math skills and reading for information. He spent two afternoons a week in the local public library, where he signed out records and reclassified returns. With supervision he was learning to type out orders for new recordings, chosen by the librarian. Although not considered a work placement, this was a learning experience with the potential for developing work skills for a possible summer job. Jeff also spent several hours a week of school time on a project, which involved selecting simple recipes from newspapers and magazines and converting them to formats requiring very little reading. With the help of a parent he had developed several rubber stamps that designated quantity and substituted for hand-drawn pictures, which he could not make well because of his hemiplegia. His dream was to publish a looseleaf cook book for handicapped persons.

The creative ways in which Jeff's school capitalized on his interests stands in marked contrast to the experience of many pupils with similar handicaps. Often they are assigned to the "slow" tracks of vocational courses, which lack any appeal or usefulness for them. Jeff might have been placed in a shop course, where his poor manual coordination would have made the teacher uncomfortable and Jeff's projects very mediocre.

Under current regulations, students with developmental disabilities are entitled to publicly funded education until their 22nd birthday. This means that students who formerly were encouraged to drop out at age 16, or to accept a special diploma at age 18, must now be offered an appropriate program to prepare them for adult life and employment. Schools are meeting this new challenge with varying degrees of success. When a program is unappealing to young adults, most will not participate, but parents and involved professionals must advocate for needed program options.

The Student with Cerebral Palsy and Mental Retardation

Students with mild to moderate mental retardation, in addition to their other handicaps, will usually be placed in self-contained special classes. Often they do not fit comfortably in the EMR class, where most pupils have intact motor and sensory abilities. The specialized therapies and interdisciplinary services that they require may not be available, or parents may be asked to spend many hours each week coordinating services, transporting the child, and conveying recommendations and suggestions from one professional to another. Some parents manage all this admirably, but many do not. Parents of a verbal child must often allow him or her to be placed with nonverbal classmates, or see a mildly retarded child placed with moderately retarded children because there is no more suitable class. In such situations, foster placement of the older child has much to recommend it. This achieves the goal of keeping the child in the community and in a home atmosphere, while not depriving him or her of needed services. It is an alternative that should be developed further, and parents should be helped to see its advantages, as compared to placement in a large institution. Adolescence may be a turning point for the family that has been coping with a nonambulatory child. Physical and emotional needs may change at the same time that family circumstances are changing. A marriage may have ended, older siblings may have left home, and a mother may find herself with limited personal

and financial resources to meet the handicapped young person's needs (see the case studies below).

Carol, aged 14 years with spastic quadriplegia and moderate mental retardation, was seen for evaluation and program recommendations because a residential placement had become necessary. Her mother's illness and Carol's social isolation and depression were particular issues, but Carol had also spent seven years in the same educational program, where she was the oldest and highest functioning pupil. She was a verbal and charming adolescent, but an appropriate placement near her home community was unavailable. Carol was not mentally handicapped enough to qualify for one program, but was too retarded to win a place in another. The best alternative appeared to be a group or foster home in a community that had a suitable public school program for Carol.

David, a boy of 12 yr, with multiple handicaps had always been in a self-contained special class. He functioned at a mid-second-grade level academically, and his verbal intelligence fell at the bottom of the mildly retarded range. His personality and humor were very appealing to adults but were less appreciated by the other special class pupils, and he was a lonely child. His parents were loving and effective advocates, but they had difficulty recognizing and acknowledging his depression and dependence on them. They wondered if the school was meeting all his needs, since he did not seem to have made much progress.

The Student with Severe or Profound Mental Retardation

The last children to win public educational services were, not surprisingly, those with the most devastating handicaps. Before 1960, few special educators were trained to work with them or had any desire to invest themselves in children considered hopeless and unteachable. As the so-called trainable classes became an accepted part of public school services, however, it was inevitable that attention should turn to the still unserved handicapped children. The federal grovernment subsidized personnel preparation and funded model programs to demonstrate what could be accomplished. At this time, knowledge of these students' educational needs and strategies for teaching them remain incompletely understood, but their education is recognized as a public responsibility. Classes are housed in public school buildings, developmental centers, state institutions, and a variety of other structures. In the best programs, home and school collaboration is stressed for setting priorities and maintaining consistency.

With the severely and profoundly impaired, a concern is sometimes raised that the educational program will subject a particular child to undue stress. It is suggested that he or she may be overstimulated, fatigued, exposed to infection, or subject to weight loss as a consequence of attending class. These fears should be dissipated, if, in fact, the child does not show negative effects of participation after an initial adjustment period. A sensitive teacher will observe all pupils for indications of stress and will modify the program appropriately. A child who does not tolerate noise well, for example, can be placed in a carpeted area, with acoustic tile or other sound-reducing features. Rest periods may be provided for a child who shows signs of fatigue.

The following case study provides an example of this type of student.

Timmy is a profoundly retarded boy with cerebral palsy who resides in a pediatric nursing home. Since he is seven, the director requested modest funding for a stimulation program. The school district investigated the situation and concluded that Timmy was below the level at which any improvement in function could be expected. The parents retained a lawyer, and the school was required to provide funds.

What, in fact, can be offered to the child with such devastating handicaps as Timmy's? Who should deliver the services, and what should be the goals? Physical therapy will be important in developing his muscles and in presenting contraction deformities. The physical therapist will assist other team members by planning how Timmy will be positioned for various activities and what special equipment should be employed. A teacher or supervised aide should work with him to develop social responses and attending behavior. A child who has not been placed in a sitting position has usually been unable to profit from the visual environment; he or she may have had only a ceiling to look at and may be quite indifferent to the relationships between visual and auditory stimuli. Spending several hours a day in a sitting position may enable the child to learn many new associations with practical applications to daily life. He or she will be aware of caretakers who can be followed visually; he or she will understand that the appearance of table utensils signifies a meal. The caretaker will respond differently to a child who opens his or her mouth at the approach of a spoon or who retains food and liquids better because of improved positioning. Other educational goals will involve stimulation of the eyes and ears with art materials, recordings, and educational toys, the training of eye contact and a social smile, and the lengthening of attention span for auditory and visual materials. If available, a developmental occupational therapist will help the teacher

and other staff to plan appropriate tasks and strategies. The mastering, where possible, of self-feeding and other self-help skills can have far-reaching effects on the child's future, since group and foster homes are more apt to have admission criteria based on such skills than an IQ scores.

Learning to listen and observe are important leisure activities. The child will take pleasure in the sounds of voices on radio and television when not receiving direct attention. For children who have significant sensory impairment, it is important to provide glasses or hearing aids. Others may not appreciate this reasoning that the child could not make good use of vision or hearing anyway, but for these most handicapped persons, every possibility for help must be explored, particularly during infancy and early childhood, so that they will not withdraw from the world around them. The well-known finding of Fraiberg is but one example of the devastating impact of a sensory handicap.[4] The risks are correspondingly higher when the child has additional neuromotor handicap. Some parents, as Fraiberg found, seem born with the ability to take care of a handicapped child. They intuititvely modify approaches to the child and recognize the signals that the child sends relative to developmental needs. Many, perhaps most, however, need assistance in rearing the profoundly impaired child. Early education programs help such parents develop confidence in their abilities as they learn how to work with their child. Interaction with other parents can help them to deal with the powerful feelings aroused by their dilemma.

IMPLICATIONS OF SENSORY HANDICAPS

An important factor in the exclusion of children with cerebral palsy from educational programs is the high incidence of sensory and perceptual handicaps. The implications of these handicaps for education are enormous. Visual impairment severe enough to require educational accommodations is a low-incidence handicap, affecting only about 0.1 percent of the school-aged population. The options for educating these pupils, if they have no other educationally significant handicap, are private or state residential schools or an adapted curriculum in the local public school. The children with cerebral palsy do not fit comfortably into either arrangement because of their other handicaps. Their visual limitations may be almost ignored in the search for an appropriate placement based on their diagnosis (see below).

Howard, aged 7, attended a public school class for physically handicapped pupils in an urban school district. He had completed reading readiness activities, but his teacher noted how hard it was for him to see materials. In questioning his mother, the teacher learned that Howard had been seen by an ophthalmologist at a local medical center. After waiting for two hours in a crowded clinic, he had behaved very badly during the examination. The doctor noted in the record that "this severely handicapped child would never tolerate glasses." A return appointment was scheduled, glasses were obtained, and the child, who has borderline intelligence, now reads well.

The partially sighted child, who benefits from correction or whose diagnosis of legal blindness is based on a visual field limitation, will usually be educated as a print reader, using a large-type texts or a magnifying device as needed. This group includes the majority of pupils with visual impairments, whether they have cerebral palsy or not. When a child is not able to discern print, or when vision is expected to deteriorate, the child is assessed for Braille instruction. This poses special problems for the blind child with cerebral palsy. Braille is more difficult to learn than print; hence, the child with borderline intelligence or mild retardation will experience greater frustration. Additionally, the tactile perception of the Braille cell requires fingertip sensitivity, which many disabled children lack. This type of "perceptual" learning disability has minimal implications for sighted pupils but may actually preclude reading for the individual with cerebral palsy.

At adolescence, such students find prevocational and vocational opportunities restricted. Training programs for blind students traditionally assume intact abilities in other areas, while programs for cerebral palsy students may assume adequate vision. The presence of a communication handicap or mental retardation will further complicate the picture. Use of a white cane, a guide dog, or sonar devices to aid in mobility may require better motor coordination than the individual possesses. School personnel, especially if they have little experience in dealing with multihandicapped students, may avoid confronting the reality of these limitations and continue a student in a program that can do little to help. Parents are often fearful lest the school drop their son or daughter altogether; they may express the hope that the student does not realize the bleak prospects for employment.

Computer-designed aids and other complex learning devices, such as the Kurzweil reader (which reads ordinary books aloud), are extremely expensive, so that few school districts can afford them. Often the advantages of an out-of-home placement

for educational reasons must be weighted against the family upheaval that this may cause. Since other blind students tend to remain in their communities for schooling, there are more places in private and regional centers for the blind multihandicapped child. Before such a program is recommended to a family, however, it is important to check both the current entrance criteria of the school and the availability of funding.

Hearing impairment of educational significance afflicts at least 0.6 percent of the school-aged population, according to U.S. Office of Education figures. Early diagnosis and treatment have become more common in recent years; however, the child with cerebral palsy is somewhat less likely to be diagnosed early. If motor impairment of the speech mechanism is implicated, if central auditory function is thought to be impaired, or if speech delay is attributed to global cognitive deficit, the child may not be referred for audiometry until the critical years for language learning are past. Special techniques may be required to evaluate the child with severe disability who is dismissed as "too immature" even for routine school screening.

In addition to problems of auditory acuity, these children show a relatively high incidence of auditory processing, memory, and word retrieval problems. These too require the earliest possible documentation for educational treatment; however, they are more difficult to test in the child with cerebral palsy and thus may be overlooked because of other handicaps. There has also been a tendency among psychologists and educators to regard such specific learning disabilities as found exclusively in students who have normal intelligence. Experience shows, however, that they are found with greater frequency in students who also show some general or global deficit. No child should be considered too young or too low functioning to be given a trial with a hearing aid, however. The more limited the child is, the more crucial it becomes to capitalize on every aspect of his or her potential.

The history of deaf education in the United States shows that normal intelligence has been an almost invariable requirement for schooling. The American School for the Deaf, established at Hartford in 1817, introduced sign language to American deaf children, but for nearly a century there has been controversy over the most appropriate means of teaching communications. The predominant approach has been "oralism," or the auditory–oral approach. Deaf pupils were selected for oral programs on the basis of their intelligence and ability to learn lip-reading and speech.

Needless to say, few children with cerebral palsy qualified for such training. Partly as a result of the rubella epidemic of 1965–1966, attention was focused on students with hearing impairment and specific language disorder who did not succeed in oral programs. Total communication programs were developed that used a variety of communication approaches, e.g., speech training and signing. Many programs accepted students who were mentally retarded.

Those students who are dyspraxic or lack bilateral hand coordination have limited potential for signing, particularly when finger spelling is required. Instead, they need communication boards, special typewriters, and sophisticated electronic devices to speak for them. Considering the dreadful isolation that has characterized the deaf in U.S. society, it is heartening to note the expanding educational and community opportunities now available for them and the increased awareness of their presence and needs.

IMPAIRMENT OF COMMUNICATION IN STUDENTS WITH CEREBRAL PALSY (SEE CHAP. 16)

The problem of communication handicaps among children with cerebral palsy is not confined to the deaf and hearing impaired. Those with oral dyspraxia, dysarthria, problems of voice production, or central language dysfunction may also need a total communication approach. The importance of adapting methods to each learner must not be overlooked, with the range of options being greatest where the student has normal intelligence.

Signing is currently undergoing considerable popularity as an alternative communication strategy for nonverbal, mentally retarded children. Teachers with only one or two pupils for whom signing is appropriate take a beginners course and may encourage their other pupils to pick up some signing. This situation, although better than nothing, is less than ideal. A better course is the placement of students who use signing in a separate program. Signs will always be paired with verbal communication for students able to hear speech. In many cases, the students will also use "pairing," since their acquisition of speech, however limited, is a high priority. Parents may be reassured that using signs and gestures will not prevent their child from developing speech but will reduce the frustration that the child experiences when he or she cannot be understood.

A serious limitation of signing at this time is the lack of uniformity among users of different methods. Fristoe and Lloyd, in a study of nonspeech systems used with mentally retarded pupils in public schools, found that respondents lacked sophistication in their knowledge of signed systems; they most often chose a system on the basis that it was the only one that they knew, rather than on its merits for the student.[5] They also indicated that they had incomplete understanding of the system that they claimed to be employing. In addition to several systems of manual communication, the respondents reported using several nonspeech, nonmanual communication systems with these students, including Bliss Symbolics, Rebus, pictographic language, and a method based on Premack's plastic chip system.

There are instances when severely retarded, nonverbal students with cerebral palsy are taught approximations of a few signs. It is understood that these will have little value outside of the home or school environment, but they do allow the student to indicate basic needs.

The problem of assigning responsibility for the nonspeech communication program of the child with cerebral palsy remains unresolved. Except for those instances where a speech–language professional is the teacher or works in the classroom daily, programs tend to be fragmented, with therapy for two to four hours a week and incomplete carryover to classroom and home. Work loads may preclude regular communication between the teacher and therapist or parent; sometimes one or both are resistant to the therapist's suggestions. One possibility for improving this situation would be the training of some special educators to offer expanded communication services, perhaps with the consultation of a therapist.

BEHAVIORAL ISSUES AT SCHOOL

Early writers on the education of children with cerebral palsy insisted that "psychosocial handicaps resulted from the impact of society's reaction to physical deviation, from the child's interpretation of this reaction to his limitations, and from discrepancies between his aspirations and capacities."[3] There was recognition that in adolescence, the more capable individual would experience anger and depression because of his or her limited social and educational opportunities and the prospects for adult life. Although the emotional problems of children with cerebral palsy and mental retardation were not discussed, they were surely a concern to the children and to their families. Currently, options for helping handicapped children and their families are more varied and available. Schools and mental health centers offer individual and family counseling and group therapy for parents, handicapped adolescents, and even siblings. A most helpful practice in some school districts is the use of a behavioral consultant to assist both parents and teachers when a student exhibits a serious behavior problem (see the following case studies).

Sam, aged eight years, had occasional toilet accidents at school; he was also emotionally labile, crying if his teacher seemed displeased with his work. Although of near-normal intelligence and reading achievement, he was kept in a self-contained class because the regular class teacher did not feel that she could cope with his immature demands for attention. Counseling at a child guidance center did not prove helpful, but short-term behavior therapy showed good results.

Peter, aged nine years and severely retarded with cerebral palsy, had developed the habit of spitting on others and then laughing. His teachers found the behavior unacceptable and disruptive of class activities, but his parents managed the behavior by putting a bib on their son and laughing at what they termed his silliness. After tactful persuasion they agreed to use ignoring and temporary isolation, as recommended by the behavioral consultant. The spitting was soon extinguished.

When a child exhibits a behavior problem only at school or only at home, it is helpful for the parent and teacher to examine the possible percipitating or reinforcing variables in a manner that does not suggest that one or the other is mismanaging the child. The cooperation of the parents should, of course, be enlisted before a behavioral program is begun.

In the past, children with multiple handicaps and severe handicaps were often left alone for extended periods and tended to develop interfering behaviors that made them harder to work with and less acceptable to others. Self-abuse, including head banging, eye gouging, self-induced vomiting, and hand biting, were frequently seen in the institutionalized population. Stereotyped self-stimulation, such as rocking, rumination, and finger flicking, while less concerning, do interfere with attempts at training other behaviors, e.g., establishing eye contact, instituting self-feeding regimens, and manipulating educational materials. The experiences of the last decade, when most children were kept at home, suggests that interfering behaviors may be averted if the child receives appropriate stimulation and if the parents are guided in ways to help the child when he or she begins

to show problem behaviors. The practice of keeping children with severe disabilities in the community ensures that most of them will receive a quality and quantity of stimulation that is not available in a large institution. Usually the child will learn to establish eye contact, look at objects, and attend to sounds. Such behaviors help to ensure that he or she will receive the caring and respect often denied to persons who are less responsive (see below).

Keith, an adolescent with multiple handicaps, had been institutionalized from birth. At age 17 he was transferred to a community residence. His "autisticlike" behaviors kept his teachers and others at a distance; even after a year of intensive programming, he was responsive only to his favorite caretaker.

Jessie, another institutionalized young adult, was attractive and had always been a favorite of the staff. Because of her severe handicaps she had never been enrolled in the school program, but she benefited greatly by her contacts with staff. She could follow simple conversations and show social responsiveness. Unfortunately, she had never even been taught a means for indicating yes or no, but she at least was open to teaching.

In each of these cases, the individual had suffered extreme environmental deprivation. Jessie, however, had been given a powerful tool with which to forge a better environment for herself.

PUBLIC OR PRIVATE OPTIONS

Only a careful review of available local programs and the needs of a particular child can suggest which of several options is the most appropriate. The decision should be made by parents, involved professionals, and school personnel as a team. Frequently parents bring their child to a developmental clinic requesting assistance in getting the child into a private school; they are disappointed when told that the staff can not circumvent school authorities or require the district to pay the child's tuition at a private school, if there is an available public school program. This is the case even when the the private program appears to be superior.

Because the child with cerebral palsy is frequently multihandicapped and requires many services, districts are somewhat more likely to allow private day placements, especially for the preschool child and the older adolescent. At the preschool level, programs sponsored by United Cerebral Palsy or Easter Seal may be the only ones that can meet the child's needs; public school early education class may be heterogeneous, and the nonambulatory child may be at physical risk if integrated with a very lively group. Also, parents who must transport their child to various medical and therapeutic appointments are enormously helped when all the needed services can be coordinated under one roof.

For the child aged 6–13 yr, options for educational programming will usually be broader. The long-established private schools can offer much to children with normal intelligence. What they do not offer, of course, is the opportunity to participate in activities with children who are normal. Commuting time is often lengthy, and the child's friends live at a great distance, making social contacts very awkward. In addition to public and private alternatives, many school districts have collaborative arrangements with other districts, so that children with low-incidence handicaps are pooled. Such programs may be housed in public schools or in separate plants; they usually have the services of a physical therapist, occupational therapist, speech therapist, and various consultants. Such programs offer high quality education and better home–school coordination than many local schools.

Pediatricians and other clinicians who work with children with cerebral palsy need to be aware of what each program in their community can offer and also what state laws govern the choice and funding of private programs. In most states, private tuition will only be provided if the school has no adequate placement for a pupil. Demonstrating the inadequacy of a local program, as opposed to proving its inferiority, may be quite difficult. A pediatrician sometimes realizes that parents cannot cope with their child at home and presses for a residential placement; however, local school personnel may insist that outside funding be found for the child's living expenses when the need for placement is unrelated to lack of an educational program. Because cerebral palsy requires more medical supervision and treatment than many other handicaps, parents are more likely to ask the physician for educational advice or advocacy on obtaining services. If he chooses to accept this role, he must be prepared to invest considerable time in familiarizing himself with programs and developing good working relationships with school personnel. Otherwise, the parents should be referred to a public or private agency that can help them. Referral to a psychologist will help the physician to make better predictions about the child's ultimate achievement (see below).

Marta's parents bitterly resented her placement in a special class for most of her school day. She was a cheerful, talkative child who, nevertheless, scored low in the mildly retarded range. Her physician had assured the parents that, on the basis of Marta's speech and social skills, she was not mentally retarded and should not be placed with retarded children.

Carl, a boy with athetoid cerebral palsy of prenatal origin, appeared mentally retarded because of his abnormal facies and slow development as a preschooler. When he was four, his neurologist suggested to his parents that he be placed in an institution. Three years later he was discharged, having learned to speak intelligibly and having earned an IQ score of 90. In retrospect, his placement with severely retarded children was inappropriate and could have been avoided if his parents had been better advised.

THE FUTURE

In the past, children with cerebral palsy have suffered extreme educational and societal neglect; their potential has often been tragically wasted. The question of what to teach is a major consideration now that they are guaranteed an appropriate education. If there can be a single answer, it must be what the student can learn, beginning with the highest priority behavior that he or she can master. For one child that may be learning to make eye contact; for another, it may be reading Shakespeare, with the help of an automatic page turner. Programmed instruction and computer aids offer great promise. Unless school personnel investigate the possibilities, including means of financing them, they will not be used. The choice of a communication system for a nonverbal cerebral palsy student must take into consideration communication needs as well as all attributes relevant to communication. These include intelligence, memory, visual and auditory skills, manual coordination, and emotional characteristics.

If the error of other times was that infants with handicaps were snatched from the bosoms of their families at an age when all children are helpless and placed in environments that could not meet their developmental needs, the error of these times may be that society assumes that every "good" parent will be able to cope indefinitely with a severely handicapped son or daughter. There should be acceptable alternatives when home care is not possible, and these should provide the same educational and social opportunities as the young person would have enjoyed in his or her own community.

The litigation of the 1960s and the legislation of the 1970s, to the extent that they are not set aside by the economies of the 1980s, ensure that all children whatever the nature of their handicaps, will have a free and appropriate education. It is up to parents and professionals to see that students with cerebral palsy and other developmental disabilities receive those services that should be their birthright.

REFERENCES

1. Best GA: Individuals with Physical Disabilities. St. Louis, Mosby, 1978
2. Blatt B, Kaplan F: Christmas in Purgatory. Boston, Allyn and Bacon, 1966
3. Cruickshank W, Johnson G: Education of Exceptional Children and Youth. Englewood Cliffs, N.J., Prentice-Hall, 1958
4. Fraiberg S: Insights from the Blind. New York, Basic Books, 1977
5. Fristoe M, Lloyd L: A survey of the use of non-speech systems with the severely communication impaired. Ment Retard 16:99, 1978
6. MacMillan D, Borthwick S: The new educable mentally retarded population: Can they be mainstreamed? Ment Retard 18:155, 1980
7. Mandell C, Fiscus E: Understanding Exceptional People. St. Paul, MN, West Publishing, 1981

Gerald A. Strom
Carolyn Oppenheimer

32

Maturation and Sexual Awareness

In the last decade, adults with cerebral palsy and other chronically handicapping disorders have become vocal in requesting services. Recent surveys have shown that sex education is one area frequently ignored by professional training programs. Currently, there is no formal degree program in sex education in any college or university in the United States. Only recently could a person become certified as a sex educator through a limited program of The American Association of Sex Educators, Counselors and Therapists.[7]

Parents of disabled children and adolescents, when given the opportunity to express concerns about the curriculum in their schools, often have requested that sex education be included.[9] Alcorn found that most parents of disabled adolescents feel they should provide sex education to their children but that they do not have the proper information or ability to convey this information and also frequently see their child's disability as an impediment to sexual relations.[1] Because of these deficiencies in the educational process, it has become necessary for disabled adolescents, parents, and community leaders to form a coalition to promote programs, instruction, and research in the area of the disabled and sexuality.

Thus far, pediatric and adolescent health care providers have paid minimal attention to the needs of the chronically handicapped with respect to relationships with other handicapped and nonhandicapped people and instead have concentrated on meeting their practical and technical requirements.[11] One of the major goals of this chapter is to assist health care providers in becoming aware of the sexuality needs of their disabled clients and to allow them to deal with some of the inherent and associated issues. In addition to their sexual needs, the chron-

ically handicapped also have the problem of convincing nonhandicapped citizens that they are people with similar human desires and impulses.[10]

CONCEPTS OF SEXUALITY

In U.S. society, youth and beauty are considered essential ingredients in becoming a sexually attractive person. The communication media have promoted this concept, and adolescents, disabled or not, frequently view a lack of perfection in their physical appearance as a deterrent to success. Parents readily acknowledge that adolescents often spend a greater amount of time staring into a mirror than into a book. As feelings regarding body image become intertwined with personality, the future sexuality of the person less than perfect in appearance is greatly affected.

To discuss this negative reaction to disabilities as it relates to sexuality, a clear definition of sexuality, one that can be used by the disabled and the nondisabled, is necessary. Sexuality is one of the basic human needs and reflects the need to express one's self through the body. It is a response to the body, to thoughts, and to feelings. Sexuality can therefore be best defined as "the integration of physical, emotional, intellectual, and social aspects of an individual's personality which express maleness or femaleness."[4] This definition thus signifies that sexuality refers to more than reproductive capabilities.

Sexuality is influenced by parents during the earliest years. Touching, being held close during feedings, and fondling all influence feelings about one's self. A caring relationship, both physically and emotionally, between the adults in the home influences the child. Curiosity about the body and exploration by touch affect sexuality. How the parents react to the child's touching the genitals affects the child's feelings about the body. During the years before puberty, sexuality is influenced by the opportunities for expression of feelings about being female or male, by developing abilities to trust and love, and by becoming aware of how one fits into a family.

The following poem expresses the feeling of a mother as she relates to her handicapped child's sexuality:[3]

When you are a parent
Your child becomes a WHOLE person the moment he is born—
And a WHOLE person is aware of his boyhood
Or her girlhood
At an early age.

When you are a parent
Your child becomes a whole person the day he is born

Often his handicap does not become noticed for some time—
Even for a long time.
And what has happened in the meantime?
You have nursed, hugged, kissed, held—
And he or she has begun to know the comfort of touch and closeness—
Awareness that he had a body.
And takes pride in his body.
And this awareness of his sexuality is the basis of his total self-concept.
Sometimes—when we parents discover the fact of retardation—
We begin the long push for intellectual development—
And neglect the needs of sexuality—
Which can be expressed in so many ways:
    Dance—Art—Companionship—Friendship—
Love.
For what the child most needs is a good feeling about himself.
Which opens up avenues of hope and growth,
And he can then look to others for reinforcement—
In friendship and in love.

The severity or subtlety of a child's disability is not as relevant to a child's eventual sexuality as the child's participation in those experiences that are generic to the early sexual development of all human beings.[14] The degree to which the parents accept the handicap is of great importance. If the parents see only the handicap and not the person, this attitude will be transferred to the child and is likely to hinder future sexuality.

Psychosexual development, concepts of body image, and awareness of sexual identity should be the same for nondisabled and disabled persons, but the time span between stages may exceed that of the nondisabled (Table 32-1). The reason for these differences in psychosexual development is not always indigeneous to the specific handicap. Most parents of handicapped adolescents are able to wish for them an education, employment and a safe environment, but not that their child find a partner, lead a sexual life, or have children.[11] Many of these negative attitudes are based on anxiety regarding sexual issues such as dating, marriage, and parenting. Because of these anxiety-producing reactions to the disabled and sexuality, the sexual concerns of these individuals may be ignored, avoided, or even discouraged.[4]

SEXUALITY PROBLEMS CONFRONTING HANDICAPPED ADOLESCENTS

Several common problems surround the handicapped adolescent: sexual identity, irresponsible behavior, misinformation, and dependency.

Sexual Identity

Handicapped adolescents and adults are frequently regarded as asexual, with resultant sexual oppression.[3,11] Too often society regards them not as female or male but as neuter. When handicapped adolescents internalize these concepts, feelings of self-worth are distorted, and these teenagers often become more emotionally and psychologically handicapped then physically handicapped. Because of the recent awareness of the handicapped, there is a growing recognition that the disabled person is as much entitled to sexual expression as the general public. The physically disabled may not be able to walk, control their extremities, or hear or speak coherently, but society as a whole must increase sexual counseling, abolish sterotypes, and promote research in order to help the disabled overcome physical and social obtacles.

Irresponsible Behavior

Many believe that disabled people, especially when retarded, are oversexed with uncontrollable urges and that any sex education will result in irresponsible behavior. Often this attitude may be one of the underlying negative feelings toward group homes in residential neighborhoods. We and others have found that counseling and sex education results in responsible behavior, however.[6]

Table 32-1
Psychosexual Development of Handicapped Women Compared with
Healthy Women

Characteristic	Handicapped (%)	Normal (%)
First knowledge of sex differences before age 6	11	33
Complete sex information before age 15	11	26
Little or no preparation for menstruation	78	55
No history of masturbation	74	50
Extremely close to family	23	3
No evidence of homoerotic behavior	23	8
Never been in love	30	3
Never had dates with boys	28	1
First date before age 16	18	52
No evidence of masculine protest	43	26
Recalled a desire to be a boy in childhood	43	69
Attitude of disgust toward sex	7	21

Misinformation

Today, there are very few uninformed teenagers, but there are a great many misinformed ones who liberally share their impressions with each other.[14] Lack of proper sex education for handicapped adolescents and adults, presented in an understandable manner, thus leads to further confusion and influences concepts of self-worth. On the contrary, Timmer and associates recently documented that sexual education programs for developmentally disabled adults can be effective in eliminating this conception and improving sexual knowledge and behavior.[15]

Dependency

Many professionals as well as parents never see the handicapped child as growing into a functioning adult. All too often these children will have grown into an adolescent in a sheltered, protective environment lacking opportunities to achieve the independence that is the basis for relationships. Sexuality is associated with emancipation. Dependency is often encouraged not only by family and society, but also by the rehabilitation and medical professions.

SEXUAL PROBLEMS SPECIFIC TO CEREBRAL PALSY

Chipouras and associates have identified that sexual problems in cerebral palsy fall into three major groups: physical, communication, and psychologic.[4]

Physical Problems

Spasticity, athetosis, musculoskeletal deformities, strength, balance, and mental capabilities may all have a profound effect on the disabled person's social and sexual activities. Likewise, architectual and environmental barriers can limit mobility and the chance to interact with others.

Communication Problems

Speech problems, vision and hearing impairments, and mental retardation can severely impair an individual's social and sexual interactions because communication is necessary to develop personal relationships. Communication disorders can also limit an individual's ability to obtain social skills as well as sex education.

Psychologic Problems

Psychologic problems occur primarily from society's attitude toward individuals with physical or mental handicaps and an individual's concept of self-worth.

COMPREHENSIVE SEXUALITY PROGRAMS

In order to assist adolescents achieve maximum developmental potential and find success in expressing their sexuality, various experiences or opportun-

Table 32-2

Opportunities Necessary in Sexual Development

Understanding of an individual's disability
Association with nonhandicapped peers
Independent living experiences
Education on different occupations and careers
Discussion of personal problems
Work or employment experience
Participation in progressive educational programs
Performance of household tasks
Discussion on physical abilities and disabilities
Instruction in manners and social graces
Earning wages
Hobby development
Comprehensive sex education program

ities are needed. Table 32-2 gives an incomplete list of opportunities that severely disabled adults felt to be important in satisfactory sexuality development.[13]

Incorporating these important opportunities, we have developed a seven-point list of educational criteria for a comprehensive sexuality program:

1. Growth and development, which includes awareness and understanding of body changes during puberty and the emotional changes that occur
2. Reproduction, intercourse, pregnancy, fetal development, and birth
3. Appropriate behavior, i.e., time and place
4. Relationships
5. Family planning
6. Socially transmitted diseases
7. Marriage and parenting

Counseling and information on socialization should also be included, since this area is one of the greatest needs of the disabled. We recently conducted a sexuality program for the United Cerebral Palsy Association of Cleveland, in which four handicapped adult couples were assessed.[12] The area of greatest concern was loneliness, an issue too rarely addressed. One group member shared his feelings with the group by saying, "What happens to us, we are lonely. We want to be together. Does loneliness hurt? Yes, it hurts. We are fighting against loneliness and boredom. We can enjoy being together." This reaction was pervasive throughout the group.

Rights and Responsibilities

As part of any sex education program, it is important for clients to have a clear understanding of their rights and responsibilities. According to the United Nations Declaration of Human Rights, no person can be denied a right because of perceived differences, including the presence of a disability. The following list shows rights that are as necessary for disabled as for nondisabled persons:

1. The right to sexual expression
2. The right to privacy
3. The right to be informed
4. Access to needed services
5. The right to choose marital status
6. The right to have or not have children
7. The right to make decisions that affect one's life
8. The right to develop one's fullest potential

As stated in the first item, the right to sexual expression is the right of all people unless there is coercion, sexual use of children, or a possibility of unwanted children. This freedom includes for the handicapped the right to develop appropriate sexual behaviors within their capabilities.

In reference to the fifth right, we often have counseled disabled clients whose decision to marry was being questioned by parents and professionals. Although counseling and training may be helpful, the decision should rest with the couple. No one has a guaranteed marriage, so the same right for success or failure should be given to disabled couples. Along with marriage couseling, as stated in the sixth point, the capabilities and limitations of parenthood must be understood, and genetic counseling thus should be made available. As Robmault has stated, "with appropriate education, training and experience, all disabled people can have at least some level of control over their own lives. This level is almost always higher than the evaluation made by non-disabled 'caretakers'."[14]

Sex Education and Counseling

Sex education and counseling services should be available for all persons. A survey of the disabled conducted in 1975 by the Committee on Sexual Problems found that approximately 30 percent of the general population experiences some degree of sexual problem.[13] Among the disabled population, this percentage is even greater, since these individuals may also experience disability-related sexual problems. This fact was supported by a British follow-up survey of the same group.[5] This survey showed that 50 percent of those disabled persons were presently encountering sexual problems. It also showed that 90

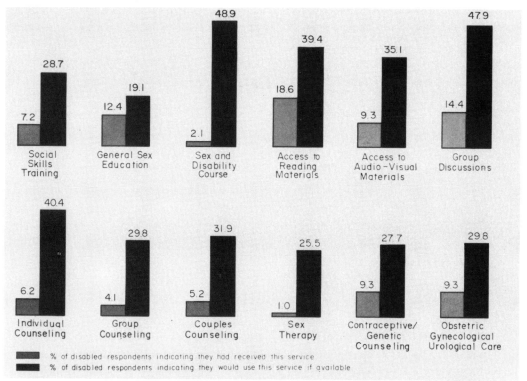

Figure 32-1. Results of the 1978 Sex and Disability Project: specific options. From Chipouras S, Cornelius DA, Daniels SM, et al: Education and Counseling Services for Disabled People. Washington, D.C., George Washington University, 1979. Reprinted by permission.

percent of the respondents further indicated that they would actually use the service.

The Sex and Disability Project in 1978 researched specific options in the area of sex education and counseling.[4] Disabled persons were asked which specific services they had received and which they would actually use. The results of this questioning are shown in Figure 32-1. Note the large discrepancy between services received and those that would be used if available.

Social Skill Training

The area of social training shown in Figure 32-1 needs special mention because it is a misunderstood yet very important category. Before a person can become successfully integrated into the community, he or she must learn the appropriate standards for behavior. Social skill training ranges from the correct use of phrases such as "please" and "thank you," to the more complex abilities needed for dating, social interactions, and expressing feelings appropriately.

The underlying factor here is one of socialization experiences. The social skills training also affects sexuality directly in terms of dress, manners, and personal hygiene. Appropriate dress and body care are important elements in self-esteem and in a positive feeling toward one's self. Also, a knowledge of sexual norms is important in developing meaningful sexual relationships.

Sex Education Counselors

The question of who is presently providing sex education and counseling to disabled individuals and who the disabled person expects to provide such services was surveyed in 1978 by the Sex and Disability Project.[4] Disabled persons in the survey were asked the following questions:

1. Who do you think should help you with a question about sexuality?
2. Who do you think are the most appropriate providers of sex education and counseling services?

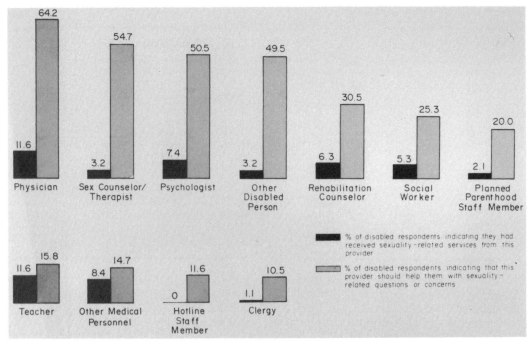

Figure 32-2.   Results of the 1978 Sex and Disability Project: sex education and counseling services. From Chipouras S, Cornelius DA, Daniels SM, et al: Education and Counseling Services for Disabled People. Washington, D.C., George Washington University, 1979. Reprinted by permission.

3. Of the services you have already received, who provided the services?

The results of this survey are shown in Figure 32-2.

The role *physicians* play in providing sex education services was found to be very important. The physician is seen by many disabled individuals as a person of knowledge and authority and thus is expected to be able to provide such services. Our concern is that if the disabled person turns to the physician, the person most often contacted concerning the body, and the physician is not open to discussing sexual concerns or questions, the patient may be discouraged from further exploration of this very necessary area. *Teachers* play a vital role and came the closest to fulfilling the expectations of those individuals surveyed. Often, the teacher becomes the sole source of information on sexuality for the disabled person. *Social workers* and *sex educators* provide direct counseling and education and have the responsibility and should have the skill to deal with such sexuality issues as social and developmental adjustment. *Parents* should play a central role in the

sex education of their children. It is important to create a home atmosphere that is open and receptive to both questions and conerns in the area of sexuality. Also, the modeling provided by parental dress and interactions sets the tone for an individual's future development.

One of the most common reasons given by professionals for not supplying sex education or counseling is "but no one asked me about it." We feel that recognition or diagnosis of sexual concerns or problems must be initiated by the professional. This hypothesis was substantiated in a 1967 study conducted by Burnap and Goldun.[4] In surveying physicians, they found that of those who asked their patients about sexual problem, 66 percent identified sexual problems in half their patients. Over 75 percent of those physicians who did not ask their patients, however, found sexual concerns in less than 10 percent of their patients. It seems apparent that one has to explore the area of sexual concerns with patients in order to offer a truly comprehensive service. An important ingredient in exploring this area is professionals own comfort with both sexuality and disability.

Permission, Limited Information, Specific Suggestions, and Intensive Therapy

In 1974, Annon developed a model to deal with concerns and questions of sexuality that might be raised by disabled individuals.[2] A structured and workable approach for helping professionals, it is called the Permission, Limited Information, Specific Suggestions, and Intensive Therapy (PLISSIT) model.

Permission

Permission is the base of any sex education program. Clients must feel free to express their thoughts, questions, and concerns without the fear of judgment or rejection. A person's thoughts and feelings always should be open for discussion. Permission to express oneself is also an important element in relieving individual anxiety, particularly in the area of sexuality. The counselor or sex educator also must be comfortable, nonjudgmental, and a good listener in order to create an atomosphere in which permission and reassurance can be offered.

Limited Information

Limited information has become the second stage in this model and requires that the professional provide additional comfort and education. This may include factual information to help the disabled individual sort through some of his or her own values. This information may be transmitted through written material, classroom teaching, or one-to-one discussion. The purpose behind conveying factual information is to answer questions and dispel myths.

Specific Suggestions

Specific suggestions include information that enables the individual to consider a behavior change or to set meaningful goals. This might also include factual information or explicit behaviors and techniques for dating, social interactions, and coital positions related to a particular disability. This level of the model is very individualized and especially effective in dealing with personal concerns such as appropriate behaviors and partner satisfaction.

Intensive Therapy

Intensive therapy is the fourth and final level of this model. A very individualized program is set up to meet very specific needs and to help the disabled person deal with feelings and concerns about the specific medical condition, e.g., cerebral palsy, and how it has affected sexuality. This level of therapy should be instituted only by a trained, certified professional who can deal with both the physical and psychologic aspects of the disability and its effect on sexuality.

TREATMENT STRATEGIES IN CEREBRAL PALSY

Comprehensive sex education and counseling programs are necessary for almost all individuals with cerebral palsy. Only those with severe to profound mental retardation are excluded, since sex education and other educational programs are relatively unsuccessful. In unclear situations, picture tests of the male and female anatomy as described by Zelman and Tyser may be helpful in determining if the individual has enough intellectual capabilities to benefit from the education program.[16] Before entering the sex education and counseling program at our institution, the patient is given a preliminary test, which may also include pictures, to establish the level of sexual understanding and determine in what areas major deficits exist. Education and counseling are then individually provided in social skills, dating, contraception, pregnancy, veneral diseases, and marriage. A second test is given after program completion to assess the level of improved understanding and function. Counseling of adolescents is performed without the parents being present to increase spontaneity and questions. The parents are counseled separately and instructed to provide reinforcement in the home. Sexually active or potentially active disabled patients are later referred to the adolescent birth control (ABC) clinic for further instruction.

Effective sexual counseling of handicapped individuals requires certain precautions by the professional:

1. Do not get people into trouble with their religion or their morality.
2. Do not transfer your morality to the patient.
3. Do not force the patient to talk about sex.
4. Do not threaten the patient with your sexuality.
5. Do not make sex an all-or-nothing experience.
6. Do not assume that once sexuality has been discussed, it is forever resolved for the patient.
7. Do not assume that there is only one way to convey sexual information.
8. Do not expect too much from spouses in their ability to change roles.[8]

The important underlying issue addressed in the above precautions is an awareness of patients and their needs in the area of sexuality. Professionals must be aware of different backgrounds and different points of view and should not impose values on patients. Their responsibility is to understand patients' values and enable them to deal with their own values in a socially acceptable manner.

REFERENCES

1. Alcorn DA: Parental views on sexual development and education of the trainable mentally retarded. J Special Ed 8:119, 1974
2. Annon JS: The Behavioral Treatment of Sexual Problems, vols. 1 and 2. Honolulu, Enabling Systems, 1974
3. Bass M, Gelof M: Sexual Rights and Responsibilities of the Mentally Retarded. Ardmore, Pa., 1975
4. Chipouras S, Cornelius DA, Daniels SM, et al: Education and Counseling Services for Disabled People. Washington, D.C., George Washington University, 1979
5. Committee on Sexual Problems of the Disabled: Sex and the Physically Handicapped. Sussex, England, National Fund for Research into Crippling Diseases, 1975
6. Demetral GD: Does ignorance really produce irresponsible behavior? Sexual Disabil 4:151, 1981
7. Fitz-Gerald D, Fitz-Gerald M: Sexuality and Deafness. Washington, D.C., Kendall Green, 1979
8. Gochros HL, Gochros JS: The sexually oppressed. New York, Association Press, 1977
9. Gordon S: Sexual rights for the people . . . who happen to be handicapped. Syracuse, Center on Human Policy, Syracuse University, 1974
10. Mooney T, Cole R, Chilgren R: Sexual Options for Paraplegics and Quadriplegics. Boston, Little, Brown and Co., 1975
11. Nordquist I: Life Together. Stockholm, E. Olofssons Boktryckeri AB, 1975
12. Oppenheimer C, Strom G: Unpublished data, 1980
13. Porteus J, Hullinger JL: A survey of sexually disabled in Iowa—client and counselor perceptions of vocational deterrents and rehabilitation needs. RSA grant no. 065-14-605, May–June 1975
14. Robmault IP: Sex, Society and the Disabled. Hagerstown, Harper & Row, 1978
15. Timmers RL, DuCharme P, Jacob G: Sexual knowledge, attitudes and behaviors of developmentally disabled adults living in a normalized apartment setting. Sexual Disabil 4:27, 1981
16. Zelman DB, Tyser KM: EASE: Essential adult sex education for the mentally retarded. Santa Monica, The Stanfield House, 1976

William E. Kiernan
Priscilla Morrison

33

Rehabilitation and Habilitation of the Adult

By its very definition, the term *rehabilitation* implies a process of returning or going back to an earlier state of living. It is a comprehensive dynamic process. Because of the diversity of people who participate in rehabilitation, it must be highly individualized. As defined in the report to the Secretary General of the United Nations, entitled *Rehabilitation of Disabled Persons,* the ultimate goal of the rehabilitation process is "the attainment of the maximum physical and psychological adjustment of each disabled person within the limits of his or her impairment." The optimal outcome is to enable an individual to live as useful and satisfying a life as possible in the least restrictive, most normalizing environment. For some, rehabilitation is truly a relearning process, while for others, as in the case of the person with cerebral palsy, it is often a continuation of learning and adaptation and is thus more accurately termed a *habilitation* process.

TERMINOLOGY

In an effort to place the rehabilitation or habilitation process in perspective, it is important to understand the terminology most frequently encountered: impairment, disability, and handicap. Although often used interchangeably, there is a critical distinction between these terms. In fact, each of the terms can be viewed as separate and discrete, although occuring somewhat sequentially. An *impairment* in the context of a health perspective represents any loss or abnormality of a physiologic or anatomic nature. This loss can be either temporary or permanent.

A *disability* is any restriction or lack of ability to perform an activity in the manner or range considered to be normal or customary. A disability often results from an impairment that can be temporary or permanent, reversible or irreversible, and progressive or regressive. Although a disability can be a direct result of an impairment, it can also result from an individual's psychological response to the impairment. The distinction is thus that an impairment relates directly to an organ or system, while a disability relates to the individual and the individual's response to an impairment. A *handicap* is a disadvantage for an individual resulting from an impairment or a disability that limits or prevents the fulfillment of a role that is normal for that individual. The term *handicap* is concerned with the value attached to an individual's situation or experience when it departs from the norm. A handicap is often viewed as the amount of dissonance observed between the individual's behavior and the expectations placed on that individual by a particular reference or peer group. A handicap thus represents the social expression of an impairment or disability.

The relationship between these terms suggests that an impairment may lead to a disability and a disability may lead to a handicap. The important element of this analysis is, however, that not all impairments are disabilities and not all impairments and disabilities lead to a handicap. The critical factors appear to be the individual's perception of himself or herself and the appropriate reference group, particularly for an adult. During the early years, when there is insufficient time to develop compensatory strategies, an impairment can easily evolve into a disability and subsequently emerge as a significant

handicap. An example of this would be the vast number of people who, during their academic career,
require either added instruction or curriculum modification to achieve. Upon completion of their
schoooling, however, they are able to become productive contributors to society and thus should not
be considered handicapped. In addition, the impairment may persist yet may not be associated with a
lack of ability and thus cannot be viewed as a disability.

For less obvious impairments, the process of
assimilation for the individual into society or the
resolution of the handicap can often be accomplished.
For the individual with more multiple impairment or
the individual whose impairment is more obvious,
the process of assimilation is far more difficult. Although an individual may not have a disability, he
or she may, as a result of outward differences, be
viewed as disabled and correspondingly be treated as
handicapped. The true disability in this case does not
stem from the individual but, rather, from society's
tendency to focus on an individual's limitations rather
than strengths.

It follows that an adult with cerebral palsy has,
in many ways, a much more difficult course in the
rehabilitation process. Although the goal remains that
of maximizing the capacity to function in the least
restrictive environment possible, the attitudes and
perceptions of the environment may inhibit the
achievement of this goal.

HISTORICAL ASPECTS
OF REHABILITATION

The acknowledgement that there are differences
in the terms employed in the rehabilitation process
reflects the developmental stage to which concepts
of rehabilitation have progressed. In the early phases,
the focus was placed much more on the resolution of
an immediate problem, e.g., returning to work. Now
there is a growing awareness of the emotional, social,
and residential aspects of the total rehabilitation process for individuals with disabilities. This increased
awareness has resulted in increasing legislation concerning education and rehabilitation of the individual
with a chronic disability.[12,13]

Early Legislation

With the passage of the Smith–Hughes Act in
1917 and the Soldier's Rehabilitation Act in 1917,
the United States made a formal commitment to aid

individuals with disabilities in returning to gainful
employment. Although these initial efforts reflected
society's increased awareness of these individuals'
needs, the primary focus of the rehabilitation movement in the first two decades was based on an "economic rate of return" concept. These federal initiatives were the impetus for the development of individual
statewide rehabilitation programs and resources. Although there was general enthusiastic acknowledg-
ment that the country had an obligation to disabled
persons, it took 35 yr from the passage of the Sol-
diers' Rehabilitation Act before all states and terri-
tories had rehabilitation programs.

In 1936, with the passage of the Ran-
dolph–Shepard Act, the nation established a prefer-
ential treatment procedure for disabled persons in
seeking employment. The Vocational and Rehabilitation Act of 1943 (Public Law 78–113) expanded
the focus of service to include mentally handicapped
and mentally ill persons as eligible for rehabilitation
services. This represented a major shift in rehabilitation in that services could now be directed toward
individuals who were disabled regardless of prior history of employment. Although the emphasis continued to be on employment, there was recognition of
the need for not only relearning but learning, and a
concept of habilitation was thus evolving.

Recent Legislation

Vocational Rehabilitation Act

The Vocational Rehabilitation Amendment of
1954 (Public Law 83–565) brought about major
changes in the administration and focus of rehabilitation activities nationally. Emphasis was now being
placed on training of staff and expansion of resources.
A key concept of this law was its focus on research
and demonstration projects. There was now a recognition that the development of new service and
training technologies was essential, since more and
more disabled individuals were seeking vocational
rehabilitation services.

Vocational Rehabilitation Act
Amendment

As the scope of vocational services continued to
expand, so also did the demand for these services.
The Vocational Rehabilitation Act Amendment of
1965 (Public Law 89–333) had, as its primary ini-
tiative, services for severely disabled persons. Along
with an expansion of the eligibility criteria for ser-

vices came a recognition that not all disabled persons could achieve gainful employment.

This law then broadened the definition of gainful employment to include not only competitive but sheltered and home-bound employment as well. Eligibility criteria for vocational rehabilitiation services now asserted that there must be a reasonable expectation of achieving gainful employment. The evaluation process to determine eligibility for full vocational rehabilitation services could then be extended to 18 mo. The act created the National Commission on Architectual Barriers in an effort to adapt not only the individual to the environment but the environment to the individual. The rehabilitiation process thus was expanded to include the provision of services to the most severely disabled over a longer period while employing a more reasonable definition of the outcome measure. Also, the rehabiliation process was looked on as somewhat of a partnership, with adaptation required not only by the individual but by the environment as well.

Rehabilitation Act

Although a somewhat symbolic change, the Rehabilitation Act of 1973 (Public Law 93–112), for the first time in the history of vocational rehabilitation, did not have as part of its title the word *vocational*. Although the title reflected a further broadening of the scope of rehabilitation, there continued to be a major focus on the achievement of gainful employment for disabled persons. As in the Vocational Rehabilitation Amendments of 1965, the focus was placed on the provision of services to more severely disabled individuals.

Rehabilitation, Comprehensive Services, and Developmental Disabilities Amendments

By far the most significant of all pieces of legislation relating to vocational rehabilitation was the passage of the Rehabilitation, Comprehensive Services, and Developmental Disabilities Amendments (Public Law 95–602). This act accomplished what the Rehabilitation Act of 1973 had intended to accomplish in that it redefined and significantly expanded the scope of rehabilitation services. The purpose, as stated in the act, was to develop and implement, through research, training, services, and the guarantee of equal opportunity, comprehensive and coordinated programs of rehabilitation and independent living. The focus now would be on the provision of comprehensive services that addressed both vocational and independent living needs, thereby recognizing the interrelationship of the total life activities as opposed to the past singular focus on employment.

Title VII of the Comprehensive Services Act reflected a major change for rehabilitation. The purpose of this title was to assist the state vocational rehabilitation agencies in providing comprehensive services for independent living designed to meet current and future needs of individuals whose disabilities are so severe that they do not have the potential for employment but may benefit from vocational rehabilitation services, which will enable them to live and function independently. This title was to direct its efforts toward the provision of services to those individuals who were not being served by other portions of the act. The services provided would be directed toward enhancing an individual's ability to live independently and function within the family and community and to secure and maintain employment.

Probably one of the most significant aspects of this law was recognition that receipt of rehabilitation services was not a privilege but a right for disabled persons. Sec. 504 of the act was, and in many ways continues to be, viewed as a declaration of entitlement for disabled persons. It stipulates that no otherwise qualified handicapped individual shall solely by reason of the handicap be exluded from participation in, be denied benefits of, or be subjected to discrimination under any program or activity receiving federal financial assistance or conducted by any executive agency. Combined with Sec. 503, which requires any contract awarded by the federal government in excess of $2500 to have an affirmative action plan and advance in employment for qualified handicapped individuals, the emphasis of PL95–602 was clearly an action with a capacity for corrective steps to be taken in the event of discrimination.

Current Results of Legislation

It is apparent that the U.S. perspective of vocational rehabilitation services has evolved from an industrial and economic to a comprehensive and employment one.[6] In the early days, vocational rehabilitation service focused on a retraining or a relearning mode with the program justification based on the economic return achieved as the disabled individual returned to competitive employment. Through the years, although there continued to be strong emphasis on employment, there was a recognition that fulltime comprehensive employment was not the only type of gainful employment that should be pursued. There gradually emerged an acknowledgement that the more severely disabled individual would benefit from vocational rehabilitation services and that, in fact, the service was more a habilitative than rehabilitative. More recently there has been a recognition that vocational rehabilitation services cannot just focus on employment but, rather, must consider the individual's comprehensive needs. The vocational rehabilitation movement has progressed from a univariant to a multivariant focus, which has the capacity to respond to a wide range of needs.

SCOPE, SERVICE, AND NEED

If one is to accept the tenets of the principles of normalization, the scope of service needs of the adult with cerebral palsy should be no different than the scope of service needs of the adult without cerebral palsy. What may be different is the intensity or technique of service provision in light of some of the physical, cognitive, or social differences that may exist between the adult with cerebral palsy and the person without a disability.

One of the most effective methods to identify major categories or groups of activities, which should be available to persons with disabilities, is to look at how the nondisabled community spends its time. The earlier review of the historical development of vocational rehabilitation services clearly places a major emphasis on employment, however, assuming an average work week of 40 hr, less than 25 percent of an individual's weekly time is spent "on the job." The balance of the week is spent in a variety of activities, including activities of daily living, recreation, transportation, sleep, and a wide variety of personal enrichment activities, e.g., reading, watching television, personal interactions, and many more.[7]

The basic week has a total of 168 available hr. Depending on individual preferences, fiscal resources, personal capabilities, and geographic location, the specific time allocations to individual activities may vary greatly, but most can be clustered into three major groups: vocational, residential, and recreational. For the nondisabled individual, the question is often, Which specific activity should I engage in? For the disabled person, the question is more frequently, Which activity will I be allowed or able to engage in? In the former case, although there may

be restrictions in the range of options available, more often than not the factors causing the restriction are, to some extent, if not entirely, determined by the individual. In the latter case, the individual often cannot mediate the restrictions, e.g., inaccessibility due to physical or attitudinal barriers, nonexistence of options, or physical or cognitive requirements beyond the individual's ability. It is thus often not an issue of motivation but an issue of lack of opportunity that limits options for the disabled person.

Beyond the specific health care needs that certain groups of disabled individuals may have, there is little difference between the needs of various groups of individuals for vocational, residential, and recreational opportunities. What may differ is the extent to which individuals can effectively take advantage of the resources and the degree to which specific modifications may have to be made to accommodate to each individual. Too often, when planning services for groups of disabled individuals, there is a tendency to look on a diagnostic classification as homogeneous when, in fact, this is not the case. A striking example of this is the wide range of abilities, both cognitively and physically, which are present within a group of persons with the diagnosis of cerebral palsy. In light of this and in an effort to reflect the wide range of abilities within such a group, no single service delivery model would seem to be appropriate in planning goals.

Vocational Programs and Goals

Employment Program Options

The area that has received the most attention in planning and training for the disabled adult is the area of employment.[2,8] In recent years, however, there has been an increased recognition that certain disabled individuals, particularly those with severe motor and cognitive impairment, would have great difficulty succeeding in a competitive employment setting. In the past the only option was that of a sheltered workshop, but there has been some recognition that this type of environment may not be suitable for all disabled individuals.[3,15] For the adult with cerebral palsy the sheltered workshop environment is often extremely frustrating because of the labor-intensive nature of the facility and the manual requirements of the job.

Typically, the work done in a training and evaluation facility, sheltered workshop, or work activity

Table 33-1
Vocational Day Program Options*

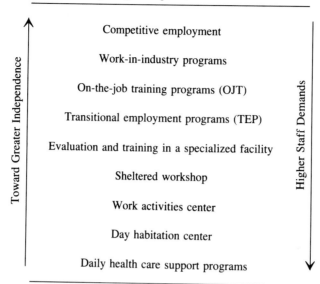

*Programs are listed in order of greatest independence.

center is of a routine and repetitive nature, e.g., bench work, collating, inserting, folding, and other manual tasks. For the adult with cerebral palsy, many of these gross and fine motor activities focus directly on his or her deficits and accentuate an inability to perform. By the very nature of these programs, many of the participants may have cognitive deficits and thus be responding on a more concrete level than those individuals with cerebral palsy, who do not have such limitations. The concern often expressed by the individual with a physical impairment and normal intelligence is one of isolation, apprehension, and despair in programs of this nature because of the physical demands and lack of appropriate peer interaction. Concerns such as "people will think I am retarded if I go there" or "I don't have anyone I can talk with" or "I am bored" are often voiced. For those individuals who do have cognitive deficits, these programs may be appropriate for their social needs but again reinforce the existing physical deficits.

More recent alternatives to sheltered workshops and work activity centers have emerged (Table 33-1). Work in industry and on-the-job training programs have opened new areas of training. These programs tend to focus on the normal work environment, providing training and activities that require both physical and social abilities. Many of the service activities, including receptionist, clerical, food service,

maintenance, and communication, allow the individual to receive training in an environment that closely approximates or, in fact, is the actual environment in which the job is to be performed.

The work in industry program of the sheltered enclave uses the normal working environment, at the same time recognizing that certain disabled individuals will not be able to achieve a satisfactory rate of productivity because of physical or cognitive deficits. This would allow for a payment rate that reflects the rate of individual productivity, as in the sheltered workshop situation, but provides employment in a much more normalized environment. Competitive employment, however, remains the goal in most training programs.

Because of the diversity of the population, it is extremely difficult to identify specific career clusters in which an individual with cerebral palsy can succeed. Cohen reported that types of employment opportunities for the adult with cerebral palsy depend heavily on the extent of the disability and the attitude of prospective employers.[1] A number of studies show that 25–50 percent of adults with cerebral palsy can achieve sufficient skills to maintain a job in the competitive labor market.[5,9,11,14] No specific career cluster has emerged as being more appropriate than another, but the jobs that were obtained reflected the individual's abilities and not the diagnostic classifications.

Habilitation Program Options

There remains a group of adults with cerebral palsy who, because of the severity of their disability and extent of associated limitations, are not able to succeed in any type of employment setting. In these cases a day habilitation program may be more appropriate. In these programs, the focus is more on sensory stimulation, training in activities of daily living, and basic self-help and self-care skills. For certain individuals this type of program can provide as much a sense of accomplishment as competitive employment would for others. It is a highly structured program that helps develop a greater degree of independence through self-awareness and awareness of the environment. For some, this will be a stepping stone to a work activities center; for others, this will represent a long-term activity.

Daily Health Care
Program Options

To complete the range of service options for vocational and habilitation day programs, recognition must be made of the needs of those individuals who have compelling daily health care requirements. As can be seen in Table 33-1, the daily health care support program is the most heavily staffed program option, with the least amount of independent activity. In each state this type of option varies from a pediatric nursing home to a chronic care facility to an institution; however, the major focus remains on the provision of direct services to the adult with cerebral palsy. In most instances the nature of the disability is so severe that, without this type of support, the situation could be considered life threatening for the individual. These programs, although they provide total care, in nature, should be considered habilitative rather than custodial.

The vast array of vocational and habilitation day program options reflects the wide spectrum of skills of adults with cerebral palsy. No one option is best for any group of individuals, although one option is clearly best for a specific individual. The determination of which option is best will require input from a range of professionals and the individual as well as from the family when appropriate. Once a program is determined to be appropriate, care must be taken to ensure that a monitoring system is established so that as gains are made, modifications can be undertaken and changes instituted. Because rehabilitation is a developmental process that is constantly changing, an individual rehabilitation plan must be modified to reflect the individual's abilities as growth and development occurs.

Residential Programs and Goals

As in the case of the vocational and day options, a number of residential program options have evolved. The options, however, have only been available for the past decade or two. These options can be organized according to the degree of independence that each offers a resident (Table 33-2). Although the natural home environment often provides a source of stability, needs change as the child moves into adolescence and adulthood. In the development of any rehabilitative or habilitation plan, the residential environment must be an integral component. All too often the focus is placed on vocational goals while the residential environment is neglected. Ambivalence on the part of the disabled individual, the parents and family, and society in general are often present in considering residential needs in the future. Historically, large institutions have reduced the need for some individuals to look at anything other than this type of option. The changes of the past decades, however, have shown that institutional settings may not be the most appropriate and may, in fact, be regressive settings.

The residential needs of the adult with cerebral palsy are no different than those of any disabled adult. At times, specific modifications in the environment must be made to accommodate unique physical constraints, while in other cases more intensive supervision may be required because of social and cognitive limitations.

Intermediate Care Facilities

For those adults with cerebral palsy who need continued supervision and support, the resources of an intermediate care facility (ICF) for the mentally retarded (ICF type A or B) may be made available. In these cases a high degree of structure with extensive staffing resources are required. Contrary to opinions at the turn of the century, the size of the ICF is critical. The large warehousing approaches of the past have proved to be ineffectual in providing humane and acceptable residential services. Regulations that pertain to the ICF are responsible to individuals' needs and thus are client centered and developmentally oriented. The nature of the ICF is dictated by the residents' capacity for self-preservation (Type B) and non-self-preservation (Type A) skills, with an individual service plan developed for each resident. By definition, the adult who would benefit from such a program would have a significant degree of mental retardation associated with his or her diagnosis of cerebral palsy.

Table 33-2
Residential Program Options*

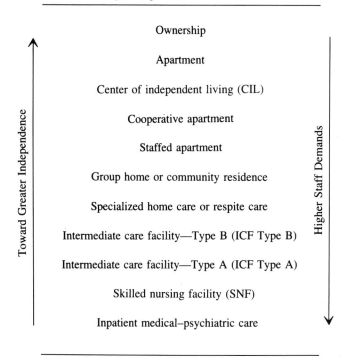

Toward Greater Independence →

Ownership

Apartment

Center of independent living (CIL)

Cooperative apartment

Staffed apartment

Group home or community residence

Specialized home care or respite care

Intermediate care facility—Type B (ICF Type B)

Intermediate care facility—Type A (ICF Type A)

Skilled nursing facility (SNF)

Inpatient medical–psychiatric care

Higher Staff Demands ↓

*Programs are listed in order of greatest independence.

Skilled Nursing Facility

In certain instances, based on age, a skilled nursing facility (SNF) would be viewed as a residential option. Most SNFs, however, will not have the staffing resources to respond to the physical needs of the geriatric person with cerebral palsy. To date, few resources other than large institutions have been viewed as appropriate for the needs of disabled individuals in this age group. Some new initiatives are looking at the use of the ICF model as a type of residential option. Additionally, large SNF programs have begun to look at modifying the more traditional approaches to the geratric community and establishing programs, as well as staff resources, which can deal with physical needs and personal and emotional levels of functioning. This resource, however, has been slow in developing.

Inpatient Resources

On a short-term basis, the services of an inpatient resource may be necessary. In these situations, because of medical or psychiatric needs, short-term stays in inpatient units may be necessary. The services of such a resource should, however, be directed at assisting the individual in returning to a more normalized residential setting.

Home and Respite Care

Specialized home care and respite care programs provide services to medically stable individuals who are in need of a highly structured, supportive, and nurturing environment. Respite care is generally short term, serving as an adjunct to the natural home environment. This type of program provides support and, at times, relief for the immediate family. The nature of these programs is transitional, with the goal directed toward assisting the disabled individual to acquire greater self-care skills and an increased capacity to respond socially and emotionally in an appropriate fashion.

Community Residences

The group home and community residence are, by far, the most popular of the residential options. These programs have the capacity to provide residential services for a specific number of individuals in a neighborhood setting. Although the optimal number of individuals who should reside in group home varies, the most frequent number of individuals in a residence ranges from 8 to 10. This type of program provides an environment that gives continuous assistance and supervision with ongoing emphasis on the development of self-care and self-help skills directed toward increased social competence. The supervisors of house managers do not serve as surrogate parents but, rather, as sounding boards to community perception and help the residents learn the skills to interrelate with nondisabled persons.

Centers for Independent Living

With the incentives offered through the Department of Housing and Urban Development (HUD), a number of apartment buildings, both new and substantially renovated, now contain a specified number of units for disabled person. As the move toward greater independence is achieved, the individual may progress to a staffed apartment, a supervised apartment, or a center for independent living (CIL) program. Each of these options varies according to the degree of supervision required. In the first instances, as in group homes, the staff is in residence much, if not all, of the time, providing both supervision and instruction. In a supervised apartment, the staff provides only limited support, with the residents performing most of the activities of daily living in an independent fashion. Often the supervision provided relates to monitoring of budgets, development of nutritional programs, and general assistance with problems or issues encountered in the community.

The CIL programs, part of the Rehabilitation, Comprehensive Services, and Developmental Disabilities Amendments of 1978, direct their efforts toward provision of services to those individuals whose disabilities are so severe that they do not presently have the potential for gainful employment. Such programs provide assurances that these handicapped individuals are substantially involved in policy direction and management of the program. This type of program provides a wide range of services, including peer counseling, advocacy, independent and group social and recreational activities, attendant care, and training of personnel to provide such care. Supervision in CIL programs, as in staffed and cooperative apartments, will vary; however, the staffing pattern more often reflects the physical rather than the cognitive needs of the individual resident. For the adult with cerebral palsy, the apartment and CIL resources open up new opportunities for living a more normal life. In both, consistent and sufficient fiscal resources are required. Often, when one thinks of these options, the disabled individual is eliminated automatically, yet in those instances where the disabled person is gainfully employed, these options are quite attainable. Reluctance on the part of certain financial institutions to grant loans to disabled individuals has made ownership more difficult.

As in the case of the vocational and day options, residential options reflect a wide range of facilities that are potentially available for disabled people. In those instances where cognitive or physical constraints require greater assistance or supervision by staff, resources such as group homes and ICFs may be able to meet the need. For some, this type of environment is too restrictive, and a type of apartment, CIL program, or ownership option would be more appropriate. In all instances, no one option should be viewed as fixed but, rather, considered through regular review with progress toward a less restrictive option.

Recreation

The last, but not the least, of the human service needs is recreation. Often recreation is viewed as a frill rather than as an essential part of individual growth and development. The opportunity to relate to others and to engage in group and individual leisure time pursuits provides the variety and diversity that enables an individual to function more effectively at work and with others in the place of residence. Because of the diverse residential and vocational needs of disabled individuals, the importance of recreation is often overlooked or minimized.

Recreation takes on a variety of different aspects, ranging from independent or free play to structured group activities. For the nondisabled individual, within broad limits, the issue is not one of access but of personal preference. For the disabled individual, however, the issue frequently is one of access—social or environmental. The range of choices is limited, more often than not, because of external rather than internal limitations. Concerns about health and safety, inability to follow rules, or fear of ridicule are often expressed by those in charge when considering the involvement of a disabled individual in a "nondisabled" recreational activity. Self-contained programs dealing exclusively with disabled persons have frequently been viewed as the means to address the recreational needs of disabled people. This approach unfortunately does not allow for peer interaction with nondisabled persons and, in many ways, eliminates one of the most effective methods of reducing social barriers by segregation and highlighting differences rather than similarities among people. An isolated program ignores the fact that, although capacity to respond may vary, degree of interest and enthusiasm may be quite similar.

It would be inconsistent to list the types of recreational options that should be available to the disabled individual while emphasizing that these individuals should be viewed as having the same needs and desires as their nondisabled peers. The types of recreational options that one has access to depends on personal preference, developmental state, peer pressure, available resources, and countless other factors. The essential element is that sufficient options be available so that the individual, disabled or nondisabled, can satisfy his or her preferences. The choice is individual, and options should be diverse enough to reflect all tastes. Prohibitions on certain options should be based on reasons other than the presence of a disability or a handicap.

SUPPORTIVE SERVICE OPTIONS

In addition to the vocational, residential, and recreational options, at times there is a need to provide additional assistance to compensate for certain individual disabilities. For any disabled adult, a number of supportive services should be available (Table 33-3). The focus of these services is to provide assistance in achieving the goal of maximum independent function within a community setting. The extent of the independent functioning and the nature of the community setting will depend on the abilities and preferences of the disabled individual.

Each category in Table 33-3 provides a list of resources that may be assessed by the disabled adult. Although, again, certain modifications may need to be made in some areas, e.g., education and transportation, in other instances caution must be exercised so that the service does not become too structured or overprotective, e.g., specialized health care, case management and outreach, and social–interpersonal skill development. In the former case, the activity may not be phsyically accessible, while in the latter case, wholly specialized services may emphasize the differences rather than the similarities of disabled and the nondisabled persons.

Many of these services can be located through state departments of health, mental health, and education. Several of the services may be integrated into residential and vocational and day programs. In each community, advocacy groups and develop-

Table 33-3
Ancillary or Supportive Service Options

Educational
   Higher education opportunities
   Adult education opportunities
   Career—vocational education services

Health and habilitative
   Daily health care
   Specialized health care
   Routine habilitative services (dental, speech, physical and occupational therapy)

Mental health services
   Counseling and guidance
   Crisis intervention

Transportation
   Independent travel (mobility training)
   Use of public transportation

Case management
   Information and referral
   Monitoring
   Legal assistance
   Financial entitlement assistance

Social–interpersonal skill development
   Sex education
   Peer group activities
   Community education

mental disabilities councils can provide specific information on the availability of resources and the location of service providers. In some instances, the services will focus exclusively on the needs of the disabled person, while in other cases the service will be generic to the community. In all instances, the disabled individual must express interest, motivation, and a willingness to follow through if the provision of the service is to be meaningful.

ATTITUDES AND PERCEPTIONS

No service or resource will be effective unless it is viewed as relevant and necessary by the consumer. The rehabilitation process is a partnership process, one in which all involved have agreed that the plan and associated services are appropriate.[4,8] The involvement of the disabled individual in the planning as well as the delivery of the service is critical. In light of this, it would be beneficial to review some of the perceptions of various people involved in the development of a total rehabilitation plan.

As discussed earlier, the general public often perceives the adult with cerebral palsy as a member of a homogeneous group. Because there is often a problem in communication, the average individual assumes that there is also difficulty in cognitive ability, perception, and general affect. The greater the physical manifestations of cerebral palsy, the more likely it is that the general public will underestimate, be apprehensive of, or even discriminate against the individual.

Societal Responses

Because of difficulties in motor coordination there is a varied but definite response among individuals and society in general. At times this response can be supportive to a fault, as in the case of overprotection, and at other times it can be detrimental, as in the case of apprehension or fear. In an effort to obtain life insurance, for example, a disabled person's application may be initially denied because of so-called high-risk. Although subsequent legislation in many states has responded to this type of discrimination, the concept of the child or adult with cerebral palsy being a "bad risk" is not uncommon even today.

One would assume that this example reflects a stereotypic response by those who are not familiar with disabled individuals. This, unfortunately, is not always so, as the following case report shows:

A woman with cerebral palsy found that her co-workers, although extremely supportive, remained reluctant to involve her in all of the "shop talk." Special efforts had been made by the staff to involve her in all social activities. An excellent comraderie had developed to the point that several workers would go that extra step to ensure that the restaurant was accessible and that transportation was available. Any conversation regarding heterosexual relationships was, always conducted in private, however. Although there was acceptance at one level, there was the feeling that because of the nature of this woman's disability, relationships or even feelings about sexuality were not a reality.

In this instance, it is clear that the disability was viewed as a significant handicap, emotionally and physiologically, by the group. Not infrequently, the disabled individual is assumed to be either unaware or impervious to usual adult desires and feelings. Although not discriminatory or malicious, this type of behavior can cause feelings of disappointment, uncertainty, and even anger. It is again an example of how the disabled individual is viewed as deviant and not as a fully franchised citizen in U.S. society.

On a day-to-day level, typical responses occur in the general public concerning adults with cerebral palsy. Society often responds to a disabled person as a person with major limitations, not an individual with specific abilities. Trips to the supermarket, for instance, frequently bring on curious stares and concerns at store managers that normal business may be disrupted. Although the example may seem rather trivial, it is these social attitudes that impede the ability of the adult with cerebral palsy to progress toward greater independence.

Professional Responses

The professional world is not without its biased responses either. It is not uncommon that inquiries about current or historical events be addressed to the parents or a nondisabled companion in the presence of the adult with cerebral palsy. When dealing with children such an approach is quite acceptable, yet for the adult this type of overprotection or underestimation of capacity can be both frustrating and demoralizing. The inconsistent message is clear: you should be big enough to dress yourself, feed yourself, or practice your therapies, yet you are not old enough to receive instruction or be given a chance to ask questions. Among health care professionals there is a greater tendency to look at the diagnosis or impairment of the individual rather than at the abilities of the whole person—physically, socially, emotionally, and vocationally. The continuous line of appointments with professionals can lead to sheer physical exhaustion and, at times, confusion. Coordination among helping professionals is frequently absent, especially for the person with multiple needs.

Family Responses

Attitudes and perceptions reflect both the belief structure and the views of an individual. The family plays a key role in the development of goals and expectations in the child and adult with cerebral palsy. For the parents during the early years, the emotional trauma associated with having a disabled child and the continuous tasks of coping with the child's health, educational, and social needs can be overwhelming. For the siblings, apprehension, fear, and embarassment at having a brother or sister with cerebral palsy as well as decreased attention from parents can have long-term effects. (see Chap. 29) For the child with cerebral palsy, the constant focus on developmental landmarks, physical achievements, and communication skills can be so compelling that affective response to the handicapping conditions can easily be supressed.

During the academic years, all family efforts are focused on achievement, with the desire, on the part of the parents, to have this experience be a positive one. There is a tendency to overprotect, to shield, and to frequently underestimate the child during this period. Expectations are low so that success can be ensured. This concept sets the stage for the cyclic process of the self-fulfilling prophecy. It is imperative during this time that movement toward independence is encouraged. The child should be given choices, encouraged to make decisions, and allowed the responsibilities related to those decisions. Overprotection eliminates the valuable learning experiences associated with risk taking and failure. Learning can occur effectively through failure, yet parents often feel that this is not good.

Individual Responses

For the child with cerebral palsy, the emphasis on attainment of developmental landmarks overshadows necessary emotional adjustments. The apparent discrepancies between sibling and peer performance become more pronounced as the years progress. Questions about peer relationships, family support structure, and future options are often the concerns of all, yet are seldom addressed. Parental concerns about future residential options are frequently suppressed out of fear and of ambivalence toward increased independence for their son or daughter. Beliefs about continued family support by siblings are expressed by the parents, but seldom is this issue or its implications on the future of others discussed. Because of the investment of the parents in the growth and development of their disabled child, siblings are not as regularly involved in care and decision making for their brother or sister and may have limited experience dealing with day-to-day needs and concerns.

It is not only the parents and siblings who have questions about the future but the affected individual as well. Plans for the future are often made without consideration of the child's feelings and desires. This attitude, although intended to be supportive, can often be detrimental. Overprotection is, at times, interpreted by the child as a lack of confidence, a reaffirmation that his or her problems are, in fact, quite severe or that cerebral palsy is something people should

not talk about. For both the parent and child, many of these issues reflect the ongoing ambivalence about the future and the desire to protect those who are perceived as not being able to protect themselves. Overprotection and ambivalence about greater independence and separation are not uncommon for all children, yet for the disabled child the magnitude of these issues is greater. The personal resources, past experiences, and range of options are less well defined for the disabled than for the nondisabled child.

The lack of experience, or limited knowledge of the world, is an issue that can and should be addressed by the child and family throughout the developmental years. Broader exposure to the community and its resources, a varied educational experience that reflects both vocational and academic subject matter, and a chance to develop skills of daily living will provide the child with cerebral palsy the foundations for making informed choices in the future. The range of service options must continue to expand in both magnitude and scope so that the social, vocational, and residential needs of the adult with cerebral palsy can be met. Choices cannot be made if options do not exist.

REFERENCES

1. Cohen J: Vocational guidance and employment, in Cruckshank WM (ed): Cerebral Palsy, A Developmental Disability. New York, Syracuse University Press, 1976
2. Dalton Jr RA, Latz A: Vocational placement: The Pennsylvania Rehabilitation Center. Rehabil Lit 39:336, 1978
3. Floor L, Rosen M: New criteria of adjustment for the cerebral palsied. Rehabil Lit 37:268, 1976
4. Floor L, Rosen M, Peet D: Follow-up Services for the Cerebral Palsied: A three year Research and Demonstration Project (SRS project no. 15-P-55903/3/01). Elwyn, Pa., Elwyn Institute, 1975
5. Karlsson B, Gardeström L, Nordquist IL, et al Cerebral palsy in young adults. A socio-medical study with special regard to employment problems. Dev Med Child Neurol 7:268, 1965
6. Kiernan WE, Rehabilitation planning, in Magrab P, Elder JO (eds): Planning for Services to Handicapped Persons; Community, Education, Health. Baltimore, Paul H. Brooks, 1979
7. Kiernan WE: Habilitation: A dynamic system, in Bellamy GT, O'Connor G, Karan OC (eds): Vocational Rehabilitation of Severely Handicapped Persons. Baltimore, University Park Press, 1979
8. Machek O: Rehabilitiation of the cerebral palsied adult: Preparation for adulthood. Rehabil Rec 5:9, 1961

9. Magyar CW, Nystrom JB, Johansen N: A follow-up of former cerebral palsy students at a school for neuro-orthopedically disabled children. Rehabil Lit 38:40, 1977

10. OlShansky, S, Beach D: A five year follow-up of physically disabled clients. Rehabil Lit 36:251, 1975

11. Reynolds KM: in Lynch KP, Kiernan WG, Start JA (eds): Prevocational and Vocational Education for Special Needs Youth: A Blueprint for the 1980's. Baltimore, Paul H. Brooker (in press)

12. DHEW: A Summary of Selected Legislation Relating to the Handicapped. Washington, D.C., U.S. Government Printing Office, 1975

13. DHEW: A Summary of Selected Legislation Relating to the Handicapped. Washington, D.C., U.S. Government Printing Office, 1977

14. Wigfield ME: Cerebral palsy: Altered sensation, stereognosis and sensory perception in relation to vocational training and job performance. Clin Orthop 46:93, 1966

Index